Clinical Protocols in Pediatric and Adolescent Gynecology

Clinical Protocols in Pediatric and Adolescent Gynecology

Second Edition

Edited by

S. PAIGE HERTWECK MD

Chief of Gynecology
Norton Children's Hospital
Clinical Professor, Pediatrics, Obstetrics, Gynecology & Women's Health
University of Louisville School of Medicine
Louisville, Kentucky, United States

MAGGIE L. DWIGGINS MD, MS

Co-Director, Pediatric and Adolescent Gynecology Fellowship
Norton Children's Hospital
Clinical Associate Professor, Pediatrics
University of Louisville School of Medicine
Louisville, Kentucky, United States

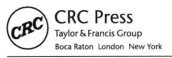

CRC Press
Taylor & Francis Group
Boca Raton London New York

CRC Press is an imprint of the
Taylor & Francis Group, an **informa** business

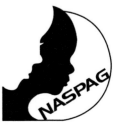

First edition published 2006
by CRC Press
6000 Broken Sound Parkway NW, Suite 300, Boca Raton, FL 33487-2742

and by CRC Press
2 Park Square, Milton Park, Abingdon, Oxon, OX14 4RN

© 2022 Taylor & Francis Group, LLC

CRC Press is an imprint of Taylor & Francis Group, LLC

ISBN: 978-0-367-48311-1 (hbk)
ISBN: 978-0-367-48309-8 (pbk)
ISBN: 978-1-003-03923-5 (ebk)

DOI: 10.1201/9781003039235

Typeset in Times
by KnowledgeWorks Global Ltd.

Contents

Preface

This book provides a comprehensive review of the common and less commonly encountered Pediatric and Adolescent Gynecology (PAG) conditions that present in an ambulatory as well as surgical settings. By design, we list conditions in an alphabetized table of contents to facilitate quick reference in an office or emergency room setting, allowing clinicians to locate information in an expedited fashion. We have placed information in a bulleted text format listing key points about each condition, followed by what to ask for in history taking, then what to look for on physical examination, and concluding with how to manage conditions. We have included helpful photographs, figures, algorithms, and some patient questionnaires where pertinent to assist both the student and the medical practitioner in their care for a PAG patient.

In this second edition, we have included as authors current and past fellows in PAG, along with their mentors and PAG colleagues. A third of the proceeds from this book will support the North American Society for Pediatric and Adolescent Gynecology (NASPAG) Fellowship Research Committee to enhance research in the field of PAG.

We are grateful for CRC Press/Taylor & Francis for assisting us with this second edition and thankful to the authors and our families who supported us while we had the privilege to put this edition together.

Contributors

Virginia Ramsey Aldrich, MD
University of Louisville School of Medicine

Patricia Amorado, MD
University of Arkansas for Medical Sciences

Amy Boone, MD
Children's of Alabama and University of
    Alabama at Birmingham

Charis Chambers, MD
Piedmont Healthcare

Krista J. Childress, MD
Emory University and Children's Healthcare of
    Atlanta

Ariel Cohen, MD
Eunice Kennedy Shriver Institute for Child
    Health and Human Development, Children's
    National Hospital

Christina N. Davis-Kankanamge, MD
Texas Children's Hospital

Melina L. Dendrinos, MD
Michigan Medicine

Jennifer E. Dietrich, MD, MSc
Texas Children's Hospital

Tania Dumont, MD
Children's Hospital of Eastern Ontario

Dana Elborno, MD
Northwestern Medicine Regional Medical Group

Y. Frances Fei, MD
Michigan Medicine

Rachael L. Fisher, DO
Advocare Center for Specialized Gynecology

Kelsey Flood, MD
University of Cincinnati Medical Center

Kylie Fowler, MD, MS
Children's Minnesota

Amanda French, MD
Tufts Children's Hospital

M E Sophie Gibson, MD
Queen's University School of Medicine

Yuan Yuan (Jackie) Gong, MD
Norton Children's Medical Center

Frances Grimstad, MD, MS
Boston Children's Hospital

Kaiane Habeshian, MD
Children's National Hospital and George
    Washington University School of Medicine

Angie Hamouie, MD
Texas Children's Hospital

Katherine Hayes, MD
University of Utah Health

Tina Ho, MD
Boston Children's Hospital

Laura Hollenbach, MD
University of Arkansas for Medical Sciences and
    Arkansas Children's Hospital

Kim Hoover, MD
Children's of Alabama and University of
    Alabama at Birmingham

Kimberly Huhmann, MD
Norton Children's Medical Group

Wendy L. Jackson, MD
University of Kentucky

Lauren A. Kanner, MD
University of Iowa Hospitals and Clinics

Chelsea A. Kebodeaux, MD
Texas Children's Hospital

Sari Kives, MD
The Hospital for Sick Kids and University of Toronto

Marc Laufer, MD
Boston Children's Hospital

Ashli Lawson, MD
University of Missouri at Kansas City

Kalyani Marathe, MD
Cincinnati Children's Hospital and University of
  Cincinnati College of Medicine

Allison Mayhew, MD
Pediatric Specialists of Virginia and Children's
  National Hospital

Kate McCracken, MD
Nationwide Children's Hospital

Sarah McQuillan, MD
University of Calgary

Ann Marie Mercier, MD
University of Arkansas for Medical Sciences

Diane F. Merritt, MD
Washington University School of Medicine

Swetha Naroji, MD
Eunice Kennedy Shriver National Institute of
  Child Health and Human Development
Children's National Hospital

Sameen Nooruddin, MD
OBGYN Medical Center Associates

Katherine L. O'Flynn O'Brien, MD
Children's Minnesota

Christine Osborne, MD, MS
Canmore Obstetrics and Gynecology

Benjamin L. Palmer, DO
University of Iowa Hospitals and Clinics

Melissa Parks, DO, MPH
Phoenix Children's Hospital

Christine M. Pennesi, MD
Cincinnati Children's Hospital

Shashwati Pradhan, MD
University of Chicago

Elisabeth H. Quint, MD
University of Michigan Medical School

Ellen Rome, MD, MPH
Cleveland Clinic Foundation

Kelsey Shnaekel, MD
OBGYN Associates of Jonesboro

Jessica Shim, MD
Boston Children's Hospital

Judith Simms-Cendan, MD
University of Central Florida

Kathryn Stambough, MD
Arkansas Children's Hospital and University of
  Arkansas for Medical Sciences

Julie Strickland, MD
University of Missouri-Kansas City School of
  Medicine

Jacqueline Sugarman, MD
Children's Advocacy Center of the Bluegrass and
  University of Kentucky Albert B Chandler
  Medical Center

Vikki Tulchinskaya, MD, MSCR
University of Louisville

Alla Vash-Margita, MD
Yale School of Medicine

Amy Williamson, MD
Phoenix Children's Hospital

Olivia Winfrey, MD, MPH
University of Kentucky

Jennie Yoost, MD, MS
Marshall University School of Medicine

Andrea Zuckerman, MD
Tufts Medical Centre

1

Abnormal Uterine Bleeding (AUB)

S. Paige Hertweck and Maggie L. Dwiggins

Key Points

- In the adolescent, abnormal uterine bleeding (AUB) is usually due to anovulatory cycles (non-structural etiologies)
- Important to consider the possibility of pregnancy, sexual trauma, and infection regardless of the sexual history that the patient provides
- Must rule out pelvic inflammatory disease and ectopic pregnancy before considering the PALM-COEIN differential (**p**olyp; **a**denomyosis; **l**eiomyoma; **m**alignancy and **h**yperplasia; **c**oagulopathy; **o**vulatory dysfunction; **e**ndometrial; **i**atrogenic; and **n**ot yet classified)

Normal Menstrual Cycles in Adolescent Girls

- Normal menarche: Age 12–13
- Normal cycle interval/length: 21–45 days
- Normal flow length: 2–7 days
- Normal menstrual product use: 3–6 pads/tampons per day

Differential Diagnosis

- PALM-COEIN (structural-nonstructural)
- PALM (rare in adolescents only 1.3% of population have these)
  - **P**olyps
  - **A**denomyosis
  - **L**eiomyomas
  - **M**alignancies
    - Rhabdomyosarcoma, hormonally active tumors (i.e. granulosa cell tumor of ovary)
- COEIN (more prevalent in adolescents)
  - **C**oagulopathies
    - 20% of adolescents with heavy bleeding have underlying bleeding disorder
    - Von Willebrand disease is most common of bleeding disorders
    - Platelet aggregation disorder
  - **O**vulatory disorder
    - Anovulation due to
      - Immature hypothalamic-pituitary-ovarian axis (present in 95% of adolescents)

DOI: 10.1201/9781003039235-1

- – Polycystic ovarian syndrome (PCOS)
- – Hypothalamic issue (i.e. stress, chronic medical illness, eating disorder)
- **E**ndometrial disorders
- **I**atrogenic
  - – Includes medications such as anticoagulants, hormonal medications like oral contraceptives, or medications that interfere with ovulation like antipsychotics
- **N**ot yet classified

Diagnosis

History

- Menstrual history
  - Date/age of menarche
  - Frequency of menstrual cycles
  - Date/length of most recent menses
  - Number of pads/tampons per day used
- Evaluate for coagulation defects (If "Yes" to several of the below)
  - Menses longer than 7 days
  - Changing pad or tampon every 1–2 hours
  - Passing blood clots larger than a quarter size
  - History of soiling clothes due to heavy menstrual bleeding
  - History of anemia
  - History of epistaxis, gingival bleeding
  - History of bleeding after hemostatic challenge (i.e. tooth extraction, surgery)
  - Family history of bleeding disorders
  - Family history of need for blood transfusion
- Medications
  - Hormonal contraceptive use
  - Antipsychotic medications
  - Anti-epileptic medications
- Confidential sexual history
  - Chlamydia can cause AUB
- Related health changes that may affect ovulation
  - Weight change
  - Nutrition history
  - Exercise history
  - Weight concerns
  - Chronic medical problems

Physical Examination

- Vital signs
  - Pulse, blood pressure check (signs of anemia, orthostatic)
  - Height, weight, body mass index (extremes of weight associated with anovulation)

- General
  - Look for signs of androgen excess (acne, hirsutism, acanthosis nigricans)
- Thyroid
  - Palpate for enlargement
- Breast exam
  - Assess sexual maturity rating
- Abdomen
  - Assess for tenderness or mass
- Pelvic exam (consider use of thinnest bladed speculum)
  - Assess for anatomic/traumatic cause of bleeding
    – Rule out vaginal foreign body
    – Rule out reproductive tract laceration
  - Assess cervix
    – Rule out inflammation, lesion
    – Test for gonorrhea, chlamydia
  - Assess uterine/adnexal size
    – Rule out pregnancy, ovarian mass
- Pelvic ultrasound
  - If unsure of adequacy of pelvic exam
    Or
  - Concern of adnexal mass on exam
    Or
  - If bleeding persistent despite medical management (rule out Müllerian anomaly i.e. perforated hemivagina with uterine didelphys)

Laboratory Evaluation

- Baseline
  - Urine pregnancy test
  - CBC with platelets (hgb > 11 g/dL)
  - Ferritin (ideally should be >30 ng/dL)
- Recurrent/severe bleeding since menstrual onset
  - Coagulation testing
    – Prothrombin time
    – Partial thromboplastin time
    – Von Willebrand panel
      – Von Willebrand-ristocetin cofactor activity
      – Von Willebrand antigen
      – Factor VIII activity
  - Thyroid-stimulating hormone level
- If chronic anovulation/irregular bleeding noted
  - Follicle-stimulating hormone level
  - Prolactin level (rule out prolactinoma)
- If AUB with severe acne, hirsutism
  - Total/free testosterone

- Dehydroepiandrosterone sulfate level (DHEAS)
- 7 am 17 hydroxyprogesterone (17OHP) level
- If concern for primary ovarian insufficiency (POI), female athlete triad, or disordered eating (based on history)
  - Estradiol

Management

- Based on
  - Presenting signs/symptoms
  - Examination and laboratory findings
  - Presence/absence/severity of anemia

When pregnancy, infections, structural causes, thyroid conditions have been ruled out, medical management can be tailored based on patient preferences/medical conditions.

- Acute AUB
  - Mild cases (bleeding 20–60 day intervals, hemoglobin > 11 g/dL, low ferritin)
    - Reassurance
    - Educate on keeping menstrual calendar (mobile apps can be helpful)
    - Iron supplementation
    - If sexually active, offer contraception
    - If not sexually active but wants treatment
      - Offer hormonal treatment (see Table 1.1)
        Or
      - Offer nonhormonal treatment
        - Tranexamic acid 1300 mg every 8 hours for 5 days
  - Reevaluate in 3 months

TABLE 1.1

Hormonal Management for Chronic Abnormal Uterine Bleeding

Therapy	Route	Dose	Frequency	Method of Use
Combination OC	Oral	10- to 50-mcg ethinyl estradiol in combination with various progesterone	Daily	Cyclic or continuous
POP	Oral	4-mg drospirenone	Daily	Cyclic or continuous
POP	Oral	35-mcg norethindrone	Daily	Continuous
POP	Oral	5- to 15-mg norethindrone acetate	Daily	Continuous
Combined patch	Transdermal	0.12-mg etonorgestrel /35-mcg ethanol estradiol/d	Weekly	Cyclic or continuous[a]
Combined ring	Vaginal	0.12-mg etonorgestrel/15-mcg ethinyl estradiol/d	Monthly	Cyclic or continuous
Injectable	IM or SC	150–mg IM or 104-mg SC DMPA	Every 3 months	Continuous
Implant	SC	68-mg etonorgestrel	Every 3 years Up to 5 years[b]	Continuous
IUD	Intrauterine	13.5- to 52-mg levonorgestrel	3–7 years	Continuous

Abbreviations: OC, oral contraceptive; POP, progesterone-only pill; IM, intramuscular; SC, subcutaneous, DMPA, depot medroxyprogesterone acetate; IUD, intrauterine device.

[a] Caution with continuous use in patients with BMI > 30.

[b] Ali M, Akin A, Bahamondes L, et al.; WHO study group on subdermal contraceptive implants for women. Extended use up to 5 years of the etonogestrel-releasing subdermal contraceptive implant: comparison to levonorgestrel-releasing subdermal implant. Hum Reprod. 2016; 31(11):2491–2498; McNicholas C, Swor E, Wan L, Peipert JF. Prolonged use of the etonogestrel implant and levonorgestrel intrauterine device: 2 years beyond the Food and Drug Administration-approved duration. Am J Obstet Gynecol. 2017; 216(6):586.e1–586.e6.

- Moderate-severe cases that are hemodynamically stable (hemoglobin 8–11 g/dL)
  - Educate regarding keeping menstrual calendar
  - Rule out bleeding disorder/treat STI if suspected or detected
  - Iron supplementation in conjunction with vitamin C to help absorption
  - *If actively bleeding* (see Table 1.2 for all therapeutic options)
    - Recommend treatment with medroxyprogesterone acetate due to improved compliance, decreased adverse side effects, and safety of use:
      - Start with 20 mg every 8 hours for 7 days
      - Continue 20 mg daily for the next 3 weeks
        - ***NOTE***: Expect some bleeding when decreasing dose after 7 days
      - After initial 28 days of treatment, consider long-term alternative (see below)
    - Determine if contraindications to estrogen
      - Severe cardiac conditions
      - Uncontrolled hypertension
      - Thrombotic conditions
      - Migraines with aura
      - Hepatic dysfunction
        - If none, consider combination estrogen/progesterone pill
        - If present, consider medroxyprogesterone acetate or norethindrone
          - ***NOTE***: Norethindrone acetate is metabolized to ethinyl estradiol
          - (20 mg of norethindrone acetate equivalent to 30-mcg ethinyl estradiol)
  - *If not actively bleeding*
    - Determine if contraindications to estrogen (see above)
      - *If yes*: Use one of the following progesterone therapies
        - Cyclic progestin therapy with
        - Medroxyprogesterone acetate 10 mg × day 1–10 of each month
          Or
        - Daily use of one pill of norethindrone 0.35 mg
      - *If estrogen not contraindicated* Use
        - Monophasic oral contraceptive pill (suggest 30-mcg estradiol)
    - Reevaluate three cycles
- Acute hemorrhage (hypotension or hemoglobin < 8 g/dL)
  - Fluid resuscitation and stabilization of patient vital signs
  - Admit to hospital
  - Rule out coagulopathy, STD
  - Start iron replacement
  - Obtain hematology consult
  - Consider transfusion if symptomatic
  - Begin hormonal therapy (see Table 1.2)
    - Determine if contraindications to estrogen (see above)
      - *If yes:* Use one of the progesterone therapies
    - Use IV if unable to tolerate oral medication
    - Goal of therapy is bleeding cessation within 24–48 hours
    - If bleeding is not under control within that time frame, consider additional use of anti-fibrinolytic medications (see Table 1.2)

- Surgical intervention is used as a last resort
  - Consider suction dilatation and curettage (D&C)
  - Consider the placement of 30 mL Foley balloon in intrauterine cavity for tamponade effect
    - Leave in place for 24 hours and then slowly decrease volume from balloon
  - If these methods fail, endometrial ablation or hysterectomy are last resort options in this population

TABLE 1.2

Medical and Hormonal Therapies for Acute Heavy Menstrual Bleeding

Therapy	Dose	Route	Initial Frequency
Conjugated estrogen	25 mg	IV	Every 4–6 hours
50-mcg ethinyl estradiol combined pill[a]	1 tablet	Oral	Every 6 hours
30- to 35-mcg ethinyl estradiol combined pill[a]	1 tablet	Oral	Every 6 hours
Medroxyprogesterone	10–20 mg (maximum 80 mg/d)	Oral	Every 6–12 hours
Norethindrone 0.35 mg	1 tablet	Oral	Every 8–12 hours
Norethindrone acetate[b]	5–10 mg	Oral	Every 6 hours
Tranexamic acid	10 mg/kg	IV	Every 6–8 hours
Aminocaproic acid	100–200 mg/ kg (maximum 30 g/d)	IV or oral	Every 4–6 hours

Abbreviation: IV, Intravenous.

Source: Adapted from Santos M, Hendry D, Sangi-Haghpeykar H, Deitrich JE. Retrospective review of norethindrone use in adolescents. J Pediatr Adolesc Gynecol. 2014; 27:41–44.

[a] High doses of ethinyl estradiol may cause nausea, consider concurrent use of antiemetic.

[b] 20 mg of norethindrone acetate equivalent to 30-mcg ethinyl estradiol due to peripheral conversion.

BIBLIOGRAPHY

Chu M, Zhang X, Gentzschein E, Stanczyk FZ, Lobo RA. Formation of ethinyl estradiol in women during treatment with norethindrone actate. J Clin Endocrinol Metab. 2007; 92:2205–2207.

Haamid F, Sass AE, Dietrich JE. Heavy menstrual bleeding in adolescents. J Pediatr Adolesc Gynecol. 2017; 30(3):335–340.

Hernandez A, Deitrich JE. Abnormal uterine bleeding in the adolescent. Obstet Gynecol. 2020 March; 135(3):615–621.

Management of acute abnormal uterine bleeding in nonpregnant reproductive-aged women. American College of Obstetricians and Gynecologists Committee Opinion No. 557. Obstet Gynecol. 2013; 121:891–896.

Menstruation in girls and adolescents: Using the menstrual cycle as a vital sign. American Academy of Pediatrics Committee on Adolescence, American College of Obstetrics and Gynecologists Committee on Adolescent Health Care. Pediatrics. 2006; 118:2245.

Munro MG, Mainor N, Basu R, Brisinger M, Barreda L. Oral medroxyprogesterone acetate and combination oral contraceptives for acute uterine bleeding: a randomized controlled trial. Obstet Gynecol. 2006; 108(4):924–929.

Use of hormonal contraception in women with coexisting medical conditions. American College of Obstetricians and Gynecologists Practice Bulletin No 206. Obstet Gynecol. 2019; 133:e128.

2

Adolescent Pregnancy

Ariel Cohen

Key Points

- The pregnant adolescent may initially present with vague complaints; clinical suspicion should be high for all sexually active adolescents.
- Pregnant adolescents should be counseled on all pregnancy options: Continuing the pregnancy, placing the infant for adoption, or pregnancy termination. They will unlikely be able to make a firm decision initially.
- Obstetrically, these patients are at increased risk for low birth weight (LBW) infants, preterm birth (PTB), sexually transmitted infections (STIs), and hypertensive disorders of pregnancy (gestational hypertension, preeclampsia, and eclampsia).
- Pregnancy more likely to be complicated by congenital anomaly, including central nervous system, gastrointestinal, or musculoskeletal.
- Postpartum, adolescents have at 2–3× increased risk of postpartum depression (PPD) and are less likely to breastfeed their infants.
- Risk factors for adolescent pregnancy include interfamilial (parent who was an adolescent parent, sibling who is a teen parent, familial dysfunction), individual (early menarche, depression), or sociocultural (peers who are adolescent parents, history of sexual abuse, educational failures, media messaging, pressures from male partner, older sexual partners, lack of access to reproductive healthcare).
- Research suggests that comprehensive adolescent pregnancy programs contribute to the prevention of psychosocial complications and the promotion of good outcomes. Examples include group prenatal care and early intervention for adolescents with depression.

Diagnosis

- Patients can present specifically for a pregnancy test but more often present with other vague chief complaints (vaginal and urinary symptoms, abdominal pain, fatigue, syncope, nausea and vomiting, depressive symptoms).
- Check urine pregnancy test (UPT) for any sexually active adolescent who is not on reliable contraception and any adolescent presenting with oligo- or amenorrhea.

History

A confidential interview is recommended, as this is a sensitive topic

- Gynecologic history with menarche and regularity of periods
  - When were your last menstrual period (LMP) and prior period? Were they normal?
    - Adolescents may be falsely reassured by first trimester bleeding from embryo implantation or a ruptured corpus luteal cyst (CLC)

DOI: 10.1201/9781003039235-2

- Are you sexually active? With boys, girls, or both? In which sexual activities do you participate?
- How do you prevent pregnancy? How do you prevent sexually transmitted infections?
- Is there any chance you may be pregnant?
- What would you do if a pregnancy test were positive?
    - Exploring the adolescent's perceptions about parenthood/pregnancy prior to completing diagnostic testing can be helpful since adolescents are developmentally more likely to be concrete thinkers
    - The adolescent's perception of the implications of pregnancy frequently bears little resemblance to reality
- Depression screening
  - There is an increased rate (2–3×) of PPD
  - Early therapeutic interventions have shown reductions in PPD
- Medication history
  - Teratogenic medications should be noted, for example, isotretinoin (Accutane®), methotrexate, testosterone

Physical Exam

This should be directed toward symptoms, screening for STIs, and hypertension

- Vital signs
- Breast examination, if indicated: May find engorgement with dark pigmentation to areola
- Abdominal examination: Tenderness, possibly palpable uterine fundus. Acute abdominal exam may be suggestive of ectopic pregnancy
  - Uterine fundus is below the level of symphysis pubis prior to 12 weeks' gestation; approximately midway between symphysis and umbilicus at 16 weeks; approximately at umbilicus at 20 weeks
  - Symphysis pubis tenderness is common from progestational effect
- Pelvic examination: Recommended by American College of Obstetricians and Gynecologists (ACOG) for all new prenatal patients for endocervical STI testing
  - Among patients who will not assent to pelvic examination, vaginal swab self-collection or urine specimen collection for nucleic acid amplification testing (NAAT) is another option in patients engaging in oral and/or anal sex, pharyngeal and/or rectal swabs can similarly be collected or self-collected.
  - A uterine size less than estimated gestational age (EGA) and/or adnexal tenderness/enlargement may be suggestive of ectopic pregnancy. Further evaluation will be necessary (see "Laboratory Tests")

Laboratory Tests

A clinical diagnosis of pregnancy must be confirmed by laboratory testing

- Confirmation of pregnancy by a human chorionic gonadotropin (hCG) assay
  - UPT: Qualitative, yes/no/indeterminate
  - Quantitative serum hCG: Quantitative, needs clinical correlation, potential serial lab draws, and imaging (see "which hCG test to order")
- Pelvic ultrasound to confirm intrauterine location of the pregnancy
  - This can be at approximately 4–5 weeks' gestation by LMP dating (on endovaginal ultrasound) and when serum hCG 1500–3200 mIU/mL
  - Imaging should be performed imminently if the patient is experiencing pelvic pain to evaluate for ectopic pregnancy

Which hCG test to order

- UPT should be the *first* test
  - This tests urine hCG levels as low as 5–10 mIU/mL (assay-dependent). Results will be positive, negative, or indeterminate
  - Repeat at least 14 days after last sexual intercourse to be certain of negative result
  - Only confirms the presence of hCG hormone, not location of pregnancy
  - False results are possible in severe renal disease, high immunoglobulin levels, and low serum protein
- A serum quantitative hCG
  - This has a lower discriminatory threshold for serum levels of hCG and provides a numerical measurement. It can be helpful in the assessment of pregnancies of unknown location (PUL), ectopic pregnancy, or resolution of spontaneous abortion (SAB)
    - Discriminatory zone for determining the presence of intrauterine pregnancy on endovaginal ultrasound: 1500–3200 mIU/mL
    - Serum hCG values trended over 48 hours should roughly double in normal intrauterine pregnancies
    - Serum hCG values should decrease serially following SAB
  - Different assays may yield different results, and if trending hCG values, using the same assay and laboratory is optimal.
  - Notably, gestational trophoblastic neoplasia, such as hydatidiform moles, are more common at extremes of age. This diagnosis will be made if the hCG is over 3200 mIU/mL and ultrasound with a mixed echogenic pattern ("snow storm" appearance). This should prompt immediate referral to a gynecologist for management.

Other testing

- STI screening
  - Gonorrhea and chlamydia NAAT
  - Trichomonas NAAT or wet mount
  - Serum non-treponemal testing (e.g. rapid plasma reagin, RPR) and HIV antibody/antigen
- Prenatal panel
  - Type and screen
  - Rubella and varicella IgG
  - Hepatitis B surface antigen (HBVsAg) and Hepatitis C virus antibody
  - Urine culture (if EGA >10 weeks)

Management

Decision-making regarding the outcome of pregnancy

1. After confirming pregnancy, inform the adolescent of the test result
   a. Elicit thoughts and feelings about the test result
   b. Ambivalence, apathy, fear, tearfulness, or shock are common
   c. Providing emotional support is **key**
   d. Find out how the adolescent wants to go about informing their parent(s)/guardian and the other parent of the baby

2. Provide factual information regarding the estimated date of delivery (EDD), prenatal care, and course despite her initial plans
   a. Schedule close follow-up as adolescents are often unable to reach firm decisions regarding the pregnancy initially
3. If the provider does not provide pregnancy counseling or prenatal care, refer to the provider with pregnancy counseling
   a. Discuss options (parenthood, adoption, and termination) in a non-judgmental manner
      i. Offer referral to each resource
   b. Care provider should check in with the adolescent about one week after the scheduled referral. This can help ensure appropriate follow-up

Follow-up and referrals

1. Parenthood and adoption
   a. Refer to prenatal care
      i. Providers should be familiar with caring for adolescents in pregnancy
      ii. Nutritional services: Pregnant adolescents are at risk for poor weight gain and require adequate nutritional support and weight gain throughout the entirety of the pregnancy. Food security may be a concern
      iii. Social service assistance, financial support services, and educational services (pregnancy classes)
      iv. If available:
         A. Group prenatal care has shown to be beneficial
         B. Evening clinical hours so that visits do not interfere with school
   b. When to refer to a subspecialist (perinatologist)
      i. Preexisting medical conditions: Diabetes mellitus, epilepsy, cardiac disease, sickle cell anemia or hemoglobinopathies, cancer, or history of teratogenic medication use
      ii. When suspicion is high for congenital anomaly
2. Pregnancy termination
   a. Adolescents choosing termination should be aware that some states require parental notification for a legal abortion (AB)
   b. A judicial bypass system also exists if the judge determines that the adolescent is a mature minor or if termination of pregnancy is in the minor's best interest
   c. No legal requirement to notify the father of the baby prior to the termination
3. Mental healthcare
   a. Early intervention is the best option to prevent PPD

Early Pregnancy Complications

Bleeding or spotting occurs in 20–25% of pregnancies; approximately half of these pregnancies will miscarry

- If Rh-negative blood type, will require intramuscular prophylactic Rho(D) immune globulin (RhoGAM) within 72 hours of the bleeding event (spotting, miscarriage, uterine evacuation) to prevent anti-Rh isoimmunization

- Abnormal pregnancies and abortion (AB)
    - Spontaneous AB: Cramping, bleeding, passage of products of conception (POC) over a limited period of hours
        - If there is bleeding without passage of POC
            - Threatened AB: Closed cervix, pregnancy still viable. Adolescents may think this is falsely "reassuring" that they had a period and they are not pregnant
            - Incomplete AB: Open cervix, pregnancy no longer viable. Treatment with uterine evacuation
    - Septic AB: Fever and uterine tenderness. As this is life-threatening, it requires emergent evaluation and treatment (antibiotics, uterine evacuation)
    - Missed AB: Nonviable gestational sac on ultrasound. See Doubilet criteria for radiologic guidelines. Treat with uterine evacuation or expectant management (many will have spontaneous AB within 1–2 weeks)
    - Complete AB: Mostly resolved bleeding, closed cervix on exam, minimal tissue on ultrasound. Manage expectantly
- Ectopic pregnancy and pregnancy of unknown location (PUL)
    - PUL: Positive pregnancy test and hCG below discriminatory zone (of 1500–3200 mIU/mL), without evidence of intrauterine pregnancy on ultrasound.
        - Needs follow-up imaging and serum hCG to confirm normal pregnancy. Refer to a gynecologist for management. Many are normal pregnancies
        - Give precautions to present for emergency evaluation if in acute abdominal pain
    - Ectopic pregnancy: Abdominal pain and bleeding is an ectopic pregnancy until proven otherwise (see Chapter 52, "Tubal Mass" for management)
        - Adolescents at increased risk, especially if history of chlamydia or gonorrhea
        - Evaluate with ultrasound and serum quantitative hCG
        - If meeting criteria for PUL, and no evidence of ruptured ectopic pregnancy or hemodynamic instability on examination and imaging, follow with a serial hCG draw in 48 hours
        - Referral to gynecologist for treatment of ectopic pregnancy. Treatment is with surgical management (uterine evacuation, salpingectomy, or salpingostomy for tubal ectopics) or IM methotrexate per ACOG guidelines
        - Rare ectopic pregnancies (cervical, interstitial, ovarian, and abdominal) may require management at a tertiary referral center

BIBLIOGRAPHY

Cox JE. (n.d.). Teen Pregnancy. In Emans SJ and Laufer MR (Eds.), *Emans, Laufer and Goldstein's Pediatric and Adolescent Gynecology* 2020 (7th ed., pp. 664–679). Philadelphia, PA: Wolters Kluwer.

Cypher RL. Collaborative approaches to prenatal care: strategies of successful adolescent programs. J Perinat Neonatal Nurs. 2013 Apr–Jun; 27(2):134–144. doi: 10.1097/JPN.0b013e31828ecc40

Doubilet PM, Benson CB, Bourne T, Blaivas M; Society of Radiologists in Ultrasound Multispecialty Panel on Early First Trimester Diagnosis of Miscarriage and Exclusion of a Viable Intrauterine Pregnancy, Barnhart KT, Benacerraf BR, Brown DL, Filly RA, Fox JC, Goldstein SR, Kendall JL, Lyons EA, Porter MB, Pretorius DH, Timor-Tritsch IE. Diagnostic criteria for nonviable pregnancy early in the first trimester. N Engl J Med. 2013 Oct 10;369(15):1443-51. doi: 10.1056/NEJMra1302417.

Panzarine S, Slater E, Sharps P. Coping, social support, and depressive symptoms in adolescent mothers. J Adolesc Health. 1995 Aug; 17(2):113–119. doi: 10.1016/1054-139X(95)00064-Y

Phipps MG, Raker CA, Ware CF, Zlotnick C. Randomized controlled trial to prevent postpartum depression in adolescent mothers. Am J Obstet Gynecol. 2013 Mar; 208(3):192.e1–e6. doi: 10.1016/j.ajog.2012.12.036

Soper JT. Gestational Trophoblastic Disease: Current Evaluation and Management. Obstet. Gynecol. 2021 Feb; 137(2): 355–370. doi: 10.1097/AOG.0000000000004240

3

Ambiguous Genitalia and Differences of Sexual Development (DSD)

Amy Williamson

Definition

Differences of sexual development (DSD) are defined as "congenital conditions in which development of chromosomal, gonadal, or anatomic sex is atypical" in a consensus statement on the management of intersex disorders.

Key Points

- May be discovered at any time, including prenatally, at birth, during infancy, during adolescence, or during an evaluation for infertility
- There is controversy regarding surgical intervention for children with DSD prior to their ability to give assent or consent for irreversible treatments
- Due to the heterogeneity of presentations, options for management, and paucity of long-term data on psychological and outcome data, multidisciplinary care should be provided, including pediatric and adolescent gynecology, pediatric urology, pediatric surgery, pediatric endocrinology, pediatric radiology, genetics, psychology/psychiatry, adolescent medicine, neonatology, social work, nursing, ethicists, and legal experts

AMBIGUOUS GENITALIA

Definition

Variation in the appearance of the external genitalia that is not clearly male or female.

Newborn

1. This is a medical and social emergency in the newborn
2. 75% of these cases have life-threatening salt-wasting nephropathy that, if unrecognized, can cause hypotension, vascular collapse, and death
   a. Ensure electrolyte/endocrine abnormalities are corrected
   b. Establish the most probable cause

DOI: 10.1201/9781003039235-3

   c. Defer making a gender assignment

      i. Reassure the parents that they have a healthy baby, but the appearance of the external genitalia is atypical. Testing will be performed to determine the cause of the genital findings

      ii. Refer to the child as "your baby or your infant" rather than as a girl or a boy

      iii. Involve a mental health professional to help educate the family about sexual development and coach them on how to deal with grandparents, siblings, and babysitters

      iv. While the child's karyotype may be identified early, their gender identity can be more difficult to predict and should be deferred until the child has input into the decision

Diagnosis

1. 46,XX DSD

   a. Disorders related to androgen synthesis or action resulting in androgen excess with normal ovaries

      i. *Congenital adrenal hyperplasia (CAH)*: Most common cause of ambiguous genitalia

         A. Highest frequency in people of European Jewish, Hispanic, Italian, or Slavic ancestry

         B. Results from enzymatic defect in conversion of cholesterol to cortisol

         C. 95% of cases are due to 21-hydroxylase enzyme deficiency (CYP21A2 6p21.33) resulting in

            a. Elevated 17-hydroxyprogesterone (17-OHP)

            b. Low cortisol

            c. Elevated adrenocorticotropic hormone (ACTH)

            d. Can result in life-threatening salt-wasting

         D. Less commonly

            a. 11-beta-hydroxylase deficiency (CYP11B1 8q24.3) resulting in elevation of 11-deoxycorticosterone

            b. 3-beta-hydroxysteroid deficiency (HSD3B2 1p13.1) in elevation of 17-hydroxypregnenolone

            c. POR (P450 oxidoreductase 7q11.23)

            d. Aromatase deficiency (CYP19 15q21.2)

            e. Glucocorticoid receptor (NR3CI 5q31.3)

   b. Maternal androgen excess from adrenal/ovarian tumors or administration of androgenic medications

   c. Disorders of ovarian development (rare)

      i. Gonadal biopsy required

      ii. Usually presents with testis or ovotestis and absent Müllerian structures

      iii. *Typical mutations*: SRY (Yp.11.3), SOX9 (17q24), SOX3 (Xq27.1), NR5A (SFI 9q33.3), RSP1 (Ip34.3), and WNT4 (Ip36.12)

   d. Other

      i. Vaginal atresia; (see Chapter 58, "Vaginal Tract Anomalies")

      ii. Vaginal agenesis (Mayer-Rokinansky-Kuster-Hauser syndrome); (see Chapter 56, "Uterovaginal/müllerian agenesis")

2. 46,XY DSD: Undervirilizing, testes present (***those listed in italics are not likely to be seen by PAG providers but are included for completeness***)
    a. Disorders of androgen response
        i. AR (Xq12) Androgen receptor defect
            A. Complete/partial androgen insensitivity
            B. Normal testis/female or ambiguous genitalia (see Chapter 5, "AIS")
    b. Disorders of testicular development
        i. WT1(11p13)
            A. Dysgenetic testis, +/− Müllerian structures, female or undervirilized male external genitalia
            B. Frasier syndrome, Denys-Drash syndrome with Wilms tumor
        ii. NR5A1 (SF1 9q33.3)
            A. Dysgenetic gonads, +/− Müllerian structures, undervirilized male external genitalia
            B. Accompanied by adrenal insufficiency
        iii. SRY (Yp11.3), SOX9 (17q24), NROB1 (DAX1 Xp21.3)
            A. Dysgenetic testis or ovotestis, +/− Müllerian structures, typically female or undervirilized external genitalia
        iv. GATA4 (8p23.1)
            A. Dysgenetic testis, absent Müllerian structures, typically female or undervirilized external genitalia
            B. Associated cardiac defects (ASD/VSD/TOF)
        v. ZFPM2 (FOG2 8q23.1)
            A. Dysgenetic gonads, +/− Müllerian structures, typically female or undervirilized male external genitalia
            B. Associated cardiac defects, diaphragmatic hernia
        vi. MAP3K1 (5q11.2)
            A. Dysgenetic gonads, +/− Müllerian structures, typically female or undervirilized male external genitalia
        vii. DMRT1 (9p24.3)
            A. Dysgenetic gonads, Müllerian structures absent, typically female external genitalia
        viii. DHH (12q13.1), SAMD9 (7q21.2), ARX (Xp22.13)
            A. Dysgenetic gonads, Müllerian structures absent, typically female or undervirilized male external genitalia
        ix. *MAMLD1 (CXORF6 Xq28)*
            A. *Dysgenetic gonads/normal male internal genitalia/undervirilized male external genitalia*
    c. Disorders of androgen synthesis or action
        i. LHCGR (2p16.3)
            A. Normal testis, female or undervirilized male external genitalia
        ii. *DHCR7 (11q13.4)*
            A. *Normal testis, normal to undervirilized male*
            B. *Smith-Lemli-Opitz syndrome (microcephaly, classic facies, cleft palate, syndactyly, and/or polydactyly)*
        iii. STAR (8p11.2), CYP11A1 (15q24.1)
            A. Normal testis, female or undervirilized male
            B. Lipoid CAH (primary adrenal insufficiency), delayed or absent puberty

        iv. HSD3B2 (1p13.1)
            A. Normal testis, female or undervirilized male
            B. CAH (primary adrenal insufficiency), elevated delta 5:4 ratio
        v. CYP17A1 (10q24.3)
            A. Normal testis, female or undervirilized male
            B. CAH with hypertension due to increased deoxycorticosterone
        vi. *POR (P450 oxidoreductase 7q11.2)*
            A. *Normal testis, normal to undervirilized male*
            B. *CAH*
        vii. HSD17B3 (9q22.23), SRD5A2 (2p23.1)
            A. Normal testis, female to undervirilized male
            B. Virilization may occur shortly after birth or at puberty, increased testosterone(T) to dihydroT ratio
     d. Structural DSD
        i. *AMH (19p.13.3)*
            A. *Normal testis, Müllerian structures internally, normal male external genitalia*
        ii. *AMH (12q13.13)*
            A. *Normal testis, Müllerian structures internally, normal male external genitalia with bilateral cryptorchidism*

3. Sex chromosome DSD: Karyotype not 46,XX or 46,XY
     a. Ovotesticular DSD
        i. Over 50% genotype 46,XX, 33% chimeric 46,XY/46,XX, or mosaic 46,XY/47XXY or 45,X/46,XY
        ii. Genitalia, most often ambiguous but can be male or female
        iii. Both ovarian and testicular tissue present
     b. Mixed gonadal dysgenesis (MGD*)*: Sex chromosome mosaicism
        i. 45,X/46,XY mosaicism
        ii. 50% of patients with MGD are born with ambiguous genitalia
        iii. Common one dysgenetic testis (non-sperm-producing) and one streak gonad
        iv. Unilateral unicornuate uterus/fallopian tube on streak gonad side

Diagnostic Workup

History

1. Family history
     a. Ambiguous genitalia, infertility, unexpected changes at puberty
        i. Recessive traits appear in siblings and X-linked abnormalities tend to appear in males who are scattered sporadically across the family history
     b. Consanguinity: Increases the likelihood of autosomal recessive disorders (CAH)
     c. Neonatal deaths may suggest a previously missed diagnosis of CAH
     d. Maternal virilization may suggest a maternal androgen-producing tumor
2. Pregnancy history
     a. Prior pregnancies with ambiguity
     b. Prior pregnancies that ended in fetal demise/early death
     c. Consanguinity
     d. Hormonal ingestion/pharmaceutical exposure during pregnancy, particularly androgens or progestational drugs
3. Maternal symptoms of androgen excess

Physical Exam

General

1. Abnormal facial appearance, dysmorphic features suggesting a multiple malformation syndrome (intrauterine growth retardation, abnormal body proportions)
2. Urine output, weight, blood pressure
3. Skin hyperpigmentation of the areola/genital skin due to elevated ACTH
4. Signs of salt-wasting such as decreased skin turgor, no tears with crying

Gonadal exam

1. Palpate inguinal canal, labioscrotal folds, or scrotum for the presence of gonadal tissue
   a. Abduct the thighs. Start with fingers at the line of inguinal canal and sweep down the canal on each side above the inguinal line. Any gonad that is nudged down toward the scrotum should be gently grasped by the other examining hand, noting the size, and the consistency of the gonad
   b. Palpable gonads below the inguinal canal are almost always a testicle and **exclude** diagnoses of gonadal females (CAH, Turner syndrome, and pure gonadal dysgenesis), and may indicate XY DSD, XX ovotesticular DSD, or testicular DSD
   c. Non-palpable gonads in a virilized female infant should raise the possibility of a severe 46,XX DSD, such as CAH

External genitalia

1. Consider using the Prader staging to describe virilization of female genitalia (Figure 3.1) and Quigley staging to describe incomplete masculinization

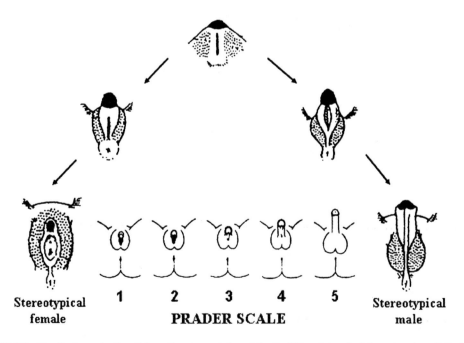

FIGURE 3.1   The Prader scale. Top: Schematic representation of the "indifferent stage" of the external genitalia that is common to XX and XY fetuses early in development. Middle: Schematic representation of the sexual differentiation of the external genitalia during the first trimester of fetal life. Bottom: The Prader scale assigns values ranging from 1 to 5, where 1 is a stereotypical female and 5 is a stereotypical male. Values ranging from 2 to 4 denote an intersex phenotype. (From Jorge JC, et al. J Sex Med. 2008; 5(1):122–131, with permission.)

Prader 1: Slightly virilized female, mild clitoromegaly with no labial fusion

Prader 2: Presence of posterior labial fusion with an anogenital ratio greater than 0.5 (distance from anus to fourchette divided by the distance from anus to base of clitoris). Clitoromegaly and small vaginal opening with separate urethral opening

Prader 3: Complete fusion of labia with single urogenital sinus

Prader 4: Looks more male than female, with empty scrotum and a phallus the size of a normal penis with possible chordee. A single small urethral or vaginal opening at the base or on the shaft of the phallus would be to consider hypospadias in males but is urogenital sinus

Prader 5: Complete male virilization with a normally formed penis with a urethral opening at or near the tip. The scrotum is normally formed but empty

2. Clitorophallus: Note the length and width. Variations can represent clitoromegaly or hypospadias
   a. Mean stretched penile length in a full-term male is 3.5 ($\pm$0.4) cm
      i. Measure the stretched penis from the pubic ramus to the tip of the glans and also note the mid-shaft diameter
      ii. Rough rule, a full-term male should have a penile length > 2.5 cm
   b. Newborn clitoral size 2.0–8.5 mm in length and 2.0–6.0 mm width
3. Urethral meatus: Note position (on the glans, shaft, or at the perineum)
4. Labioscrotal folds
   a. Note degree of fusion, rugosity
   b. Rugose scrotal or labioscrotal folds with increased pigmentation suggest the possibility of increased corticotropin levels as in CAH
   c. Asymmetric labioscrotal folds with unilateral gonad make mixed gonadal dysgenesis more likely (normal testis on one side/streak gonad on the other)
5. Presence of hernia (may contain uterus, ovary, or testis)
6. Vaginal opening or urogenital sinus
7. Rectum: Evaluate for patency and note if a palpable cervix and uterus present on recto-abdominal exam
   a. Confirms internal Müllerian structures. The uterus is relatively enlarged in the newborn due to maternal estrogenization

NOTE: Presence of hypospadias, small clitorphallus, and/or bilateral cryptorchidism needs DSD evaluation

Laboratory Evaluation

1. Assess and follow serum electrolytes daily if abnormal or CAH suspected
   a. CMP for hyperkalemia, hyponatremia, and metabolic acidosis
   b. Salt crisis does not occur until 4–15 days of life
2. Additional labs
   a. Karyotype, FISH (Fluorescence in situ hybridization for SRY on Y Chromosome) LH, FSH, testosterone, DHEA, androstenedione, DHT, and 17-OHP
3. 17-OHP level should be drawn after 24 hours of life if gonads not palpable
   a. Normally elevated in cord blood
   b. Newborn screening includes 21-hydroxylase deficiency screening in all 50 states
   c. Decreases to 100–200 ng/dL after 24 hours of life
   d. 17-OHP levels of <1,000 ng/dL is considered normal and >10,000 ng/dL is diagnostic of 21-hydroxylase deficiency CAH
   e. If 17-OHP elevated but not diagnostic, repeat in a few days and monitor fluids and electrolytes

4. If 46,XX DSD present and etiology is unclear, order the following:
   a. ACTH (cosyntropin) stimulation test
   b. 11-deoxycorticosterone
   c. 11-deoxycortisol
   d. 17-hydroxypregnenolone

Laboratory Findings

1. 46, XX karyotype
   a. Elevated 17-OHP → 21-hydroxylase deficiency
   b. Normal 17-OHP and unclear etiology for ambiguous genitalia, perform an ACTH stimulation test and evaluate 11-deoxycorticosterone, 11-deoxycortisol, and 17-hydroxypregnenolone to determine if another adrenal enzymatic defect is present
2. 46,XY with absent Müllerian structures and normal/elevated testosterone or elevated T:DHT ratio → 5-alpha reductase deficiency
   a. An hCG stimulation test may be useful in determining the defect in cases of 46, XY DSD
3. If normal 17-OHP and normal ACTH → sex chromosome DSD, gonadal dysgenesis

Imaging

1. Abdominal/pelvic ultrasound
2. Genitogram-retrograde injection of contrast material in the urogenital orifice
3. Consider MRI in which the ultrasound or genitogram not definitive
4. Consider endoscopic exam or urethra or urogenital sinus
5. Rarely laparoscopy/laparotomy for gonadal biopsies

Management

Multidisciplinary team approach is ideal and should include genetics, pediatric endocrinology, pediatric surgery, pediatric/adolescent gynecology, pediatric urology, and psychology.

CAH

1. Goals
   a. Replace deficient steroids while minimizing adrenal sex hormone and glucocorticoid excess
   b. Prevent virilization
   c. Optimize growth
   d. Protect potential fertility
2. Lifelong steroid and mineralocorticoid replacement required
   a. Hydrocortisone (HCT) 10–15 mg/m^2/day divided 3×/daily
   b. Use divided or crushed tablets if inability to swallow pills, oral solution not recommended
   c. Monitor baby's weight, electrolytes, fluid status, plasma renin activity (salt losing not manifested until day 4–15 days of life)
   d. Decreased serum sodium, decreased aldosterone, elevated plasma renin indicate a salt-losing condition
      i. Add salt (2–4 g/day) to formula
      ii. Fludrocortisone acetate 0.05–0.1 mg/day

    iii. Stress dosing is 2–3 times the maintenance glucocorticoid dose

    iv. Give stress dose with fever >38.3°C (>101°F), when vomiting or unable to take PO feeds, with trauma, and prior to surgery

46,XY DSD or sex chromosome DSD (see Chapter 5, "AIS")

1. If testicular tissue present within the abdomen, monitor vs excision

Surgical Care

1. Postpone immediate surgical correction of the external genitalia in the newborn unless medically necessary
2. Intra-abdominal testicular tissue is at increased risk of malignancy and requires excision/monitoring

Note: Genital appearance during childhood is less important than sexual function in the adult years.

- Early surgical intervention can impair sexual function
- Sexual development of the brain is influenced by androgens and impacts gender identity. Some CAH patients may develop a male gender identity. As such, clitoral surgery or sex assignment surgery should be delayed until puberty or until the patient can provide informed consent
- Gender identity assessments should be performed by psychology before any surgical intervention
- These decisions are best made in consultation with a multidisciplinary team skilled in dealing with these conditions

CLITOROMEGALY

Definition

1. Prepubertal clitoral size
   a. Normal: Clitoral glans diameter: 3 mm
   b. Abnormal clitoral glans diameter: >5 mm or clitoral index (glans width × length) >35 mm
2. Adolescent/adult clitoral size (average)
   a. Clitoral glans: 2–4 mm wide and 5 mm long
   b. Total clitoral length: (glans and body) 16 mm
   c. Mean clitoral index: (glans width × glans length) 18.5 mm

Key Points

- Clitoral enlargement deserves a thorough evaluation
- May be the first sign of an endocrine or disorder of sexual development, or underlying neoplasm
- Clitoral enlargement usually occurs with other signs of virilization such as hirsutism, acne, and deepening voice
- May be the presenting sign of neurofibromatosis (patients also have café au lait macules prior or at the time of clitoral enlargement)

Differential Diagnosis

1. Androgen exposure
   a. Maternal drug exposure in infants
2. Endogenous (androgen tumor)
   a. Exogenous (medications such as danazol)
3. Congenital causes/tumors
   a. Gonadal dysgenesis
   b. 46,XX disorder of sexual development
   c. 46,XY disorder of sexual development
   d. Adrenal enzyme deficiency (CAH)
   e. Neurofibroma
   f. Choristoma (aberrant or heterotopic tissue)
4. Clitoral mass
   a. Epidermal cyst
   b. Fibroma
   c. Leiomyoma
   d. Angiokeratoma
   e. Pseudolymphoma
   f. Hemangioma
   g. Granular cell tumor
   h. Neurofibroma
5. Clitoral tumors (rare)
   a. Rhabdomyosarcoma
   b. Schwannoma
   c. Endodermal sinus tumor
   d. Lymphoma
   e. Dermoid cyst

Diagnosis

History

1. Age of patient
   a. *Newborn or infant*: See evaluation for ambiguous genitalia
   b. *Children or adolescents*: Concern for late-onset adrenal enzyme deficiency or exogenous vs endogenous androgen production
2. Duration of clitoromegaly
3. Any associated symptoms
   a. Clitoral pain or irritation
   b. Facial Acne or hirsutism
   c. Abdominal pain/masses
   d. Neurofibromatosis
   e. Family history

Physical Examination

1. Height/weight (plot on growth curves)

2. Skin
   a. Café au lait spots
3. Signs of androgen excess
   a. Acne (face, chest, and back)
   b. Hirsutism
   c. Acanthosis nigricans (velvety dark-pigmented skin at the nape of the neck, axilla, and groin. Indicates insulin resistance and can be associated with severe PCOS/hyperandrogenism)
4. Abdomen
   a. Look for a male escutcheon hair pattern (ask about shaving/waxing/hair removal)
      i. Ferriman-Gallwey Hirsutism Scoring System (see Chapter 22, "Hirsutism")
   b. Palpate for hepatosplenomegaly, tumors, or masses
5. Pelvic
   a. Assess clitoral size
   b. Assess external genitalia for normal appearance
   c. Assess vagina for estrogenization
      i. *Pale pink with white mucus discharge*: Estrogenized
      ii. *Dark red hymen with thin border*: Atrophic
   d. Perform digital bimanual or recto-abdominal bimanual exam to assess for adnexal masses if patient consents

Laboratory Evaluation

1. Total testosterone
2. Dehydroepiandrosterone-sulfate (DHEAS) level
3. At 7 am, 17-hydroxyprogesterone (17-OHP) level
4. Consider karyotype

Imaging

1. Pelvic ultrasound/imaging studies of ovaries and adrenals if exam unsatisfactory or to confirm findings
2. If imaging studies negative, may need MRI of clitoris to fully visualize clitoral mass and plan treatment

Management

1. If clitoromegaly is present with other androgen excess signs, workup as a per PCOS/hyperandrogenism
2. If isolated clitoromegaly is present
   a. *If suspect mass effect from tumor*: Excisional biopsy indicated
   b. *If clitoral enlargement with normal laboratory findings*: Consult with pediatric gynecologist/surgeon/urologist, likely can be monitored without any treatment, but definitely until patient old enough to consent for any surgical procedure

See further Figure 3.2.

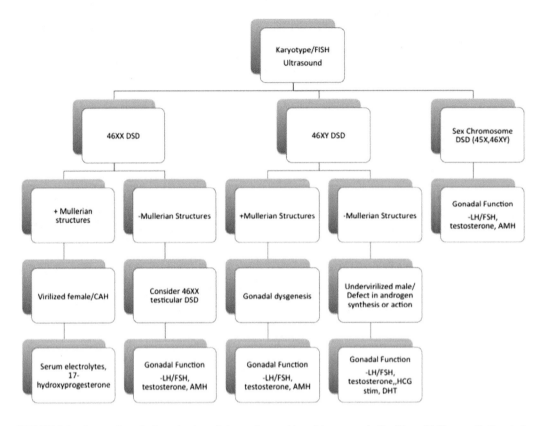

FIGURE 3.2   Approach to the investigation of the newborn with ambiguous genitalia. (From McNamara E, Swartz J, Diamond D. Initial management of disorders of sex development in newborns. Urology. 2017; 101:1–8, with permission.)

BIBLIOGRAPHY

Diamond D, Swartz J, Tishelman A, et al. Management of pediatric patients with DSD and ambiguous genitalia: balancing the child's moral claims to self-determination with parental values and preferences. J Pediatr Urol. 2018; 14:416.e1–416.e5.

Hughes IA, Houk C, Ahmed SF, et al. Consensus statement on management of intersex disorders. J Pediatr Urol. 2006; 2(3):148–166.

Jorge JC, Echeverri C, Medina Y, et al. Male gender identity in an XX individual with congenital adrenal hyperplasia. J Sex Med. 2008; 5(1):122–131.

Krege S, Eckholdt F, Richter-Unruh A, et al. Variations of sex development: the first German interdisciplinary consensus paper. J Pediatr Urol. 2019; 15:114–123.

Kremem J, Chan YM, Holm I. Ambiguous Genitalia in the Newborn and Disorders of Sexual Development. In Emans SJ, Laufer MR, Goldstein DP, eds. *Pediatric and Adolescent Gynecology* (7th ed.). Philadelphia, PA: Wolsters Kluwer, 2020.

Kremen J, Renthal N, Breault D. Congenital Adrenal Hyperplasia. In Emans SJ, Laufer MR, Goldstein DP, eds. *Pediatric and Adolescent Gynecology* (7th ed.). Philadelphia, PA: Wolters Kluwer, 2020.

Krishna KB, Houk C, Lee P. Pragmatic approach to intersex, including genital ambiguity in the newborn. Semin Perinatol. 2017; 41:244–251.

McNamara E, Swartz J, Diamond D. Initial management of disorders of sex development in newborns. Urology. 2017; 101:1–8.

Murphy C, Allen L, Jamieson MA. Ambiguous genitalia in the newborn: an overview and teaching tool. J Pediatr Adolesc Gynecol. 2011; 24:236–250.

North American Society for Pediatric and Adolescent Gynecology position statement on surgical management of DSD. J Pediatr Adolesc Gynecol. 2018 Feb; 31(1):1.

4

Amenorrhea

Allison Mayhew

PRIMARY AMENORRHEA

Definition

- No menses and no development of secondary sexual characteristics (particularly thelarche) by age 13, *or*
- No menses within 3 years of development of secondary sexual characteristics (particularly thelarche), *or*
- No menses by age 15 regardless of the development of secondary sexual characteristics

Key Points

Menstruation is dependent on

- An intact central nervous system (CNS) with appropriate hypothalamic-pituitary output
- Proper end-organ or ovarian responsiveness
- An intact and patent outflow tract

Most common causes include gonadal dysgenesis (especially Turner syndrome), Müllerian agenesis, physiologic delay (constitutional or due to chronic illness), or PCOS

- These diagnoses encompass about 80% of all patients

In order to determine the cause for primary amenorrhea, look for a defect in one of the above during evaluation with history and physical exam (e.g. check for breast development and presence or absence of uterus)

Diagnosis

History

Assess intact CNS or for any CNS symptoms

- Ask about anosmia, headaches, nausea, visual changes
- History of head trauma, CNS irradiation

DOI: 10.1201/9781003039235-4

Assess the development of secondary sexual characteristics (end-organ response)

- At what age did breast development/pubic hair begin?
  - Breast buds present on average by age 9.5 years in non-Hispanic black girls, by age 10.3 in non-Hispanic white girls
  - Pubic hair present on average by age 9.5 in non-Hispanic black girls, by age 10.6 in non-Hispanic white girls

Assess for outflow obstructive symptoms

- Does the patient have cyclic abdominal pain?

Physical Examination

Check height and weight and plot on growth curves

- Persistent height <5th percentile might indicate Turner syndrome or a growth disorder

Complete sexual maturity rate or Tanner staging with evaluation for the presence of breast tissue and pubic hair

Complete genitourinary exam for patency of outflow tract

- *Check introitus*: Is the hymen patent? (see Chapter 24, "Hymenal Anatomy")
- If initial external pelvic exam appears normal, evaluate for outflow obstructions of the upper tract such as transverse vaginal septum (see Chapter 58, "Vaginal Tract Abnormalities")
  - Place a cotton tip swab through the introitus to evaluate vaginal length
    - Typical pubertal vaginal length is 7.0–8.5 cm
  - Evaluate for transverse vaginal septum by placing single digit into vagina to palpate cervix or place small Huffman speculum into vaginal opening to visualize cervix
  - Obtain pelvic ultrasound to evaluate uterine anatomy

Assess vaginal mucosa for estrogenization

- Unestrogenized vaginal epithelium appears red, thin, and friable; estrogenized vaginal epithelium appears pink, thick, and moist

---

Management

If breasts absent/uterus present (see Figure 4.1):

- Lack of breast development indicates lack of estrogen production
- Presence of uterus indicates an intact outflow tract
  - Causes include hypothalamic-pituitary-ovarian (HPO) axis failure or gonadal failure (see Chapter 40, "Primary Ovarian Insufficiency")

If breasts present/uterus absent (see Figure 4.2):

- Breast development indicates estrogen production
- Uterine absence indicates failure of development of Müllerian structures
  - Causes include congenital abnormalities (see Chapter 56, "Uterovaginal/müllerian agenesis")

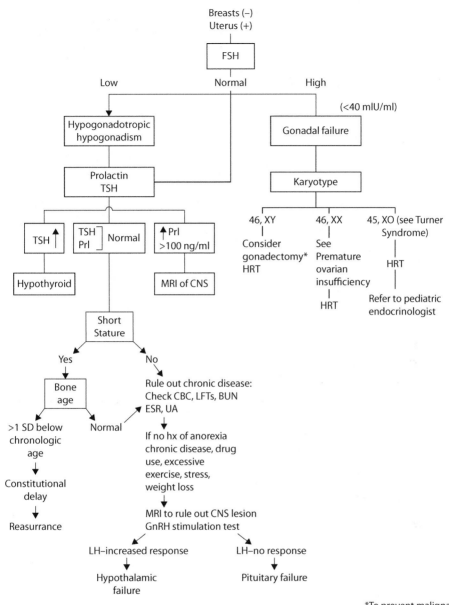

FIGURE 4.1 Management algorithm 1.

If breasts absent/uterus absent (see Figure 4.3):

- Lack of breast development indicates lack of estrogen production
- Uterine absence indicates failure of development of Müllerian structures
  - Causes include gonadal failure, agonadism, or gonadal dysgenesis

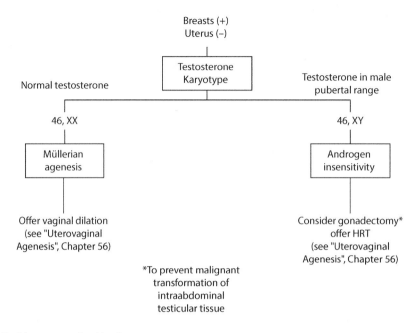

FIGURE 4.2 Management algorithm 2.

If breasts present/uterus present (see Figure 4.4):

- Presence of breasts indicates estrogen production at some point during puberty
- Presence of uterus indicates an intact upper outflow tract
    - Causes include lower outflow tract obstruction or abnormality of the HPO axis
        - If imperforate hymen, see "Hymenal Anatomy" (Chapter 24)
        - If transverse vaginal septa, see "Vaginal Tract Abnormalities" (Chapter 58)
        - If abnormality of HPO axis, follow management guidelines for secondary amenorrhea

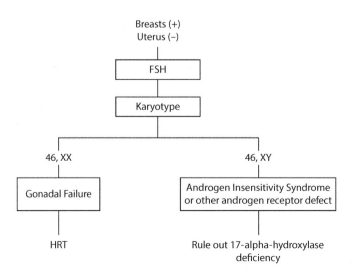

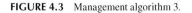

FIGURE 4.3 Management algorithm 3.

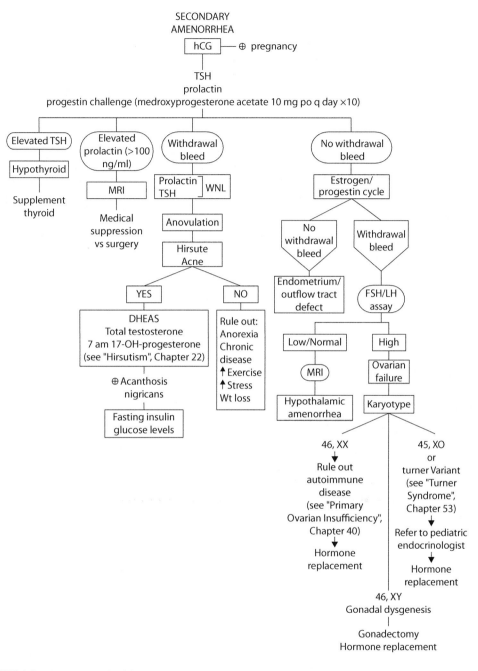

FIGURE 4.4   Management algorithm 4.

SECONDARY AMENORRHEA

Definition

Absence of menses for 3–6 months in previously menstruating adolescent

Key Points

The most common cause of secondary amenorrhea is pregnancy

- Other common causes include stress, weight loss, low energy availability (disordered eating and/or overexercise), or changes in the environment

Evaluate

- New amenorrhea lasting for more than 90 days
- Persistent oligomenorrhea (cycles >35 days) when occurring 2 or more years after menarche

Diagnosis

History

Menstrual history

- When did menarche occur? (average age menarche US 12.2–12.7 years)
- When was last normal flow?
- What were normal duration and flow of menses?
- Any history of dysmenorrhea?

Review of past history

- Any chronic diseases? (e.g. Crohn's disease)
- Any childhood illnesses?
- Any childhood radiation treatment or chemotherapy?
- Any past or current medication use?

Any past surgery?

- Any surgery on the uterus (D & C)?

Review of symptoms

- Vasomotor symptoms (e.g. hot flashes indicative of a hypoestrogenic state)
- Androgen excess signs (acne, hirsutism, etc.)
- Galactorrhea (indicating prolactin excess)
- Cyclic bloating/pain (indicating uterovaginal obstruction)
- Headaches/fatigue/palpitations/nervousness (indicate thyroid dysfunction)
- Visual changes/nausea (may be associated with CNS lesion)

Review of habits

- Nutrition/daily food diary
- Recent weight loss/gain

- Amount of physical activity
- Recent changes in life/stressors (death, divorce, move)

Confidential history

- Does patient participate in any sexual activity?

Physical Examination

Check patient's height/weight and plot on curves

- Look for significant weight increases/decreases or persistent < 5th percentile scores

Check heart rate and blood pressure

- Look for bradycardia, hypotension that may be associated with anorexia
- Hypertension may be associated with androgen excess due to Cushing disease

Evaluate for signs of hirsutism

- Acne, facial hair, acanthosis nigricans of the neck, axilla

Fundoscopy, visual field, and cranial nerve assessment

- Look for defects that may be associated with CNS tumor or lesion

Palpate thyroid

- Assess for enlargement of gland or asymmetry

Breast exam

- Determine sexual maturity rating (Tanner stage)
- Palpate and evaluate for galactorrhea

Abdominal exam

- Check for masses, pregnancy, tenderness, striae
- Check for male escutcheon pattern of hair

Genitourinary exam

- Determine sexual maturity rating (Tanner stage)
  - Excess hair may indicate androgen excess
  - Absent or sparse hair may indicate partial androgen insensitivity
- Check for clitoromegaly (sign of androgen excess)
- Evaluate for estrogen status of vagina
  - Unestrogenized vaginal epithelium appears red, thin, and friable
  - Estrogenized vaginal epithelium appears pink with the presence of thin white discharge

- If appropriate, complete bimanual exam to determine the uterine size and rule out the presence of ovarian masses
  - Pelvic ultrasound may be warranted to better assess these structures
- Look for fissures, skin tags, or perineal fistulas
  - Abnormalities may indicate inflammatory bowel disease

MANAGEMENT

Workup can be completed with serum testing and progestin challenge (see Figure 4.4)

- During progestin challenge, patients should experience menstrual bleeding 2–4 days following completion of medication
  - Some patients may require up to 10 days after completion of medication for evidence of withdrawal bleed
  - Lack of menstrual/withdrawal bleeding is considered a negative test

Principles of Management

Attempt to restore ovulatory function

- For systemic diseases and/or endocrinopathies, treat the underlying disease, and ovulatory function will return
  - Thyroid replacement with hypothyroidism
  - Normalization of serum glucose in diabetes
  - Surgical or medical treatment of prolactinoma/hyperprolactinemia
  - Replace hormone deficit in cases of pituitary destruction/inadequacy
  - Glucocorticoid replacement in congenital adrenal hyperplasia
  - Stabilization of caloric needs in eating disorders, female athlete triad, and inflammatory bowel disease

If ovulation cannot be restored, hormone therapy is usually indicated

- In those who have a withdrawal bleed following progestin challenge, indicating the presence of circulating estrogen, hormone therapy can be used to regulate menstrual cycles (see Chapter 39, "Polycystic Ovary Syndrome")
  - Combined estrogen-progestin oral contraceptive pill, *or*
  - Medroxyprogesterone acetate 10 mg daily for 10 days, used every 1–3 months
- In those who do not have a withdrawal bleeding following progestin challenge, indicating a lack of circulating estrogen, hormone therapy can be used to replace estrogen/progestin (as in the cases of ovarian insufficiency (Chapter 40, "Primary ovarian insufficiency"/Chapter 53, "Turner syndrome")
  - Combined estrogen-progestin oral contraceptive pill, *or*
  - Conjugated estrogen 0.625 mg daily with medroxyprogesterone acetate 10 mg daily for 10 days, used monthly, *or*
  - Transdermal estradiol 0.1 mcg twice weekly with cyclic use of medroxyprogesterone acetate 10 mg for 10 days or 100-mg micronized progesterone daily for 10 days

Many causes of amenorrhea require frequent reevaluation

BIBLIOGRAPHY

Emans SJ, DiVasta A. Amenorrhea in the Adolescent. In: Emans SJ, Laufer MR, eds. *Emans, Laufer, Goldstein's Pediatric and Adolescent Gynecology* (7th ed.) Philadelphia, PA: Lippincott Williams & Wilkins; 2020: 378–399.

Loveless M. Normal pubertal development and the menstrual cycle as a vital sign. In: Sanfilippo JS, Lara-Torre E, Gomez-Lobo V, eds. *Sanfilippo's Textbook of Pediatric and Adolescent Gynecology* (2nd ed.) Boca Raton, FL: CRC Press; 2020:1–10.

Menstruation in girls and adolescents: using the menstrual cycle as a vital sign. American College of Obstetricians and Gynecologists Committee Opinion No. 651. *Obstet Gynecol* 2015;126:e143–e146.

5

Androgen Insensitivity Syndrome (AIS)

Melissa Parks and Amy Williamson

Definition

Androgen insensitivity syndrome is an X-linked recessive disorder of sexual development (DSD) caused by a variety of inactivating mutations in the gene encoding for the androgen receptor (AR) in 46,XY individuals. It is classified as complete androgen insensitivity (CAIS) and partial androgen insensitivity (PAIS) based on phenotypic expression related to the level of AR dysfunction.

Key Points

- The diagnosis of individuals with CAIS should be considered in a girl presenting with primary amenorrhea, scant pubic hair, and absent uterus, or a female infant with bilateral inguinal swelling.
- The diagnosis of PAIS should be considered in a newborn with ambiguous or atypical genitalia.
- A multidisciplinary team approach is best for the management of AIS.

Differential Diagnosis

- CAIS syndrome
  - Complete gonadal dysgenesis
  - Mayer-Rokitansky-Kuster-Hauser syndrome
  - Müllerian ducts anomalies
  - Various biosynthetic androgen disorders
- PAIS syndrome
  - Chromosomal defects
    - Klinefelter syndrome
  - Genetic diseases
    - Smith-Lemli-Opitz syndrome
    - Denys-Drash syndrome
    - Fraser syndrome
  - Partial gonadal dysgenesis
  - LH receptor defects
  - Biosynthetic enzyme deficiencies
    - 12,20-lyase deficiency
    - P450 oxidoreductase deficiency

DOI: 10.1201/9781003039235-5

- 17β-hydroxysteroid dehydrogenase deficiency type 3
- 5α-reductase 2 deficiency

Diagnosis

History

- *CAIS*
  - Typically diagnosed in one of three scenarios
    - Fetal life when prenatal sex determination is a 46,XY karyotype with female external genitalia on ultrasonography
    - At birth or in childhood following workup for an inguinal mass or hernia
    - Primary amenorrhea at the time of puberty or late adolescence
  - Normal growth and development during childhood; adult height may be above average for a typical female
  - Normal onset puberty, normal breast development
- *PAIS*
  - Presentation varies depending on the degree of responsiveness of the AR to androgens
    - May present
      - In newborns as ambiguous or atypical genitalia
      - In adolescence during puberty
      - With both virilization and feminization resulting in:
        - Phenotypic female with mild virilization of the external genitalia OR
        - Phenotypic male with gynecomastia and perineoscrotal hypospadias or under virilization of the external genitalia
- *MAIS* (mild androgen insensitivity)
  - Presents as a pubertal male with gynecomastia and/or infertility in adulthood
- *Physical examination*
  - CAIS
    - Breasts may be enlarged and have subtle abnormalities, including small nipples and pale areolae
    - Axillary hair is absent or scant
    - External genitalia
      - Female in appearance
      - Underdeveloped labia minora
      - Absent or scant pubic hair
      - Vagina: Blind ending of variable length
      - Cervix: Absent
      - Uterus: Absent
  - PAIS
    - Phenotypic females with mild virilization resemble patients with CAIS
    - Breasts: Normal
    - Axillary hair: Normal
    - External genitalia
      - Partial fusion of the labioscrotal folds with or without clitoromegaly
      - Normal pubic hair

- MAIS (Reifenstein syndrome)
  - Appear phenotypically male and undervirilized
  - No facial or chest hair
  - Breasts: May have gynecomastia
  - External genitalia appearance may vary
    - Bifid scrotum and perineoscrotal hypospadias
    - Micropenis with a normal urethra to complete failure of scrotal fusion
  - Normal pubic and axillary hair
- *Diagnostic testing*
  - Testosterone normal or elevated male reference range
  - LH elevated
  - FSH normal
  - Estradiol elevated for male reference range but lower than the female reference range
  - Anti-Müllerian hormone (AMH) normal male reference range
  - Dihydrotestosterone (DHT): Useful when trying to distinguish between PAIS and 5α-reductase deficiency
  - Testosterone to DHT ratio normal in PAIS
  - Karyotype 46,XY
    - Abnormal AR sequencing
    - Multiplex ligation-dependent probe amplification (MLPA) analysis to detect deletions or duplications of exons or the entire gene: Most useful in PAIS
  - Pelvic ultrasound
    - Absent uterus, fallopian tubes
    - Gonads are testes and may be seen intra-abdominally but more commonly are located in the inguinal canals or labia majora

Management

Multidisciplinary approach recommended, including pediatric/adult endocrinologist, gynecologist, urologist, psychologist, geneticists, neonatologist/medical ethicist, and social services.

Challenges include

- Establishing diagnosis (based on clinical presentation and AR sequencing)
- Providing information about the condition in appropriate manner
- Monitoring puberty
- Considering timing and/ or need for gonadectomy based on shared decision-making
- Support of affected adults to achieve adequate sexual function and optimal quality of life

Complete Androgen Insensitivity Syndrome (CAIS)

- Psychological support
  - Directed toward full disclosure of diagnosis, reinforcement of gender identity, and discussion of sexuality
  - A majority of patients will identify as female
- Surgical considerations
  - Creation of a functional vagina
    - Progressive perineal dilation gold standard and should be considered once patients feel ready, often after age 16

- – Vaginoplasty should be used sparingly
  - – May or may not be needed depending on length of vagina
- • Possible gonadectomy (see Figure 5.1)
  - – Historically managed with bilateral gonadectomy for prevention of germ cell tumor
    - – Prepubertal risk of tumor low around 0%
    - – After age 25, risk of malignancy continues to increase with range being 0–22%
  - – A shared decision-making process should be initiated at the time of diagnosis and continued to allow for patient autonomy in the discussion to retain or remove gonads.

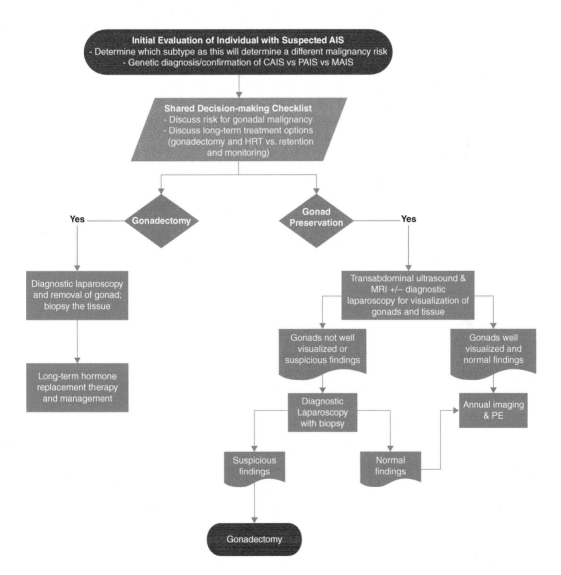

FIGURE 5.1 Gonad preservation treatment algorithm recommended for clinical process upon initial diagnosis and subsequent follow-up of individuals with AIS (HRT, hormone replacement therapy; PE, physical exam). (From Weidler EM, et al. A management protocol for gonad preservation in patients with androgen insensitivity syndrome. J Pediatr Adolesc Gynecol. 2019;32:609, with permission.)

- If a patient desires gonadectomy: Delay until after completion of puberty (16–18 years old)
  - Delaying allows for spontaneous pubertal development through the conversion of testosterone to estrogen with very little risk of malignancy
  - Hormone replacement therapy required until natural age of menopause
    - Provide hormone congruent with patient's gender identity using transdermal estradiol or injectable testosterone
    - Progesterone supplementation is not required as there is no uterus
- If gonadectomy is performed prior to puberty
  - Hormone induction with estrogen
    - Begin at 11–12 years old
    - Consider oral or transdermal estrogen in a fashion similar to pubertal induction for Turner syndrome patients
    - Begin with lowest doses and titrate up as needed
  - Hormone induction with testosterone
    - Begin by age 14
    - Initiate low doses and titrate up as needed
- If the patient elects to have a gonad retention
  - Baseline transabdominal ultrasonography and magnetic resonance imaging (MRI) should be performed to locate the position of the gonads and visualize their features
    - If normal appearing gonads, monitor annually
    - If gonads not readily seen on imaging
      - Consider completion of an examination under anesthesia to determine vaginal length coupled with a diagnostic laparoscopy to characterize the internal structures, including the gonads with possible gonadal biopsy
      - Use of laparoscopic gonadopexy and marking with surgical clip followed by ultrasound surveillance has been described
      - Any suspicious findings at time of surgery should result in gonadectomy
    - If labioscrotal or inguinal, annual monitoring via physical exam and ultrasonography
  - Tumor serum markers (hCG and LDH) are not currently recommended due to lack of evidence regarding utility

Partial Androgen Insensitivity Syndrome (PAIS)

- Psychological support
  - Psychologic distress more common in PAIS vs CAIS regardless of the gender of rearing
  - Directed toward full disclosure of diagnosis, gender identity, and sexuality
  - There is a trend toward raising patients as males, but sex rearing is not always straightforward, given the variations in phenotype
  - The degree of virilization of the external genitalia often dictates sex rearing
- Surgical management
  - As PAIS commonly presents with ambiguous genitalia in newborns, encourage parents/guardians to consider delay in surgical management to allow patient to be included in shared decision-making
  - Delaying sex assignment is an option for consideration in PAIS with strict clinical surveillance given the higher risk of malignancy
  - In male patients, surgical correction of cryptorchidism and hypospadias should occur by the third year of life

- The risk of malignancy is higher compared to CAIS at approximately 15% and may be higher (50%) in those with undescended testes
  - If choosing male social sex gender
    - Treatment of undescended testes via orchidopexy in males is crucial
  - If choosing female social sex gender
    - Laparoscopic bilateral gonadectomy before puberty is indicated to reduce the risk of malignancy and to prevent virilization
  - If a female patient chooses to retain their gonads
    - Strict surveillance with annual ultrasonography or MRI pending the location of the gonads is important given the greater risk of malignancy

BIBLIOGRAPHY

Batista RL, Costa EMF, Rodrigues AS, et al. Androgen insensitivity syndrome: a review. Arch Endocrinol Metab. 2018; 62(2):227–235.

Deans R, Creighton SM, Liao LM, et al. Timing of gonadectomy in adult women with complete androgen insensitivity syndrome (CAIS): patient preferences and clinical evidence. Clin Endocrinol (Oxf). 2012; 76(6):894–898.

Hughes IA, Davies JD, Bunch TI, et al. Androgen insensitivity syndrome. Lancet. 2012; 380:1419–1428.

Mongan NP, Tadokoro-Cuccaro R, Bunch T, et al. Androgen insensitivity syndrome. Best Pract Res Clin Endocrinol Metab. 2015; 29(4):569–580.

Patel V, Casey RK, Gomez-Lobo V. Timing of gonadectomy in patients with complete androgen insensitivity syndrome – current recommendations and future directions. J Pediatr Adolesc Gynecol. 2016; 29(4):320–325.

Taylor HS, Pal L, Seli E. *Speroff's Clinical Gynecologic Endocrinology and Infertility* (9th ed.). Chapter 8. Philadelphia, PA: Wolters Kluwer. 2020.

Weidler EM, Linnaus ME, Baratz AB, et al. A management protocol for gonad preservation in patients with androgen insensitivity syndrome. J Pediatr Adolesc Gynecol. 2019; 32(6):605–611.

6

Anesthetics in Pediatric Adolescent Populations

EMLA® (Eutectic Mixture of Local Anesthetic; Astra Pharmaceuticals, Westborough, MA)

Krista J. Childress

Definition

EMLA® is a water-oil emulsion of 1:1 mixture of 2.5% prilocaine and 2.5% lidocaine that can be used as a topical anesthetic on normal intact skin.

Key Points

- Provides pain relief during minor office procedure
- May be used on mucosal surfaces
- Use on intact skin
- Can be used before lidocaine infiltration to ease pain of injection

EMLA Cream Instructions

Gently wash area to be treated with mild cleanser and water to eliminate contaminants that may hinder absorption or efficacy of anesthetic.

Use a tongue depressor or gloved finger to apply a uniform layer of cream approximately 1/8″ thick to the desired area and cover with an occlusive dressing to facilitate absorption and achieve cutaneous anesthesia. After approximately 30 minutes, wipe the cream and proceed with the planned procedure.

Side effects/risks:

- *Mild skin reactions*: Edema, pallor, erythema, burning
- *Severe reactions*: Methemoglobinemia**, central nervous system toxicity (irritability, headache, convulsions, blurred vision or speech, numbness or tingling around mouth, metallic taste), cardiotoxicity (arrhythmias, decreased cardiac contractility, cardiac arrest)

  ** Agents associated with methemoglobinemia

  ** *Use EMLA with caution in patients using agents associated with methemoglobinemia*

Sulfonamides	Nitroglycerin
Acetaminophen	Pamaquine
Acetanilid	Para-aminosalicylic acid
Aniline dyes	Phenacetin
Benzocaine	Phenobarbital
Chloroquine	Phenytoin

  DOI: 10.1201/9781003039235-6

Dapsone   Primaquine
Naphthalene   Quinine
Nitrates and nitrites
Nitrofurantoin, phenazopyridine, dapsone, acetaminophen, nitrites, and phenobarbital

- *Dosing*: The maximum dose depends on the age of the patient, the liver and kidney function, duration of application, and size of the treated area (Table 6.1).
- *Onset of action*: Depends on anatomic location. Dermal anesthesia is achieved within 1 hour of application and continues for 1–2 hours after removal.
  - *Face/thigh*: 25–30 minutes
  - *Lips/genitals*: 5–15 minutes
- *Depth of action*: Depends on length of application.
  - *60 minutes*: 3-mm thickness
  - *120 minutes*: 5-mm thickness

Management of toxicity

- Toxicity rare if follow recommended dose and application area
- *Signs of toxicity*: Irritability, headache, convulsions, blurred vision, numbness, tingling around mouth, and metallic taste
- If suspected, wash off EMLA
- Place patient in supine position and obtain vital signs
- If patient has lost consciousness, maintain airway
- Obtain serum lidocaine levels

TABLE 6.1

Recommended Maximum Dose, Time, and Application Area for EMLA Based on Age and Weight

Age	Weight (kg)	Maximum Total Dose (g)	Maximum Total Time (hour)	Maximum Application Area (cm²)
1–3 months	<5	1	1	10
4–12 months	<5	2	4	20
1–6 years	<10	10	4	100
7–12 years	>20	20	4	200

BIBLIOGRAPHY

Sobanko JF, Miller CJ, Alster TS. Topical anesthetics for dermatologic procedures: a review. Dermatol Surg. 2012; 38(5):709–721.

Stevic M, Vlajkovic A, Trifunovic B, Rakic I, Ristic N, Budic I, et al. Topical anesthetics for pediatric laser treatment. J Cosmet Laser Ther. 2019; 21(7–8):417–421.

7

Anorectal Malformations (ARM)

Kate McCracken

Key Points

Anorectal malformations (ARM) affect 1 in 5000 live births and are a spectrum of anomalies ranging from rectoperineal fistula to cloaca in girls. There is a high incidence of associated gynecologic anomalies in girls with ARM.

Gynecologic involvement in the care of patients with ARM is important for

- Initial evaluation and surgical planning
- Pubertal evaluation, menstrual management
- Providing reproductive healthcare (i.e. contraception, family planning, optimizing obstetric outcomes)

Definitions

Rectoperineal Fistula

- Rectal fistula opens on the perineum anterior to the anal muscle complex, but with skin separation between it and the vagina (Figure 7.1)
- Most common ARM in girls
- Least severe type of ARM
- Approximately 5% of an associated gynecologic anomaly

Rectovestibular Fistula

- Rectal fistula opens in the vestibule, outside of the hymen (Figure 7.2)
- Second most common ARM in girls
- Approximately 20% have an associated gynecologic anomaly

Cloaca

- Single perineal opening into which the urinary, gynecologic, and gastrointestinal systems empty (the common channel; Figure 7.3)
- Affects 1 in 50,000–100,000 live births
- High rate of associated gynecologic anomalies (approximately 60%)

DOI: 10.1201/9781003039235-7

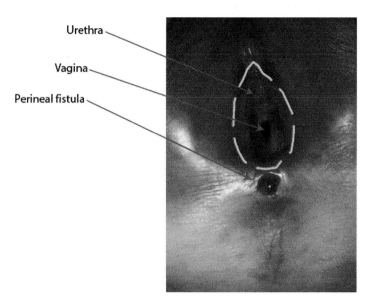

FIGURE 7.1 Rectoperineal fistula.

Rare Anomalies

Other rare ARM includes the following:

- Rectovaginal fistula (see Figure 7.4) – Rectal fistula enters the posterior vaginal wall
- Anal stenosis, rectal atresia, imperforate anus without fistula – ARM where the abnormality is confined to the GI tract, not commonly associated with gynecologic anomalies

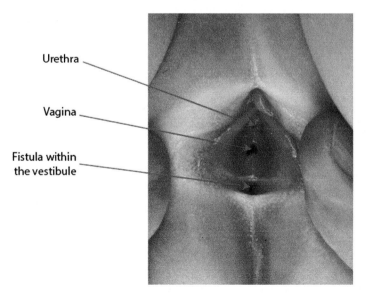

FIGURE 7.2 Rectovestibular fistula.

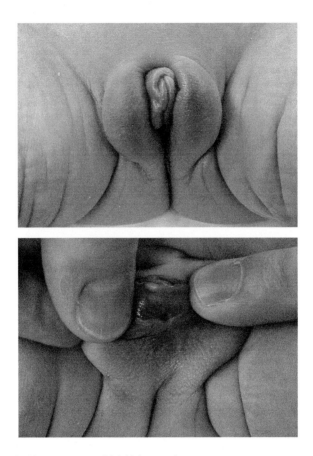

FIGURE 7.3   (a) Cloaca. (b) Cloaca: As seen with labial separation.

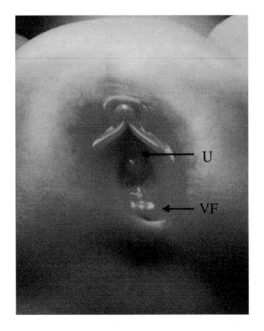

FIGURE 7.4   Rectovaginal fistula.

Diagnosis

Antenatal Diagnosis

Rectoperineal and rectovestibular fistulae are rarely detected antenatally.

Cloacal anomalies may be detected on antenatal ultrasound if the fetus develops hydro(metro)colpos that occurs when urine refluxes back from the common channel into the vagina, leading to abdominal distension. Distension of the vagina may lead to hydroureteronephrosis and renal damage.

Newborn Assessment

Standard newborn assessment includes evaluation of the perineum and anus by the pediatric team. The key to an accurate ARM diagnosis is documenting the number of perineal orifices and noting where the fistula lies in relation to the hymen.

Stabilization first

- Patients with a cloaca should have a pelvic and renal ultrasound of day of life 1.
- May need GI (and possibly urinary) diversion. Some rectoperineal or rectovestibular fistulae are managed without a colostomy if the fistula is large enough (or can be dilated) to allow the passage of stool.
- Assessment of associated anomalies – All newborns without a normal anus should have been screened for VACTERL (Vertebral defects, Anal atresia, Cardiac defects, Tracheo-Esophageal fistula, Renal and Limb) anomalies.

Initial gynecologic assessment includes the following

- Assess if there is a vaginal opening
- Assess for hydro(metro)colpos
- Assess for a longitudinal vaginal septum

Management

Newborn/Infant Period

Referral to centers with expertise in complex reconstruction is crucial. Surgical planning for reconstruction should involve a multidisciplinary team – pediatric colorectal surgery, pediatric urology, and pediatric gynecology.

Treatment of associated anomalies, i.e. cardiac, trachoesophageal fistula (TEF), may be necessary prior to the definitive ARM repair.

Initial gynecologic assessment includes the following

- Labial traction to assess if there is a vaginal opening and/or longitudinal vaginal septum
- Physical exam and imaging (ultrasound) to assess for hydro(metro)colpos
- Cystovaginoscopy – performed with the colorectal and urologic teams – to determine the patient's anatomy – common channel length, urethral length, location of bladder neck and ureteral orifices, vaginal length, presence of a longitudinal vaginal septum, number of cervices (0, 1, 2)

Hydro(metro)colpos should be managed in the newborn period to reduce the risk of renal damage – either by placement of a vaginostomy tube (typically performed at the time of colostomy) or clean intermittent catheterization of the common channel until definitive repair.

TABLE 7.1

Surgical Repair of ARM

Type of ARM	Surgical Repair
Rectoperineal	PSARP
Rectovestibular	PSARP
Cloaca	PSARVUP – via either total urogenital mobilization or urogenital separation

Abbreviations: PSARP = posterior sagittal anorectoplasty; PSARVUP = posterior sagittal anorectovaginourethroplasty.

If there is not a visible vaginal opening – inspection of the Müllerian structures via laparoscopy or laparotomy should be performed prior to the primary reconstruction – to aid in surgical planning for possible neovagina creation.

Involvement of gynecology at the time of initial repair is important. Gynecologic goals of surgical treatment (Table 7.1) are as follows

- Separation of the urinary, gastrointestinal, and reproductive tracts
- Creation of a patent outflow tract for menstrual egress
- Preservation of Müllerian structures to optimize future reproductive potential

A full understanding of the patient's Müllerian anatomy may not be achieved until puberty when the uterine structures are stimulated by estrogen exposure. During the primary ARM repair, care should be taken to retain Müllerian structures in situ to maximize future reproductive potential, understanding that there may be a risk of menstrual outflow obstruction and need for additional surgery after puberty.

Puberty

Ovaries are normal in patients with ARM; if healthy and normal gut absorption, puberty timing and tempo should be similar to their peers.

Goals during this time

- Ensure patent menstrual outflow tract – Obtain pelvic ultrasound 6 months after thelarche to assess the Müllerian anatomy and risk of obstruction; may need pelvic MRI to fully delineate the Müllerian anatomy
- Evaluate the vagina – Determine if longitudinal septum needs resected; evaluate for stricture or prolapse
- Evaluate the introitus for stricture
- Evaluate the perineal body – Is the length adequate?
- Routine gynecologic care – Menstrual management, contraceptive needs, HPV vaccination, screening for sexually transmitted infections
- Successful transition of care from pediatric care to adult care

Obstetric Considerations

- Discuss reproductive potential
  - Dependent upon anatomy
  - Alternative means for creating a family
  - Provide contraception if patient does not desire pregnancy

- Encourage preconception visit/counseling with a high-risk obstetrician
  - Obtain copies of operative reports
  - Evaluation of concurrent medical conditions (i.e. renal insufficiency)
- Discuss potential for preterm labor, preterm delivery, and fetal malpresentation
  - Dependent upon Müllerian anatomy
  - Knowledge of the patient's gynecologic anatomy is crucial for counseling – Use every available opportunity to document the upper and lower tract anatomy
- Discuss recommended mode of delivery
  - Dependent upon prior repair, fecal and urinary continence
  - Shared medical decision-making; individualization of care
- Engage the appropriate collaborative teams – i.e. urology, colorectal surgery, anesthesiology
  - Surgical planning/considerations – i.e. presence of stomas
  - Consideration of other VACTERL associated conditions – i.e. spinal anomalies and anesthesia implications; cardiac anomalies and pregnancy risk to mother/fetus; renal anomalies and risk of infection/hypertension

Take-Home Points

- A longitudinal/life span approach is necessary to optimize comprehensive reproductive healthcare for individuals with ARM.
- Linking the patient to providers who have familiarity with complex anomalies may be difficult but it is crucial for best outcomes.
- Leveraging opportunities to understand Müllerian anatomy sets the patient up for success regarding menstrual outflow and future fertility (i.e. reconstructive planning, intraoperative assessment, imaging studies).
- There is a paucity of data regarding sexual function and obstetrical outcomes – this is an opportunity for ongoing collaborative research.
- Pregnancy should be managed in a multidisciplinary model.

BIBLIOGRAPHY

Pradhan S, Vilanova-Sanchez A, McCracken KA, Reck CA, Halleran DR, Wood RJ, Levitt M, Hewitt GD. "The Müllerian Black Box: Predicting and defining Müllerian anatomy in patients with cloacal abnormalities and the need for longitudinal assessment." J Pediatr Surg. 2018 Nov;53(11):2164–2169. Doi: 10.1016/j.jpedsurg.2018.05.009. Epub 2018 May 19.

Vilanova-Sanchez A, McCracken K, Halleran DR, Wood RJ, Reck-Burneo CA, Levitt MA, Hewitt G. "Obstetrical outcomes in adult patients born with complex anorectal malformations and cloacal anomalies: a literature review." J Pediatr Adolesc Gynecol. 2019 Feb;32(1):7–14. Doi: 10.1016/j.jpag.2018.10.002. Epub 2018 Oct 24. Review.

Vilanova-Sanchez A, Reck CA, McCracken KA, Lane VA, Gasior AC, Wood RJ, Levitt MA, Hewitt GD. "Gynecologic anatomic abnormalities following anorectal malformations repair." J Pediatr Surg. 2018 Apr;53(4):698–703.

8

Bartholin's Abscess

Shashwati Pradhan and S. Paige Hertweck

Definition

- Swelling resulting from the occlusion of the main duct of the Bartholin's gland (greater vestibular glands), which are pea-sized mucus-secreting glands occurring at the 5 or 7 o'clock position of the vulvar vestibule.
- These glands are not normally palpable or visible but blockage of the duct due to infection or trauma will result in symptoms.
- Bartholin's abscesses are usually accompanied by signs of infection and inflammation: Erythema, warmth, tenderness, and pain.

Key Points

- Bartholin duct abscesses can be effectively treated by office procedures under local anesthesia.
- Multiple treatment regimens have been described and include incision and drainage (I&D) alone or in combination with ablation of cavity with silver nitrate or alcohol, carbon dioxide (CO_2) incision with CO_2 ablation, fistulalization, marsupialization, and gland excision.
- Bartholin duct cysts or abscesses treated with I&D alone or needle aspiration have a higher rate of recurrence.
- Placement of a Word catheter or Jacobi ring after I&D has more acceptable recurrence rates and low complication risks.
- More invasive procedures of marsupialization or excision tend to be completed under anesthesia and reserved for more recurrent cases.

Diagnosis

- Complaints of usually unilateral vulvar swelling, discomfort, or pain most commonly in a sexually active patient.
- Physical examination and identification of fluctuant abscess at the 5 or 7 o'clock position of the vulvar vestibule, which contains purulent fluid.

Management

- While a simple I&D will provide prompt relief of symptoms, unless new duct ostium is created, the abscess can reform; therefore, the goal is not only to relieve the abscess but also to create a new epithelialized tract for drainage by one of the following techniques.

DOI: 10.1201/9781003039235-8

Word Catheter Placement

Consider use of sedation if required by patient; otherwise use local anesthesia, such as 1% lidocaine, at incision site may be adequate for the procedure.

- Use No. 11 blade to create a 3–5-mm incision on the inner surface of the cyst just outside the hymenal ring at the 5 or 7 o'clock position, which replicates the normal anatomic position of Bartholin's duct ostium (Figure 8.1).
- Consider sending culture for *N. gonorrhoeae* and *C. trachomatis* as well as other aerobic/anaerobic bacteria.
- Break adhesions with sterile Q-tip or small hemostat or forceps, taking care not to extend incision.
- Irrigate the cavity with saline and then insert deflated Word catheter (Figure 8.2).
- Inflate catheter (usually 2–3-cc saline, not air). Tuck the tail of the Word catheter inside the vagina.
- Advise patient to place nothing in vagina until catheter is removed.
- No need for antibiotic therapy unless significant surrounding cellulitis is present.

Jacobi Ring Placement

Placement of a Jacobi ring (Figure 8.3) that enters and leaves the abscess through two separate incisions is a technique for creating fistulous tract and, based on limited data, may result in less recurrence and increased patient comfort than placement of Word catheter.

There are no commercially available ring catheters. Here are described techniques to create one

1. A 7-cm length of an 8 French T tube threaded with 20 cm length of 2-0 silk suture.
2. A 5-cm piece of tubing from a butterfly blood collection set is threaded with absorbable vicryl suture through the lumen.
3. Alternatively, if neither of the above is available, simply placing a vessel loop through the caudad area of the abscess cavity and out the cephalad portion and then tying loosely together will accomplish the same process as the Jacobi ring.

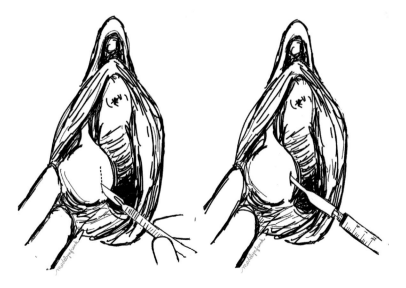

FIGURE 8.1 (a) Incising the inner surface of the cyst at the 5 or 7 o'clock position. (b) Placement of Word catheter into cyst or abscess. (Artwork by Madelyn Frank.)

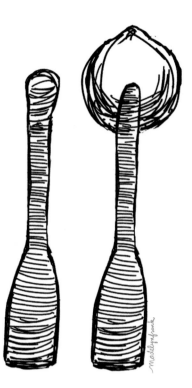

FIGURE 8.2 Word catheter: (a) deflated and (b) inflated. (Artwork by Madelyn Frank.)

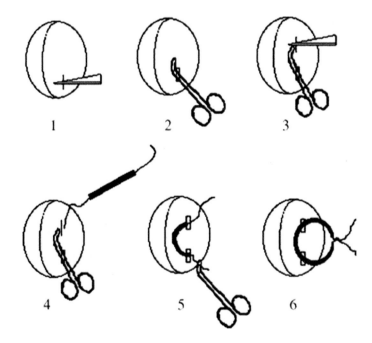

FIGURE 8.3 Placement of a Jacobi ring. (1) An incision is made into the mucosal surface of the Bartholin's abscess. Adhesions are lysed and the abscess is allowed to drain. (2) A hemostat is passed into the abscess cavity. (3) The hemostat is tunneled into the abscess cavity and a second incision is made. (4) The hemostat is used to grasp one end of the Jacobi ring. (5) The Jacobi ring is pulled through the abscess cavity with care that the suture is not pulled out of the catheter. (6) The two ends of the suture are tied, forming the closed ring. (From Gennis P, et al. Jacobi ring catheter treatment of Bartholin's abscesses, AJEM 2005; 23(3):414–415, with permission.)

Marsupialization (Creation of Window in Cyst/Abscess)

- Usually preferred in cases of failed Word catheter placement
- Involves excision of an elliptical portion of the vestibular skin and cyst wall, breaking up any loculations within cyst and suturing cyst wall edges to skin with absorbable 3-0 suture to the surrounding vestibular and introital tissue
- Usually done as outpatient surgery
- May take 2 weeks to heal
- Recurrence rate 10–15%

Follow-Up Care

- Sitz baths can be recommended for comfort with NSAIDs for pain management.
- Ring or Word catheters should remain in place for at least 3 weeks for proper epithelialization.
- Commonly, the catheter falls out before this time and there is no need to replace Word catheter if this occurs.

BIBLIOGRAPHY

Lee WA, Wittler M (Oct 15, 2019). StatPearls [Internet]. *Bartholin Gland Cyst*. Treasure Island, FL: StatPearls Publishing.

Illingworth B, Stocking K, Showell M, Kirk E, Duffy K. Evaluation of treatments for Bartholin's cyst or abscess: a systematic review. BJOG. 2020; 127(6):671–678.

Omole F, Kelsey RC, Phillps K, Cunningham K. Bartholin duct cyst and gland abscess: office management. Am Fam Physician. 2019; 99(12):760–766.

9

Breast Disorders

Amy Boone and Kim Hoover

BREAST ABSCESS

Key Points

- May result from local infection, epidermoid cysts, foreign bodies, trauma, nipple piercing, and folliculitis from shaving or plucking periareolar hair
- Although may occur in the postpartum state, non-postpartum abscesses are more common
- Most common organisms are *Staphylococcus aureus*, beta-hemolytic Streptococcus, enterococcus, anaerobic streptococci

Diagnosis

History

- Localized tenderness and induration followed by erythema and then a fluctuant mass
- History of previous breast abscess
- Associated symptoms of fever, vomiting, drainage from mass or nipple

Physical Examination

- Tender, indurated or fluctuant erythematous breast mass
- Commonly in the areolar/periareolar area
- ± Fever and or axillary adenopathy
- ± Discharge from mass/nipple

Imaging

- *Breast ultrasound:* To distinguish between cellulitis and blocked duct or abscess

Management

- Antimicrobial coverage should initially include coverage for methicillin resistant *S. aureus* (MRSA) until culture and sensitivity results are available (see Table 9.1)
- Local care with warm compresses

DOI: 10.1201/9781003039235-9

TABLE 9.1

Antibiotic Coverage for Breast Abscess

Drug	Pediatric Dose[a]	Considerations
Immune Competent, Well-Appearing, No Systemic Symptoms Treat in 7–10 Days		
Amoxicillin-clavulanate	25 mg/kg/day po of the amoxicillin component in two divided doses	
Cephalexin	25–50 mg/kg/day po divided in three to four doses (max = 2 g/day)	
Clindamycin	30–40 mg/kg/day po divided in three to four doses (max = 1.8 g/day)	Suggested in areas of increased MRSA
Immunocompromised, Ill-Appearing		
Nafcillin or Oxacillin	100–150 mg/kg/day IV in four divided doses	IV drug of choice when MRSA less likely
Vancomycin	40 mg/kg/day IV in four divided doses	Use if high concern for MRSA or life-threatening PCN allergy
Clindamycin	25–40 mg/kg/day IV in three divided doses	IV drug of choice if high concern for MRSA or life-threatening PCN allergy

[a] Above doses are not appropriate for neonates.

- Pain relief with nonsteroidal anti-inflammatory medications (NSAIDs) acetaminophen, or acetaminophen with codeine
- Should see clinical improvement within 24–48 hours
- If abscess becomes fluctuant or if symptoms progress/fail to resolve, aspirate pus for culture and sensitivity
- If continues to enlarge or fails to respond, incise and drain with consideration of packing
- Meticulous care to use small incisions with minimal tissue disruption with particular care to avoid damage to the breast bud complex, especially if Tanner stage II or less
- When afebrile 24 hours, continue treatment with oral antibiotics to complete 2 weeks of therapy
- Reevaluate in 2 weeks after completion of antibiotic therapy, and consider repeating ultrasound/exam in 6–12 weeks

Complications

- Cellulitis
- Recurrent or persistent infection (40–50%)
  - May require incision and drainage (I&D) under local or general anesthesia
- Scarring

BREAST ANOMALIES

Congenital Breast Anomalies

Accessory Nipples (Polythelia)

Prevalence: 2% of population

Diagnosis

- Additional nipples anywhere along the milk line (see Figure 9.1)

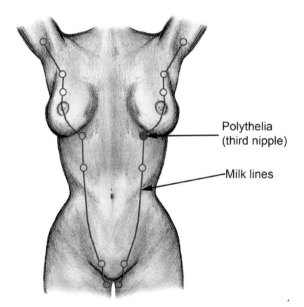

FIGURE 9.1   The 'milk line' corresponding to the embryologic mammary ridge. Accessory nipples, the most common congenital anomaly, and accessory breast tissue occur along these lines. (From the Geneva Foundation for Medical Education and Research – http://www.gfmer.ch/genetic_diseases_v2/gendis_detail_list.php?cat3=1518.)

Treatment

- If in area of frequent trauma, can be excised surgically

Accessory breast tissue (polymastia)

- May accompany polythelia
- May have engorgement with lactation

Treatment

- Consult with plastic surgeon for intervention with cyclical tenderness or irritation based on location of tissue

Absence of Nipple (Athelia): Very Rare

Treatment

- Consult with plastic surgeon

Absence of Breast Tissue (Amastia): Uncommon

- Unilateral predominance
- If associated with delayed puberty, workup for endocrinologic causes [e.g.congenital adrenal hyperplasia (CAH), hypogonadotropic hypogonadism, gonadal dysgenesis, disorder of sexual development]
- May occur with associated chest wall deformities, see Box 9.1
- May be result of exposure to radiation or traumatic loss of breast bud (e.g. prior chest tube placement at bud site)

BOX 9.1   POLAND'S SYNDROME

- Hypoplasia of pectoralis muscles, breast, and areola
- Anomalies of the rib cage, vertebral column, shoulder blade, axilla
- Symbrachydactyly (short fingers with webbing in proximal portion)
- Anomalies of the neurovascular structures of ipsilateral arm
- Hypoplasia of the hand, forearm, and arm

Treatment

- Refer to plastic surgeon to cosmetic correction

Nipple Inversion

- Normal variant, often familial
- Considered pathologic only if not present at birth
    - New onset may indicate infection or an occult tumor

Developmental Breast Anomalies

Tuberous Breasts

Definition

- Breast tissue with narrow dimensions at the base with an overdeveloped nipple-areolar complex (resembles a tuberous root plant) whereby the glandular breast tissue herniates through the areola resulting in the tuberous shape

Etiology

- Unknown
- Noted with use of exogenous hormones to treat endogenous hypoestrogenic states for pubertal induction
- May be anatomic due to fascial plane that envelopes and constricts breast development

Treatment

- Reassurance
- Consultation with plastic surgery for consideration of corrective mammoplasty

Juvenile Breast Hypertrophy (Macromastia)

Definition

- Pathologic overgrowth of breast tissue out of proportion to the body and chest size

Associated symptoms

- Back and neck pain
- Shoulder pain due to bra strap discomfort
- Intertrigo

- Psychological concerns
- *Lifestyle challenges:* Limited ability to find clothing and participate in athletic endeavors

Diagnosis

- Usually occurs near menarche
- Usually symmetric
- May be familial
- Evaluation should rule out presence of an underlying mass such as giant fibroadenoma or lymphoma (more likely if asymmetric)

Treatment

- Consultation with plastic surgeon for consideration of reduction mammoplasty in older teen or young adult once breasts achieve maturity

BREAST ASYMMETRY

Key Points

Neonatal

- Unilateral or bilateral breast enlargement
- Secondary to maternal estrogen stimulation
- May have associated clear or cloudy nipple discharge
- Spontaneous resolution within 1–12 months of life
- Persistence requires evaluation for precocious puberty
  - Consider bone age before referral to pediatric endocrinology

Adolescent

- Common complaint at the onset of breast development (thelarche) as it is often asymmetric
- Usually resolves by late adolescence
- 25% persist after age 18
- Can cause significant psychological distress

Diagnosis

History

- Onset of thelarche
- Compare thelarche temporally with onset of other sexual characteristics (e.g. pubic hair)
- Assess for symptoms of tenderness, erythema, and discharge

Assess any history of

- Prior chest surgery/trauma to breast bud complex (e.g. chest tube placement)
- Connective tissue disease/scleroderma

- Anorexia/Crohn's disease (concern for atrophy, nutritional deficiency)
- Congenital anomalies (e.g. pectus excavatum, scoliosis)

Physical Examination

- Perform breast exam in sitting and reclining position
- Check for the absence of pectoralis major muscle on hypoplastic breast side (see Box 9.1., Poland's syndrome)
- Careful breast exam to evaluate for breast mass, cyst, and abscess
- Check for nipple discharge
- Consider measuring each breast in vertical and horizontal planes for comparison with later exams (i.e. 12–6 o'clock; 3–9 o'clock)
- Check for tuberous breast shape

Treatment

- If palpable mass, consider ultrasound
- If anatomic abnormality, plastic surgery consultation
- If normal exam, reassurance with options for padded bra and periodic exams until final breast maturation (approximately age 18)
- Send for fitting for bra inserts or breast prosthesis
- Early consultation with plastic surgeon may also be helpful

BREAST MASS

Key Points

- Thelarche may be asymmetric and present as a 'breast mass'; therefore, surgical excision should be reserved for obvious pathologic processes to avoid iatrogenic amastia with excision of the breast bud
- Most common masses in this age-group are fibroadenomas, followed by fibrocystic changes
- Primary breast cancer accounts for less than 1% of all adolescent breast tumors
- Malignant breast masses more commonly from metastases of non-breast tissue origin than primary breast cancers (rhabdomyosarcoma, Hodgkin's and non-Hodgkin's lymphoma, neuroblastomas)
- Risk of breast cancer as an adult is increased for survivors of childhood malignancy and/or in those treated with thoracic radiation

Differential Diagnosis

- Fibroadenoma (firm, mobile, non-tender)
- Fibrocystic changes
- Breast cyst
- Abscess/mastitis
- Intraductal papilloma
- Fat necrosis/lipoma

- Rare lesions (e.g. hemangiomas, lymphangiomas, lymphoma)
- Lipomastia
- Mammary duct ectasia
- Cyst of Montgomery
- Malignancy
  - *Primary breast cancer:* Rare under age 18
  - Other malignancies even though rare are more likely than primary breast (e.g. rhabdomyosarcoma, lymphoma, neuroblastoma)
  - More common in patients with previous radiation to chest

Diagnosis

Physical exam and palpation of bilateral breasts in upright and supine position by provider if symptomatic

Ultrasound

- Most useful imaging modality for breast in adolescents
- Can distinguish between solid and cystic masses and help delineate abscess

Self-breast awareness/examination education

Instruct to

- Look in mirror undressed to check for asymmetry
- Examine breasts with soapy hands while standing in shower using vertical up and down movement from axilla moving toward sternum
- Re-examine breasts in same vertical method when supine in bed with ipsilateral hand behind the head, use contralateral hand to examine breast

Recommend use primarily in

- Girls with previous thoracic/chest wall irradiation (greatest risk if treated between 10 and 30 years old)
- Girls with BRCA1 or BRCA2 beginning at age 18–25 years
- Girls with history of malignancy known to present in the breast (rhabdomyosarcoma, non-Hodgkin's lymphoma, leukemia)

Mammography

- Not indicated in patients younger than 25 years
- Increased breast tissue density makes for a less sensitive test

Management (Figure 9.2)

Specific Masses

Fibroadenomas

- Most common breast mass in young girls
- Well-circumscribed, mobile, typically 1–3 cm at presentation
- Unilateral, in lateral breast quadrant
- 10% regress spontaneously
- Can be safely followed with observation if stable in size
- Recurrent or multiple in 10–25% of cases

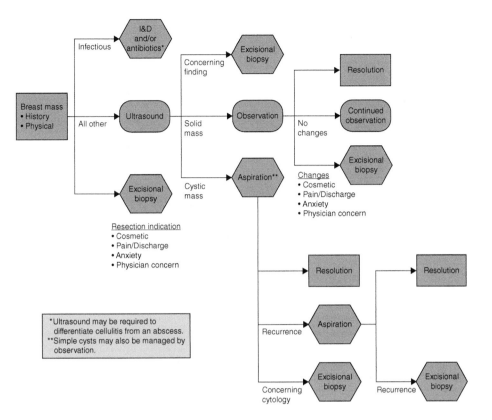

FIGURE 9.2 Breast mass algorithm: diagnosis and treatment in adolescent girls. *Ultrasound may be required to differentiate cellulitis from an abscess; **Simple cysts may also be managed by observation. (From Divasta AD, Weldon C, Labow B, The breast, in Emans SJ, Laufer MR, DiVasta AD, Emans, Laufer, *Goldstein's Pediatric and Adolescent Gynecology.* 7th edn, Wolters Kluwer, Philadelphia, 2019, with permission.)

Giant Fibroadenoma

- Rapidly increasing asymmetric mass > 5 cm
- May have distorted veins over surface
- Eventual risk of breast cancer may be slightly higher

Fibrocystic Changes

- Second most common breast abnormality in adolescents
- Defined as condition in which mastalgia and breast tenderness are associated with palpable fibrous tissue
- Symptoms fluctuate with menses

Management options:

- Oral contraceptives – 70–90% improvement
- NSAIDs

Cysts

- Small cysts (< 2 cm) will often resolve spontaneously

Phylloides Tumor

- Rare, slow-growing tumor, < 5% in those younger than 20 years
- Typically benign, but can be malignant
- *Treatment:* Wide local excision
- Malignant potential based on mitotic activity of tumor
- Tumor recurrence more common with positive surgical margins/proliferative tumor margins

Juvenile Papillomatosis

- Rare benign proliferative disorder characterized by multiple foci of intraductal hyperplasia/ cysts without atypia
- Presents as discreet mass in upper outer quadrant of breast
- Can be seen in patients with family history of breast cancer
- Has been seen with concurrent breast cancer when one of the following is present
  - Positive family history breast cancer
  - Atypical proliferative lesion
  - Bilateral or multifocal lesions
  - Recurrence of juvenile papillomatosis

Treatment: Excision and close follow-up

Contusion (Fat Necrosis)

- Results from trauma to the breast
- Presents as a poorly defined, tender mass
- Typically has resolution over several weeks to months
- Manage hematomas with analgesics, ice packs and binding of the breast (sports bra or elastic wrap)
- Post-treatment to ensure complete resolution

BREAST PAIN

Etiology

- Premenstrual hormonal/ fibrocystic changes
- Medication use (e.g. oral contraceptive pill use)
- Exercise or trauma

Evaluation

- Breast exam
- Pregnancy test

Treatment

- Reassurance
- Instruction to wear supportive bra/compressive type sports bra helpful
- Trial of NSAIDs, oral or topical
- If on oral contraceptive pill, decrease ethinyl estradiol dose
- Trial of vitamin E (1200 IU) ± evening primrose oil

NIPPLE DISCHARGE

Key Points

- Usually benign and spontaneously resolves
- Needs evaluation if unilateral, single duct, bloody, intermittent or persistent

Diagnosis

History

- May occur at any age
- Laterality and frequency
- *Characterize the discharge:* Milky, purulent, watery, serous, serosanguinous, or bloody
- Timing of discharge in relation to activity or temperature changes
- Review of medical history, medications, and social history
  - Oral contraceptives, tricyclic antidepressants, H2 antagonists, cannabis, phenothiazines, and antihypertensive agents

Physical Exam

- If palpable mass present, need imaging
- May be associated with interrupted puberty or with primary or secondary amenorrhea
- Needs evaluation if unilateral, single duct, bloody, intermittent or persistent

Galactorrhea (See Chapter 43, "Prolactin Disorders")

- Milky discharge
- Most commonly due to pregnancy/post-pregnancy, drugs (prescription or illicit), thyroid dysfunction, chest trauma or prolactin-secreting tumor
- *Labs*: HCG, prolactin, estradiol, TSH

Ductal Ectasia

- Sticky, green, serosanguinous, brown or multicolored discharge from one or both breasts
- Most common cause of bloody nipple discharge in infants
- *Ultrasound findings*: Subareolar, anechoic tubular structures that may contain debris
- Usually resolve spontaneously within 9 months
- Stasis of secretions can lead to a bacterial infection

Montgomery Tubercles

- Clear to brownish fluid through ectopic opening on the areola for several weeks
- One-third have a small subareolar lump, the remainder have acute inflammation
- Spontaneously resolves over several weeks to months
- Treat infection with oral antibiotics and NSAIDs

Intraductal Papilloma

- May have a bloody discharge
- May be solitary or multiple
- *Ultrasound findings*: Ill-defined, inhomogeneous mass with several echo-free areas observed mainly near the border of the lesion
- *Treatment*: Excision

Management

- Discharge usually resolves spontaneously; manipulation will perpetuate it
- If purulent and concerning for infection, obtain a Gram stain, culture, cell count and consider ultrasound

BIBLIOGRAPHY

De Silva NK. Breast development and disorders in the adolescent female. Best Pract Res Clin Obstetr Gyneacol. 2018; 48:40–50.

Diagnosis and management of benign breast disorders. Practice bulletin no. 164. American College of Obstetricians and Gynecologists. Obstet Gynecol. 2016;127:e141–156.

DiVasta AD, Weldon C, Labow BI. Chapter 54 The Breast: Examination and Lesions. In: Emans SJH, Laufer MR, eds, *Pediatric and Adolescent Gynecology* (7th edn.) Philadelphia, PA: Lippencott Williams & Wilkins; 2021.

Eidlitz-Markus T, Mukamel M, Haimi-Cohen Y, et al. Breast asymmetry during adolescence: physiologic and non-physiologic causes. Isr Med Assoc J. 2010;12(4):203–206.

Fallat ME, Ignacio RC Jr. Breast disorders in children and adolescents. J Pediatr Adolesc Gynecol. 2008; 21:311–316.

Greydanus DE, Matytsina L, Gains M. Breast disorders in children and adolescents. Prim Care. 2006;33:455–502.

Jayasinghe Y. Preventive care and evaluation of the adolescent with a breast mass. Semin Plast Surg. 2013;27:13–18.

Stevens DL, Bisno AL, Chambers HF, et al. Practice guidelines for the diagnosis and management of skin and soft tissue infections: 2014 update by the infectious diseases society of America. Clin Infect Dis. 2014;59:147–159.

10

Cervical Mass

Jennie Yoost

Key Points

- There is a large differential diagnosis and approach is based on type of mass
- Differential includes
  - Nabothian cyst, mesonephric cysts, cervical polyp, condyloma, ectropion, cervical pregnancy, benign Müllerian papilloma
  - Vascular lesions
    - Arteriovenous malformation
    - Hemangioma
  - Malignancy is rare but reported
    - Müllerian adenosarcoma
    - Embryonal rhabdomyosarcomas

Diagnosis

History

In child

- Abnormal bleeding, abnormal discharge, protruding mass from vagina

In adolescent

- Abnormal bleeding, menorrhagia, abnormal discharge, postcoital bleeding, or may be an incidental finding
- History of DICER-1 syndrome
- HPV vaccination status

Physical Examination

In child

- Use vaginoscopy with/without anesthesia (see "Operative Care", Chapter 31)

In adolescent

- Examination under anesthesia and vaginoscopy with biopsy can also be performed if needed
- Use appropriate speculum (see "Gynecologic Examination", Chapter 20)

DOI: 10.1201/9781003039235-10

- Pregnancy testing and screening for gonorrhea, chlamydia as indicated by history
- Pap testing if ≥21 years of age
- Consider colposcopy to evaluate with biopsy if necessary

Management

- Treatment should be diagnosis specific
- Purely cystic structures can be observed
  - Marsupialization of large cystic lesions is an option
- Vascular abnormalities should not be biopsied without appropriate consultation
  - MRI is best modality for imaging vascular lesions
  - Beta blockers (i.e. propranolol) can be used for treatment of hemangiomas
  - Consider consultation with vascular surgery regarding management
- Biopsy should be performed for solid, polypoid, or changing lesions, or if diagnosis unclear
  - Anesthesia used as needed based on patient age and type of mass
  - Biopsy indicated for pathologic assessment
  - Excisional biopsy can be performed for small lesions (i.e. polyps)
- Diagnosis of malignancy should involve consultation with gynecologic oncology
- Monitor patient for signs of recurrence

BIBLIOGRAPHY

Fleming NA, Hopkins L, de Nanassy J, Senterman M, Black AY. Müllerian adenosarcoma of the cervix in a 10-year-old girl: case report and review of the literature. J Pediatr Adolesc Gynecol. 2009; 22(4):e45–e51.

Ganti AK, Ray J, Mooney KL, Zambrano E, Hillard PJA, Fok W. Unusual cause of pediatric vaginal bleeding: infantile capillary hemangioma of the cervix. J Pediatr Adolesc Gynecol. 2019; 32(1):80–82.

McQuillan SK, Grover SR, Pyman J, Jayasinghe YL. Literature review of benign Müllerian papilloma contrasted with vaginal rhabdomyosarcoma. J Pediatr Adolesc Gynecol. 2016; 29(4):333–337.

11

Condyloma Acuminatum and Human Papillomavirus (HPV)

Vikki Tulchinskaya and Maggie L. Dwiggins

Key Points

- Human papillomavirus (HPV) is the most common sexually transmitted infection (STI) in the United States
- Transmission: Vertical, horizontal (auto- or hetero-inoculation), and sexual contact
- Condyloma acuminatum is an infection caused by HPV
  - Incubation period is generally 1–20 months, but latency periods of at least 3 years are known
  - Most common are non-oncogenic types 6, 11; isolated reports of autoinoculation of type 2 from cutaneous warts
- Vaccination against HPV is recommended by the Centers for Disease Control and Prevention (CDC) and may be given starting at age 9 years, up to age 45 years
- The pediatric and adolescent gynecologist is unlikely to screen for cervical/vaginal HPV in the immunocompetent patient

CONDYLOMA ACUMINATUM

Diagnosis

- Primarily a clinical diagnosis; may require magnification with colposcope
- Condyloma usually arises in healthy appearing surrounding skin as raised, verrucous papules of variable size
- Evaluate and document location, color, shape, texture, borders, number and distribution of lesions, as well as associated symptoms
- Most are less than 5 mm in diameter; if larger, may appear cauliflower-like
- May consider biopsy of atypical or persistent lesions
- Lesions predominate the anogenital area in prepubertal children; may occur anywhere in the genital tract in sexually active adolescents
- May present with bleeding, pruritus, and pain; can be completely asymptomatic

Management

- No data have proven that treatment is preferable to observation for spontaneous regression
- 90% of condyloma will regress within 2 years

DOI: 10.1201/9781003039235-11

- If lesions are persistent for more than 2 years, are rapidly growing, or are symptomatic, then treat
- If not sexually active, screen carefully for sexual abuse before treatment
    - Document the age when warts were first noted, mode of delivery, any history of warts or HPV in child, family, or contacts
    - Physical exam for signs of sexual abuse (see Chapter 46, "Sexual Abuse")
    - If neither conclusive, forensic interview is recommended at local children's advocacy agency
    - HPV typing should not be used to assess sexual abuse; typing methods, even new techniques (i.e. hybrid capture), have cross-reactivity as well as false-negative results; HPV types have latency and transformation characteristics still not well understood
    - In children under age 4, consider vertical transmission of HPV if no evidence of sexual abuse
- If sexually active
    - Screen for chlamydia and gonorrhea if not done within the last 3 months of the appearance of the condyloma
    - Encourage careful inspection of partner for visible lesions
- Despite successful treatment, can recur
    - If recurs, biopsy
    - With repeated recurrences screen for human immunodeficiency virus (HIV)

Treatment

Medical

- No treatment is superior; most treatments require more than one dosing
- Imiquimod is the only FDA-approved medical treatment in children 12 years or older

- Imiquimod 5% cream: Topical immune enhancer that stimulates production of interferon and other cytokines
    - Although not approved for children younger than 12 years, cure rates documented up to 75% in this age group
    - Can be very erosive to epithelium particularly in a prepubertal child
    - Apply test dose with a Q-tip to one lesion very sparingly
    - Have patient return in one week and, if no untoward effects, extend the area and frequency of treatment very slowly and check weekly
    - Do not treat more frequently than weekly in the prepubertal child and twice weekly in young adolescent; adult dosing 3 times per week at bedtime for up to 16 weeks
    - Wash off in 6–10 hours
- Imiquimod 3.75%
    - Same as above test dosing
    - Applied nightly
    - Sinecatechins 15% ointment
        - Applied to each wart 3 times per day with finger
            - Continue until complete clearance of warts, up to 16 weeks
            - Should not be washed off after application
            - Should not be used in patients with HIV or who are otherwise immunocompromised
            - Safety in pregnancy unknown
    - Intralesional interferon alpha
        - Injections are painful and cumbersome with associated fever, myalgia, lethargy, and headaches
        - Consult with pediatric dermatologist or pediatric infectious disease regarding use and dosing

- Other treatment options
  - Trichloroacetic acid (TCA) or bichloroacetic acid (BCA) 80–90%
    - Apply small amount to the wart with a toothpick
    - Lubricate surrounding skin, may use petroleum jelly
    - Allow to dry to a white coat; may wash off in an hour especially if persistent burning
    - Repeat weekly
  - Podofilox 0.5% solution or gel: An antimitotic drug that causes wart necrosis
    - Not approved for pediatric population
    - Patient or parent applies to warts twice daily for 3 days, then nothing for 4 days
    - Repeat up to 4 cycles
    - Treated wart area should be < 10 mm^3
    - Limit total volume Podofilox to 0.5 mL/day
    - Safety not established in pregnancy; would not use in children
  - Cimetidine oral tablets or suspension
    - 40 mg/kg/day in three divided doses
    - Usually treat at least 3 months since effects are rarely seen before at least two months
    - If disease persists without significant change for one month, screen with appropriate serology and tissue specimens for immunodeficiency, including HIV, and other pathologic causes and check for continued reinfection

Surgical

- Includes cryotherapy, CO_2 laser, pulsed light, electrocoagulation, and surgical excision
- Only use in recalcitrant symptomatic cases where immune deficiency and other pathologic causes are ruled out
- CO_2 laser is the preferred method
  - Advantages: More hemostatic and less tissue damage
  - Cure rate: 27–100%
  - Disadvantages: Requires general anesthesia
  - Procedure
    - Attach laser to the colposcope or microscope with a micromanipulator to best target the dermatologic planes
    - Use the super pulse mode at a low wattage – leaves minimal adjuvant tissue damage
    - Vaporized debris wiped away with 3–5% of acetic-acid-soaked gauze so that the classic white papillations can be observed
  - Postoperatively
    - Infiltrate operative sites with local anesthetic such as 0.25% bupivacaine without epinephrine
    - Prescribe narcotics and NSAIDs (see Chapter 31, "Operative Care," for dosing)
    - Apply ice pack locally for 48 hours as tolerated
    - Sitz baths QID followed by air-drying with blow-dryer on low setting and Silvadene cream applied liberally to area until healed
    - Void in bathtub or dilute urine with peri-bottle while voiding
    - Use stool softener to prevent constipation
    - If extensive resection, may need hospitalization with Foley catheter overnight

- Cryotherapy (liquid nitrogen)
  - Can be performed in office
  - Pain is common during procedure as well as after due to necrosis and blistering
  - Local anesthesia may alleviate some discomfort

Follow-Up

- Despite apparent resolution of the lesions, long-term follow-up is indicated because of the known risk of recurrence

Vaccination

- Vaccination is exquisitely effective at preventing HPV
- Available vaccine
  - HPV 9-valent vaccine against HPV 6 and 11 (responsible for 90% of cases of anogenital warts) and HPV 16, 18, 31, 33, 45, 52, and 58
- Vaccination against HPV is recommended by the Centers for Disease Control and Prevention (CDC) and may be given starting at age 9 years, up to age 45 years
- Prior to age 15 years, need 2 doses 6 months apart. After age 15, need 3 doses (0, 2, and 6 months)

Counseling/Education

- Condoms are not 100% effective at prevention of transmission due to skin-to-skin transmission of HPV; studies show that men can carry the HPV virus under their fingernails, so coital transmission not the only potential method
- Smoking and second-hand smoke inhibit viral clearing
- Transmission possible without visible lesions
- Treatment frequently may require multiple sessions and different techniques
- Male partners with visible lesions in anogenital region should be referred for management

BIBLIOGRAPHY

Centers for Disease Control and Prevention. Sexually transmitted diseases treatment guidelines 2021. MMWR July 23, 2021;70(4)
Centers for Disease Control and Prevention. HPV (human papillomavirus) vaccine: what you need to know. VIS. 2019.
Costa-Silva M, Fernandes I, Rodrigues AG, Lisboa C. Anogenital warts in pediatric population. An Bras Dermatol. 2017; 92(5):675–681.
Culton DA, Morrell DS, Burkhart CN. The management of *Condyloma acuminata* in the pediatric population. Pediatr Ann. 2009; 38:368–372.
Gibbs, NF. Anogenital papillomavirus infections in children. Curr Opin Pediatr. 1998; 10:393–397

12

Contraception

Kylie Fowler

Key Points

- A pelvic exam is not required prior to initiating almost all forms of contraception.
- Adolescent preference is important when choosing a method and improves compliance.
- Long-acting reversible contraception (LARC) methods (intrauterine devices [IUDs] and subdermal implants) are safe, highly effective, and should be considered first-line therapy for adolescent contraceptive options.
- LARC methods overall have high satisfaction and continuation rates among adolescents.
- Condoms are the only method that offers protection from sexually transmitted infections (STIs) and should be recommended to all adolescents.
- The United States Medical Eligibility Criteria for Contraceptive Use (USMEC) is a free resource offering evidence-based recommendations for use of specific contraceptive methods in patients with different medical conditions or characteristics.
- Patients who are overweight or obese have higher failure rates with use of levonorgestrel emergency contraception (EC) and the combined hormonal patches.
- Providers should be familiar with state and local regulations related to adolescent confidentiality and provision of sexual health care to minors without parental consent.

Management

Confidentiality

Explain the need for privacy and confidentiality in the adolescent years.

Reassure the parents/guardians that the provider will facilitate discussion about school, friends, drugs, and sexuality; however, confidentiality will be maintained in accordance with state and local regulations.

- Open discussion between adolescents and parents/guardians results in later onset of sexual activity and increased rates of contraception use with first sexual encounter.
- Providers should facilitate discussion between youth and parents/guardians if possible.
- Inform the adolescent and parent/guardian that confidentiality will be broken if information indicates a harmful or life-threatening situation for the adolescent or another person.
- Discuss possible breaches to confidentiality that may occur through billing or the provision of an explanation of benefits provided by health insurance companies to the insurance policyholder.

If confidentiality cannot be maintained due to billing or insurance procedures, the adolescent should be referred to a Title 10 federally funded clinic, which often includes Planned Parenthood, school-based clinics, or local health department clinics.

History

Obtain a complete medical, surgical, social, and family history.

- Medical history should include comprehensive menstrual history.
- Family history should include any bleeding/clotting disorders, gynecologic malignancies, and genetic syndromes.
- Social history should include comprehensive sexual history, including the 5 Ps
  1. Partners
     a. Gender and sex of partners
     b. Number of partners in previous 60 days
     c. Number of partners in previous 12 months
     d. Exposures (if known) of patient's partners
     e. Safety/consent with current and previous partners
  2. Practices
     a. Vaginal, oral, anal
     b. Participation in transactional sex (exchange of sex for money, housing, food)
     c. Sexual activity while under the influence of substances
  3. Pregnancy prevention
     a. Current use of contraception
     b. Previous use of contraception and why discontinued
  4. Protection from STIs
     a. Use of male or female condoms: Always, sometimes, never
     b. Use of dental dams
  5. Past history of STIs

Screen for relationship violence and counsel regarding positive consent (see Chapter 21, "High-Risk Behaviors").

- Assess for high-risk sexual activity, including multiple partners, engaging in sex while under the influence of substances, or exchanging sex for food, housing, clothing, or money.
- All information should be acquired in a nonjudgmental way with the opportunity for the patient to ask questions.

Physical Examination

- Blood pressure, height/weight, BMI
- Examination of heart, lungs, thyroid, abdomen, and extremities
- Pelvic examination should be performed for patients with symptoms such as abdominopelvic pain or vaginal discharge, or in patients planning to undergo IUD insertion

NOTE: Routine internal pelvic exam is not required for the provision of contraception.

Laboratory Tests

- STI screening should be performed in accordance with Centers for Disease Control and Prevention (CDC) recommendations. For adolescents and young adults between the ages of 15 through 24, this includes screening for *Neisseria gonorrhoeae*, *Chlamydia trachomatis* annually, and HIV at least once
- Pregnancy test

Counseling

- Discuss all available methods, including EC
- **Begin with the most effective methods, LARC, and end with the least effective methods (see the effectiveness chart from Bedsider.org)**
- Emphasize the importance of using a condom to prevent STIs
- Discuss previous methods and reasons for discontinuing that method
- Discuss myths of contraception
  - *Weight gain*: No evidence on any method other than depot medroxyprogesterone acetate
  - *Acne*: Improved on combined oral contraceptive pills (COCPs)
  - *Infertility*: No effects
  - *Cancer*: Different methods protect against uterine, ovarian, cervical, and/or colon; inconclusive evidence regarding risk of breast cancer
  - *Promotes sexual debut*: Open conversation with adults (especially parents) may actually delay sexual debut
  - *Ovarian cysts*: Prevention of physiologic cysts with methods that suppress ovulation
  - *Mood changes*: Uncommon
- Provide trusted websites where adolescents can access more information
  - *Bedsider.org*: Operated by Power to Decide, the campaign to prevent unplanned pregnancy, information in both English and Spanish, has separate website for clinicians with educational articles, materials, and CME
  - *Youngwomenshealth.org*: Operated through a partnership between the Division of Adolescent/Young Adult Medicine and the Division of Gynecology at Boston Children's Hospital, information in both English and Spanish, offers tool kits and additional resources for clinicians
  - *Plannedparenthood.org/learn/teens*: Operated by Planned Parenthood, information in both English and Spanish

Treatment

Prior to prescribing a method, the United States Medical Eligibility Criteria for Contraceptive Use (USMEC) should be referenced. It is available for free online or through a free downloadable app.

- Lists safety of contraceptives by method as well as by specific medical condition.
- The eligibility for each contraceptive method is classified into four categories:
  - *Category 1*: No restrictions exist for use of the method.
  - *Category 2*: Method can be used as benefits generally outweigh risks, closer follow-up may be required.
  - *Category 3*: Use of method is not recommended unless other methods are not available or acceptable to the patient.
  - *Category 4*: Method poses unacceptable health risk.
- When measuring the risk of contraceptive use, the appropriate risk comparison is to pregnancy NOT to nonuse. Almost all contraceptive methods have lower risk profiles than pregnancy.

Once a method is chosen, the United States Specific Practice Recommendations (USSPR) may be referenced for specific information about initiation of the method, any testing requirements, follow-up, and management of usage errors or side effects.

Any method can be started on the same day of presentation (same day start) if the clinician is reasonably sure the patient is not pregnant.

- Is ≤7 days after the start of normal menses
- Has not had sexual intercourse since the start of last normal menses
- Has been correctly and consistently using a reliable method of contraception
- Is <7 days after spontaneous or induced abortion
- Is within 4 weeks postpartum
- Is fully or nearly fully breastfeeding (exclusively breastfeeding or the vast majority [≥85%] of feeds are breastfeeds), amenorrheic, and <6 months postpartum

Perfect and typical use pregnancy rates are listed. Adolescents tend to have higher typical use failure rates.

Intrauterine Devices

Copper intrauterine device (*Paragard*®)

- Nonhormonal
- Copper exerts a spermicidal effect
- Most effective method of EC can be inserted up to 5 days after unprotected intercourse
- May lower risk of cervical cancer
- FDA approved for 10 years of use, excellent evidence for extended use up to 12 years
- *Most common side effect*: Heavier, more painful periods
- *Perfect use pregnancy rate*: 0.6%
- *Typical use pregnancy rate*: 0.8%
- *Effective*: Immediately

Levonorgestrel intrauterine devices

- Progestin-only method
- Thickens cervical mucous to prevent sperm from accessing uterine cavity and oocyte
- Thins the lining of the uterus, which offers noncontraceptive benefits, including lighter menses/amenorrhea, decreased menstrual pain, decreased risk of uterine cancer
- Effective method of EC can be inserted up to 5 days after unprotected intercourse
- *Most common side effect*: Irregular bleeding especially in the first 3–6 months of use
- *Perfect and typical use pregnancy rate*: 0.1%
- *Effective*: Immediately

Levonorgestrel 52 mg

- *Mirena*®: FDA approved for 7 years of use
- *Liletta*®: FDA approved for 6 years of use, excellent evidence for extended use up to 7 years
- Both devices have the highest rate of amenorrhea among the hormonal IUDs

Levonorgestrel 19.5 mg

- *Kyleena*®: FDA approved for 5 years of use, no data on extended use

Levonorgestrel 13.5 mg

- *Skyla*®: FDA approved for 3 years of use, no data on extended use

Implant

Etonorgestrel 68 mg (*Nexplanon*®)

- Progestin-only method
- Prevents ovulation and thickens cervical mucous to prevent sperm from accessing uterine cavity or oocyte
- Noncontraceptive benefits include lighter and less painful menses, decreased risk of ovarian, and uterine cancer
- FDA approved for 3 years of use, excellent evidence for extended use up to 5 years, regardless of patient weight or BMI
- *Most common side effects*: Irregular bleeding (60%)
- *Perfect and typical use pregnancy rate*: 0.1%
- *Effective*: Immediately if inserted within 5 days of last menstrual period; if inserted >5 days after last menstrual period, abstinence or a backup method is needed for 7 days

Injectable

Depot medroxyprogesterone acetate (Depo-Provera®)

- Progestin-only method
- Prevents ovulation
- Noncontraceptive benefits include lighter and less painful menses, suppression of physiologic ovarian cysts, decreased risk of uterine, and ovarian cancer
- FDA approved for up to 13 weeks, effective up to 15 weeks from last injection
- *Most common side effects*: Irregular bleeding, increase in appetite and weight gain, decrease in bone density with resolution after method stop
- Available in 150 mg intramuscular injection for in-clinic administration and 104 mg at-home subcutaneous injection kit
- *Perfect use pregnancy rate*: 1%
- *Typical use pregnancy rate*: 6%
- *Effective*: Immediately if started within 7 days of last menstrual period; if initiated >7 days after last menstrual period, abstinence or a backup method is needed for 7 days

Combined Hormonal Contraceptives

Include combined oral contraceptive pills (COCPs), transdermal patches, and intravaginal rings
Contain both estrogen and progestin

- Prevents ovulation
- Noncontraceptive benefits include lighter and less painful menses, suppression of physiologic ovarian cysts, decrease in acne, decreased risk of ovarian, uterine, and colon cancer
- Prescription of full-one-year supply is associated with improved compliance
- *Most common side effects*: Nausea, headache, and irregular bleeding
- Absolute contraindications to use include migraine with aura, known thrombotic disorder, history of venous thromboembolism (VTE) or history of VTE in the first-degree relative (consult the USMEC for comprehensive information regarding these and other medical conditions)
- *Perfect use pregnancy rate*: 0.3%

- *Typical use pregnancy rate*: 7%
- *Effective*: Immediately if started within 5 days of last menstrual period; if started more than 5 days since last menstrual period, abstinence or a backup method is needed for 7 days

Combined oral contraceptive pills

- Pills with less than 30 mcg of ethinyl estradiol should be used with caution in adolescents as bone density accrual may be impaired at lower doses
- Monophasic COCPs have consistent levels of estradiol and progestin in each pill
  - Can be used for extended cycling or continuous use by skipping placebo week
- Phasic COCPs have consistent levels of estradiol and variable levels of progestin in each pill
  - Irregular bleeding and breakthrough ovulation is more common with phasic COCPs
- In those who are overweight or obese, efficacy may be improved with no placebo or pill-free interval
- *Late (<24 hours) or missed (24–48 hours) pills*: Take dose as soon as possible even if that means taking two pills on the same day, no backup or EC is necessary
- *Two or more missed pills (>48 hours)*: Take dose as soon as possible even if that means taking two pills on the same day, abstinence or backup method is needed until 7 days of consecutive hormonal pills are completed; if pills were missed in days 15–28 of a 28-day pack, skip the placebos and start a new pack to complete a full 7 days of consecutive hormonal pills, consider EC (with the exception of ulipristal acetate)
- Caution should be taken in those with concomitant use of antiepileptics:
  - Topiramate <200 mg/day dose does not decrease the efficacy of 35-mcg ethinyl estradiol pill; doses higher than 200mg may decrease pill efficacy
  - Phenobarbital, Phenytoin, and Carbamazepine decrease pill efficacy
  - Lamotrigine concentrations can be decreased by as much as 50% with concomitant use; levels must be closely monitored

Transdermal patch

- Available in 30-mcg estradiol–120-mcg levonorgestrel (*Twirla®*) and 35-mcg estradiol–150-mcg norelgestromin (*Xulane®*, *Zafemy®*) formulations
- Typical use is to apply a patch once weekly for 3 weeks followed by a patch-free week with menstrual withdrawal bleed
- Can be used in extended manner by applying a patch every week with no patch-free weeks
- USMLE category 2 (benefits generally outweigh risks) in women with a BMI >30 due to possible decreased efficacy and increased risk of VTE
- Potential for local skin reaction

Vaginal ring

Etonogestrel 11.7 mg–ethinyl estradiol 2.7 mg (*Nuvaring®*)

- Inserted for 3 weeks and removed for 1 week to have withdrawal bleed; however, a single ring is effective for up to 6 weeks
- Can be used for extended cycling by replacing the ring once a month with no ring-free interval
- Rings that will not be used within 4 months need to be stored in the refrigerator (may cause privacy concern for adolescents)
- Designed to stay in place during sex; however, it can be removed for up to 3 hours.
- If the ring is removed for more than 3 hours, abstinence or a backup method is necessary until it has been replaced for 7 days. If the ring is out for more than 3 hours during the third week of use, it should be removed on day 21 and a new ring immediately inserted, skipping the ring-free week

Segesterone acetate 103 mg–ethinyl estradiol 17.4 mg (*Annovera*®)

- Inserted for 3 weeks and removed for a 1-week interval during which time a withdrawal bleed occurs. The ring is cleaned and stored in a provided case during this week. The same ring is reinserted and can be used for a total of 13 cycles
- Can be used for extended cycling by keeping the ring in the vagina with no ring-free interval. However, should be removed once a month for brief cleansing with warm water and a gentle cleanser
- Designed to stay in place during sex; however, it can be removed for up to 2 hours
- If the ring is removed for more than 2 hours, abstinence or a backup method is necessary until it has been replaced for 7 consecutive days

Progestin-Only Pills

Norethindrone 35 mcg "Minipill"

- More sensitive to user error, pills should be taken within 3 hours of the same time each day for maximum efficacy
- Taken in a 28-day continuous fashion with no set week for menses
- Thickens cervical mucous, prevents ovulation in about half of cycles
- Noncontraceptive benefits include lighter and less painful menses, decreased risk of ovarian, uterine, and colon cancer
- *Effective*: Immediately if taken within 5 days of last menstrual period. If >5 days since the last menstrual period, abstinence or a backup method is needed for 48 hours
- Late (<24 hours) or missed (24–48 hours), abstinence or a backup method is needed for 48 hours after resumption of pills
- *Most common side effect*: Irregular bleeding
- *Perfect use failure rate*: 0.3%
- *Typical use failure rate*: 7%

Drospirenone 4 mg (*Slynd*®)

- *Designed for 24/4 use*: 24 days of active medicated pills and 4 days of inactive placebo pills
- FDA approved to treat acne
- Should be used with caution in patients with renal impairment due to diuretic and electrolyte disturbances; potassium levels should be checked after one cycle in patients with potential for electrolyte abnormalities
- Thickens cervical mucous, prevents ovulation in about half of cycles
- Noncontraceptive benefits include lighter and less painful menses, decreased risk of ovarian, uterine, and colon cancer
- *Effective*: Immediately if <7 days from last menstrual cycle. If >7 days from the last menstrual cycle, abstinence or a backup method is needed for 7 days
- *Late (<24 hours) or missed (24–48 hours) pills*: Take dose as soon as possible even if that means taking 2 pills on the same day, no backup or EC is necessary
- *Two or more missed pills (>48 hours)*: Take dose as soon as possible even if that means taking 2 pills on the same day, abstinence or backup method is needed until 7 days of consecutive hormonal pills are completed; if pills were missed in days 15–28 of a 28-day pack, skip the placebos and start a new pack to complete a full 7 days of consecutive hormonal pills, consider EC (with the exception of ulipristal acetate)
- *Most common side effect*: Irregular bleeding

- *Perfect use failure rate*: 0.3%
- *Typical use failure rate*: 7%

Spermicides

- Available in many formulations, including creams, gels, foams, and suppositories
- Nonoxynol-9
  - Decreases sperm motility
  - Available over the counter
  - Can be used with any other method
- Lactic acid 1.8%, citric acid 1%, and potassium bitartrate 0.4% vaginal gel (*Phexxi®*)
  - Maintains acidic pH of the vagina to decrease sperm motility
  - Prescription only
  - Cannot be used with a vaginal ring
- Nonhormonal
- Low efficacy and are recommended to be combined with other methods
- Increases susceptibility to HIV and other STIs
- Intercourse must take place after 10 minutes but within 60 minutes of insertion
- *Common side effects*: Local irritation of both sexual partners
- Must be used with each sexual act
- *Perfect use failure rate*: 18%
- *Typical use failure rate*: 28%

Emergency Contraception

- EC is used to prevent pregnancy after unprotected sexual intercourse.
- The sooner they are initiated, the more effective they are at pregnancy prevention. The methods of EC will be described in the order of most to least effective.
- EC methods are not recommended for repeat use as they are not as effective as regular preventive contraceptive methods.

Copper intrauterine device (*Paragard®*)

- If inserted within 5 days (120 hours) of unprotected intercourse, it lowers pregnancy rates by over 99%

Levonorgestrel 52 mg—intrauterine device (*Mirena®, Liletta®*)

- As effective as copper IUD for EC

Ulipristal acetate (*Ella®*)

- One dose formulation available by prescription only
- Many pharmacies do not keep this medication in stock and can only order it (acquiring it within 48–72 hours, which may impact efficacy)
  - Clinicians should be familiar with pharmacies that regularly stock it, call the patient's preferred pharmacy ahead of time, or encourage patients to keep a dose on hand if they are at risk of needing it

- Available via online pharmacies with expedited (24 hours or less) delivery in some states
- *Most common side effects*: Nausea, irregular menses after use

Oral levonorgestrel 1.5 mg (*Plan B® One Step®, Next Choice® One Dose®, My Way®*)

- Previously divided into two doses, however similar efficacy with one-dose regimen
- Take as soon as possible up to 5 days (120 hours) after unprotected sex
- Available over the counter without age restrictions
- *Most common side effects*: Nausea, irregular bleeding
- Efficacy decreased by as much as 33% in patients who are overweight or obese

The Yuzpe regimen

- Many combined hormonal contraceptive pills can be used as EC by combining doses, which are then taken 12 hours apart. Doses range from taking 2 to 5 pills at one time
- Efficacy is highest if doses are initiated within 72 hours of unprotected sex; however, they may be started up to 120 hours after unprotected sex
- *Most common side effects*: Nausea, irregular bleeding
- Specific EC doses for different forms of COCPs can be found at https://ec.princeton.edu/questions/dose.html

Barrier Methods

Condoms

- Should be recommended for all adolescents regardless of other contraceptive methods used
- Available in male (external) and female (internal) designs
- Commonly made of latex, but available in non-latex materials such as nitrile or polyurethane
- Non-latex lambskin condoms block sperm but **do not** block STI transmission
- Adolescents should be instructed not to use more than one condom per sex act (i.e. do not use an internal condom with an external condom) as this decreases, rather than increases, efficacy
- Latex condoms require water or silicone-based lubricants (oil-based lubricants will degrade the latex and decrease efficacy)
- *Common side effects*: Minimal
- *Perfect use failure rate*: 2%
- *Typical use failure rate*: 13%
- Provide condoms to all adolescents in a discreet manner

Cervical cap (*FemCap®*)

- Requires fitting
- Made of silicone
- Needs to remain in place for 6 hours after sex, can be left in place for up to 48 hours
- More effective if used with spermicide
- *Common side effects*: Difficulty with insertion or removal, vaginal irritation
- Less effective if user has previously given birth
- *Perfect use nulliparous failure rate*: 9%
- *Typical use nulliparous failure rate*: 14%

- *Perfect use parous failure rate*: 26%
- *Typical use parous failure rate*: 29%

Diaphragm

- Requires fitting
- Made of silicone
- Needs to remain in place for 6 hours after sex, can be left in place for up to 24 hours
- More effective if used with spermicide
- *Perfect use failure rate*: 6%
- *Typical use failure rate*: 18%

Sponge (*Today Sponge®*)

- Blocks sperm and releases continuous amount of spermicide
- Available over the counter
- Needs to remain in place for 6 hours after sex, can be left in place for up to 24 hours
- Less effective if user has previously given birth
- *Perfect use nulliparous failure rate*: 9%
- *Typical use nulliparous failure rate*: 16%
- *Perfect use parous failure rate*: 20%
- *Typical use parous failure rate*: 32%

BIBLIOGRAPHY

Adolescents and long-acting reversible contraception: implants and intrauterine devices. American College of Obstetrics and Gynecology Committee Opinion #735. Obstet Gynecol. 2018 May; 131(5):e130–e139.

Bedsider.org and Bixby Center for Global Reproductive Health, How well does Birth Control work? Available at: https://beyondthepill.ucsf.edu/sites/beyondthepill.ucsf.edu/files/Tiers%20of%20Effectiveness_English-043019.pdf.

Committee on Adolescence. Contraception for adolescents. Pediatrics. 2014; 134(4):e1244–e1256.

Curtis KM, Jatlaoui TC, Tepper NK, et al. U.S. selected practice recommendations for contraceptive use, 2016. MMWR Recomm Rep. 2016a; 65(RR-4):1–66.

Curtis KM, Tepper NK, Jatlaoui TC, et al. U.S. medical eligibility criteria for contraceptive use, 2016. MMWR Recomm Rep. 2016b; 65(RR-3):1–103.

Diedrich JT, Klein DA, Peipert JE. Long-acting reversible contraception in adolescents: a systematic review and meta-analysis. Am J Obstet Gynecol. 2017; 216(4):364e1–364e12.

Noncontraceptive uses of hormonal contraceptives. American College of Obstetrics and Gynecology Practice Bulletin #110. Obstet Gynecol. 2010; 115(1):206–218.

Turok DM, Gero A, Simmons RG, et al. Levonorgestrel vs copper intrauterine device for emergency contraception. N Engl J Med. 2021; 384:335–344.

13

Depression

Virginia Ramsey Aldrich and Maggie L. Dwiggins

Key Points

- In youth aged 9–17 years, one in five has a diagnosable mental health disorder that causes some degree of impairment. Two-thirds of these youth do not receive the necessary treatment.
- Of youth aged 15–24 years, suicide is the second leading cause of death. There are 13.9 deaths by suicide in this population every day. The rate of suicide attempts is 100–200 times greater than completions.
- Patients with depressed mood may have decreased motivation to practice safe sex, resulting in pregnancy and/or sexually transmitted infections (STIs).
- Early identification, prompt referral, and care coordination of mental health disorders can reduce morbidity and mortality in the adolescent; therefore, every youth 12 and above should be screened with confidential screening tool annually and when depression suspected.

Risk Factors

- Personal and/or parental history of mental health disorders
- Stressful academic, social, or family environment
- Early or significant loss (parental death, divorce, termination of a relationship)
- History of bullying (including cyberbullying)
- History of neglect or physical, mental, or sexual abuse
- History of alcohol or substance abuse
- Internet addiction
- Sleep deprivation
- Problems with sexual orientation, gender identity

Comorbidity

- Substance abuse
- Anxiety disorders
- Attention-deficit/hyperactivity Disorder
- Physical abuse
- Trauma
- Eating disorders
- Learning disorders

DOI: 10.1201/9781003039235-13

Diagnosis

Differential diagnosis of mental illnesses in adolescents: Anxiety, mood, and behavior disorders.

Major Depressive Disorder (DSM-V)

- **Five or more** of the following symptoms present during a two-week period with at least one symptom being either depressed mood or loss of interest
  - Depressed most of the day, nearly every day by patient report or observation by others
  - Markedly diminished interest or pleasure in all or most activities most of the day, nearly every day
  - Increased or decreased appetite nearly every day, or significant weight loss or weight gain when not dieting (change of 5% body weight in one month)
  - Insomnia or hypersomnia nearly every day
  - Psychomotor agitation or retardation nearly every day observable by others
  - Fatigue or loss of energy nearly every day
  - Feelings of worthlessness or excessive or inappropriate guilt nearly every day
  - Diminished ability to think or concentrate, or indecisiveness, nearly every day
  - Recurrent thoughts of death, recurrent suicidal ideation with or without a specific plan, or a suicide attempt

Mild, moderate, and severe forms of major depressive disorder can be diagnosed based on symptom count, intensity of symptoms, and/or level of impairment.

History

Every patient aged 12 years and above should be screened for mental health disorders annually using validated standardized instruments and non-stigmatizing questions.

Standardized instruments
- Patient Health Questionnaire-2 (PHQ2)
- Patient Health Questionnaire-9 (PHQ9)
- Diagnostic Interview Schedule for Children-IV (DISC-IV)
- Columbia Depression Scale
- Mood and Feelings Questionnaire

Non-stigmatizing questions
- *Everyone I know gets sad sometimes, what kind of things make you sad?*
- *Sometimes adolescents dealing with similar issues or problems get very down and start to question life itself. Does this happen to you?*
- *Have you ever thought about suicide or harming yourself?*
- *Are you thinking about suicide now?*
- *Do you have a plan for suicide?* (If the patient answers affirmatively, ask for details of the plan and whether the patient has ever attempted suicide in the past)
- Evaluate in the context of precipitants, stressors, academic, social, and family function

Physical Examination

Examine skin for non-suicidal injury (cuts or scars on the breasts, abdomen, arms, or legs).

Management

If suicidal, immediate psychiatric intervention and hospitalization is necessary!

- Educate patient's family and involve them in care
- Communicate across all care providers
- Consult with mental health specialist for counseling or medical management
- Routine tracking of the patient progress with short interval, appropriate follow-ups as needed

Psychopharmacologic Medications

Medical treatment should be pursued with caution by knowledgeable and trained professionals.

- *Antianxiety Drugs*: SSRIs, sertraline*, fluoxetine*, duloxetine*, benzodiazepines, diazepam, lorazepam, and alprazolam
- *Antihistamines*: Hydroxyzine
- *Antidepressants*: SSRIs, fluoxetine*, sertraline*, citalopram*, escitalopram*, tricyclics*, bupropion*, and venlafaxine*
- *Mood stabilizers*: Lithium carbonate, carbamazepine, valproic acid, and lamotrigine
- *Antipsychotic drugs*: Risperidone, olanzapine, aripiprazole, quetiapine, asenapine, and haloperidol
- *Psychostimulants*: Methylphenidate, amphetamines, lisdexamfetamine, and atomoxetine
- *Adjuvants*: Clonidine and guanfacine

* Clinical trials show a twofold increase in suicidal ideation and attempts by adolescents and young adults; however, the benefits likely outweigh the risks for adolescent patients with depressive mood and anxiety disorders.

BIBLIOGRAPHY

Cheung AH, Zuckerbrot RA, Jensen PS, et al. Guidelines for adolescent depression in primary care (GLAD-PC): Part II. Treatment and ongoing management. Pediatrics. 2018; 141(3):e20174082.

Concerns regarding social media and health issues in adolescents and young adults. American College of Obstetricians and Gynecologists Committee Opinion No. 653. Obstet Gynecol. 2016; 127:e62–e65.

Mental health disorders in adolescents. American College of Obstetricians and Gynecologists Committee Opinion No. 705. Obstet Gynecol. 2017;130:e32–e41.

Zuckerbrot RA, Cheung A, Jensen PS, et al. Guidelines for adolescent depression in primary care (GLAD-PC): Part I. Practice preparation, identification, assessment, and initial management. Pediatrics. 2018; 141(3):e20174081.

14

Dysmenorrhea

M E Sophie Gibson and Tania Dumont

Definition

- Pain during menses; can have associated nausea, vomiting, and diarrhea
- **Primary:** Painful menstruation in the absence of specific pathologic conditions; more likely if presents later in the menstrual years with onset of ovulatory cycles
- **Secondary:** Painful menstruation in the presence of pathologic conditions of the pelvic organs, such as endometriosis, salpingitis, obstipation, adhesions, or obstructive congenital anomalies of the Müllerian system; more likely if presents early in the menstrual years particularly at the beginning

Key Points

- The most common cause of dysmenorrhea in adolescents is primary dysmenorrhea
- The most common cause of secondary dysmenorrhea is endometriosis
- Both primary and secondary dysmenorrhea are likely to respond to medical therapy; therefore, establishing a diagnosis is not required before initiating therapy
- A pelvic examination is not required prior to treating unless patient is not responding to conventional therapy or history suspicious for organic pathology
- NSAIDs are first line in treating primary dysmenorrhea
- Hormonal therapy should be considered if NSAIDs are not effective

Diagnosis

History

- Menstrual: Age at menarche; menstrual pattern
  - Relationship between menarche and onset of dysmenorrhea
  - Timing of pain in relation to menses and amount of menstrual flow
  - Description of menstrual pain and other associated symptoms (i.e., nausea, vomiting, diarrhea)
  - Presence/description of vaginal discharge
  - School performance and school absenteeism associated with menstrual problems
- Sexual: Sexual activity with inquiry of any sexual abuse history
  - Contraceptive and condom use
  - History of sexually transmitted diseases
- Previous treatments: Including dose, duration of use, side effects, and treatment response
- Family (particularly mother's) history: Menstrual problems and/or endometriosis

DOI: 10.1201/9781003039235-14

Physical Examination

- Check height, weight, and blood pressure
- Examine thyroid for goiter
- Examine breast for galactorrhea
- Examine abdomen to rule out any masses (obstructive Müllerian lesions) or tenderness
- Elicit any trigger points of rectus or iliopsoas muscles with musculoskeletal exam (see Chapter 38, "Pelvic Pain")
- Vaginal speculum and bimanual examination optional given age; can offer rectoabdominal instead of vaginal examination
- There is no evidence to indicate routine use of ultrasound in the initial evaluation of dysmenorrhea but may be useful in cases refractory to treatment

Rule Out Other Causes

- Pathologic lesions
  - Ultrasound to rule out obstructive Müllerian anomaly if concerned based on examination or presentation
- Infections
  - Testing for chlamydia and gonorrhea

Management

Conservative

- Encourage exercise modifications, increasing amount of weight bearing exercise one week before menses
- Eat well-balanced meals
- Perform stress reduction techniques

NSAIDs

- Blocks prostaglandin buildup that causes vigorous contraction of the uterus
- Preferred initial treatment in nonsexually active adolescents or as adjuvant in adolescent who also desires contraception
- Can cause gastric upset, take with small food portions
- Begin with loading regimen 48 hours before the dysmenorrhea (onset of menses) and continue at regular dose until menses becomes very light or ceases
- Suggested treatment
  - Ibuprofen 200–600 mg every 6 h or 800 mg every 8 h (maximum daily dose 2400 mg, dosage is weight based with 10 mg/kg)
  - Naproxen sodium 440–550 mg initially, followed by 220–550 mg every 12 h (depending on formulation); maximum daily dose 1000 mg
  - Mefenamic acid 500 mg initially, followed by 250 mg every 6 h
  - Celecoxib 400 mg initially, followed by 200 mg every 12 h
- Very individual response; if one type does not work, try another
- Use cautiously in renal and hepatic insufficiency, may be contraindicated with coexisting bleeding disorders

Topical Heat

- Synergistic effect when used with NSAIDs such as ibuprofen
- Various methods available, including electric heating pads, pads that can be warmed, or topical adhesives
- Caution against use of electric or adhesive varieties during sleep as may cause burns

Complementary Treatment Options

- High-frequency transcutaneous electrical nerve stimulation for patients unable/unwilling to use other conventional therapy
- Acupoint stimulation
- Ginger (750–2000 mg during first three days of menses)

When NSAIDs Cannot Be Used

- Consider acetaminophen alone, or in combination with caffeine or Pamabrom (mild, short-acting diuretic)
  - Regular strength acetaminophen 650 mg every 4–6 h; maximum daily dose 4000 mg
  - Extra strength acetaminophen 1000 mg every 6 h; maximum daily dose 4000 mg

When NSAIDs Fail Try Hormonal Treatment

- Be sure no contraindications to estrogen before initiating therapy.
  - Combination oral contraceptive pills (COCs)
    - Prefer monophasic
    - Continuous or extended cycle use offer superior treatment for dysmenorrhea compared to cyclic use
  - Intravaginal ethinyl estradiol/etonorgestrel ring
  - Transdermal ethinyl estradiol/norelgestromin patch
  - Systemic progestins
    - Depot medroxyprogesterone acetate (DMPA)
    - Norethindrone acetate and norethindrone
    - Drospirenone
    - Etonorgestrel implant
  - Local progestins – 52-mg levonorgestrel-containing intrauterine system (LNG-IUS)

When Hormones Fail after 3–6 Months of Treatment

- Laparoscopy to rule out endometriosis and/or structural abnormality and/or other cause
- Consider leuprolide acetate or dienogest if over the age of 18 years for empiric treatment of endometriosis (see Chapter 16, "Endometriosis")

BIBLIOGRAPHY

Burnett M et al. No. 345 Primary dysmenorrhea consensus guideline. J Obstet Gynaecol Can. 2017; 39(7):585–595.

Dysmenorrhea and endometriosis in the adolescent. ACOG Committee Opinion No. 760. American College of Obstetricians and Gynecologists. Obstet Gynecol. 2018; 132(6):e249–e258.

Harel Z. Dysmenorrhea in adolescents and young adults: an update on pharmacological treatments and management strategies. Expert Opin Pharmacother. 2012; 13:2157–2170.

15

Eating Disorders (EDs)

Ellen Rome

Key Points

- Weight is not the only marker for eating disorders (EDs) — Many with EDs can look healthy but be extremely ill
  - 66% of individuals with EDs are normal weight at onset of disorder
  - 33% of individuals with EDs are obese at onset of their ED
- Patients with EDs carry an increased risk for both suicide and medical complications
- Transgender youth may be at more risk: 16% vs 2% cisgender
- 80% of patients with anorexia nervosa (AN) recover but high hospital relapse rates occur in 35%–65% of patients with AN and 42% with bulimia nervosa
- Family-based treatment is the best evidence-based means to treat AN in children and adolescents; blame and shame have no role in FBT, and weaving parents into the solution helps both parents and child
- Cognitive behavioral therapy and family-based treatment are helpful in treatment of bulimia nervosa in adolescents
- Adolescent patients with EDs who are sexually active need contraception and cannot rely on menstrual cycle to predict ovulation. Long-acting reversible contraceptives (LARCs) remain the most reliable contraceptive method and should be considered. If oral contraceptive therapy is preferred, 30- to 35-ucg ethinyl estradiol containing pills are better than lower dose at protecting bone

DSM-5 Definitions

Anorexia nervosa

- Restriction of energy intake relative to energy needs leading to a significantly low body weight in the context of age, gender, growth trajectory, and physical health
- Intense fear of becoming fat or gaining weight or persistent behavior that interferes with weight gain, even though already being at a significantly low weight
- Disturbed body image or disturbed perception of one's shape, with undue influence of body weight or shape on self-evaluation or persistent lack of recognition of the seriousness of the current low weight

Two Subtypes

- **Restricting type**: Within the last 3 months, no recurrent episodes of bingeing or purging behaviors (vomiting, laxatives, diuretics, diet pills)
- **Binge-eating/purging type**: During the last 3 months, having recurrent episode of binge eating or purging behavior (self-induced vomiting, misuse of laxatives/diet pills/diuretics)

DOI: 10.1201/9781003039235-15

Atypical anorexia nervosa

- Has all the features of AN including fear of being fat and distorted body image but remains above a minimum weight for age; may or may not have lost weight already

Bulimia nervosa

- Recurrent episodes of binge eating, characterized by both:
  - Eating a substantially larger amount of food in a discrete period of time than would be eaten by most people
  - A sense of lack of control over eating during the binge
- Inappropriate compensatory behaviors to prevent weight gain (e.g. self-induced vomiting, laxative, diuretic or diet pill use, fasting, excessive exercise)
- Binges/behaviors occur at least once a week for at least 3 months
  - Self-evaluation is overly influenced by body shape or weight
- The disturbance does not occur exclusively during episodes of AN

Avoidant/Restrictive food intake disorder

- Eating or feeding disturbance characterized by significant weight loss or failure to achieve expected weight gain, significant nutritional deficiency, dependence on nutritional supplement or marked interference with psychosocial function due to persistent failure to meet appropriate caloric and/or nutritional needs
- Absence of weight or body concerns
- Includes excessively picky eaters, those avoiding abdominal pain associated with eating, fear of choking or vomiting, disrupted appetite cues, sensory processing difficulties, or other anxiety regarding consequences of eating

Binge-eating disorder

- Binge eating without compensatory behavior that occurs at least once a week for 3 months or more
- Associated with rapid eating even when not hungry, to point of extreme fullness, and/or to point of depression, shame, or guilt

Other Terms Not in DSM-5

- Orthorexia: Families may present using this lay-person's term, which in the 1990s through early 2000s meant excessive exercise with insufficient intake. Now the term has evolved to mean overly healthy eating.
- Relative energy deficiency in sport, or RED-S (replaced the term "Female athletic triad" in 2007): This term is used to describe athletes impacted by low energy availability, or the amount of energy remaining after exercise that is available for other physiologic functions of the day. Low energy availability leads to menstrual irregularities and hypogonadotropic hypogonadism with resultant decreased bone mineral density.

Diagnosis

History

Key questions on the history can include the SCOFF Questionnaires

1. Do you make yourself **S**ick because you feel uncomfortably full?
2. Do you worry you have lost **C**ontrol over how much you eat?
3. Have you recently lost more than **O**ne stone (14 lb/6.3 kg) in a 3-month time frame?

4. Do you believe that you are **F**at when others say you are too thin?

5. Would you say that **F**ood dominates your life?

Other useful, validated questionnaires include the 26 items modified Eating Attitudes Test (EAT) or the children's version (the chEAT).

Other Questions to Ask in the Office

Weight history:	What was your highest weight? How tall were you? How old were you?
	What was your lowest weight? How tall were you? How old were you?
Body image:	What do you think your weight should be? What feels too high? Too low?
	Do you do any body checking? (i.e., weighing, body pinching or checking, mirror check); What areas of your body do you worry about?
Diet history:	What did you eat yesterday? (ask amount and specifics for all meals, snacks, fluids in 24 hour period, e.g., including bites/bowls of cereal to assess quality/ quantity); Do you count calories? How much do you allow?
	Do you count grams of fat? How much do you allow?
	What foods do you avoid? Are there foods you used to eat and don't now?
	Do you ever feel guilty when you eat? How do you deal with that guilt?
	(i.e., exercising, purging, eating less)
Exercise history:	Do you exercise? What do you do? How often? How intense?
	How stressed are you if you miss a workout?
Binge eating/purging:	Do you ever binge? On what foods? How much? How often? Any triggers?
	Do you make yourself throw up? How often? How soon after eating?
	Do you use laxatives, diuretics, diet pills, caffeine? What types? How many? How often?
Menstrual history:	When was your last period? What weight were you then?
	When was the period before that?
	How old were you when you got your first period?
	Have your periods been regular?
	Do you take any hormones, birth control or medications?

The **HEADDSS** questions can also be useful (Home, Education, Activities, Drugs/Depression, Sex/ Safety) (see Chapter 21, "High-Risk Behaviors").

Of note, youth with AN may deny symptoms or seriousness of their behaviors, while youth with ARFID lack the distorted body image consistent with AN and may be actively trying to gain weight and/ or feel frustrated about inability to gain.

Review of Symptoms

General

- Marked weight loss or gain, especially when falling off expected or historical growth curve
- Weakness, fatigue

- Dizziness, syncope
- Chest pain, palpitations

GI Symptoms

- Early satiety, bloating, fullness, abdominal pain, reflux, constipation, diarrhea

Endocrinologic

- Cold intolerance
- Hair loss, easy bleeding/bruising, dry skin

Psychologic

- Changes in relationships or school/work performance
- "Hangry," irritability
- Flat affect, withdrawal; or, alternatively, constant movement

Physical Examination

NOTE: **Exam may be entirely normal!**

Findings Associated with Inadequate Energy Intake or Malnutrition

Vital signs:	Low resting heart rate or blood pressure
	Orthostatic increase in heart rate (>20 beats per minute) OR decrease in blood pressure (>10 mm Hg)
	Hypothermia
Weight/growth:	Height, weight (in gown post voiding), BMI (have patient face provider and away from scale during weight measurement)
	Deviation from previous growth curve
Psychiatric:	Flat or anxious affect
Ophthalmologic:	Rule out evidence for intracerebral process (ascertain normal neuro examination, optic discs flat, vessels intact)
Skin:	Pallor, dry sallow skin, carotenemia (particularly palms and soles)
	Cachexia, facial wasting, decreased muscle mass, thin hair, lanugo
Cardiac:	Murmur (30% will have mitral valve prolapse)
	Cool extremities Acrocyanosis
Abdominal exam:	Stool mass left lower quadrant
	Scaphoid abdomen

| *Breasts:* | Atrophic breasts |
| *Genitalia:* | Vaginal atrophy, dryness |

Findings Related to Purging

Vital signs:	Orthostatic increase in HR or decrease in BP
Skin:	Angular stomatitis, palatal scratches, dental enamel erosions
	Russell's sign (abrasion/callous on knuckle from self-induced emesis)
	Bruising or abrasions over spine (related to excess exercise or sit-ups)
Face:	Salivary gland enlargement (parotid and submandibular)
Abdomen:	Epigastric tenderness

Findings Related to Excess Energy Intake

Vital signs:	Deviation from previous growth curve trajectory
	Obesity
	Elevated blood pressure
Skin:	Acanthosis nigricans
Abdomen:	Hepatomegaly

Red Flags for Eating Disorders

- Precipitous weight change (significant weight loss or gain), especially when crosses growth chart percentiles
- Sudden change in eating habits (new vegan, vegetarian, paleo, or other meal plan labeled "healthy" by the young person, a change to gluten free, lactose free, or eliminating certain foods or food groups)
- An abrupt change in exercise patterns, including excessive exercise or extreme physical training
- Body image disturbance, a lot of "fat talk"
- Abdominal complaints, including bloating, gas, pain, early satiety
- Electrolyte abnormalities without an identified medical cause (especially hypokalemia and/or contraction alkalosis, and/or hypoglycemia)
- Bradycardia, especially when low voltage on ECG
- Irregular or absent menses
- Inappropriate use of caffeine, artificial sweeteners, sugar-free gum, prescription medications that affect weight (including insulin in patients with diabetes, thyroid medication, stimulants, and street drugs)

Laboratory Evaluation

- **Complete blood count (CBC)**: Rule out anemia; hemoglobin could be high if dehydrated; leukopenia, thrombocytopenia (happens last usually)
- **Erythrocyte sedimentation rate (ESR)**: Rule out chronic illness; will be 0–3 in the face of starvation
- **Complete metabolic panel**: Hypokalemia may indicate vomiting; elevated bicarbonate indicative of contraction alkalosis, elevated liver function tests; elevated BUN and creatinine with extreme muscle breakdown
- **Calcium, magnesium, phosphorus**
- **Human chorionic gonadotropin (HCG)** if oligomenorrheic or amenorrheic
- **Urinalysis**: Assess specific gravity; if low, consider water loading to falsely elevate weight
- **IF amenorrheic: Follicle-stimulating hormone (FSH), luteinizing hormone (LH), thyroid-stimulating hormone (TSH), prolactin, estradiol**: Rule out central causes of oligomenorrhea or amenorrhea or ovarian failure as well as polycystic ovarian syndrome
- **If acne, hirsute**: Total, free testosterone, DHEAS
- **Cholesterol** NOT usually ordered due to likelihood of being falsely elevated due to low triiodothyronineova (T3) levels that inhibit cholesterol breakdown; cholesterol-binding globulin may also be low and intrahepatic cholesterol may leak into peripheral circulation
- **TSH** as screen sufficient, as thyroid function tests likely to reveal euthyroid sick syndrome with decreased peripheral conversion of thyroxine (T4) to T3 and high or high normal reverse T3—an adaptation to starvation to reduce metabolic rate
- **Vitamin deficiencies** may be indicated on basis of nutritional history of patient (**e.g. vitamin B12, vitamin D, iron, ferritin, zinc, thiamine**)
- **Celiac screen** (total immunoglobulin A and tissue transglutaminase)
- **Bone density evaluation** if primary amenorrhea or secondary amenorrhea greater than 6 months

EKG

- Look for sinus bradycardia (HR < 50)
- Sinus tachycardia
- Low-voltage P waves and QRS complexes
- Rightward QRS axis
- Nonspecific T-wave abnormalities
- U waves
- ST segment depression
- Conduction abnormalities
- QTc interval prolongation (>450 for <18 yo, >460 for >18 yo)

NOTE: LABORATORY EVALUATION AND EKG MAY BE ENTIRELY NORMAL!

Treatment

Hospitalization

Hospitalize if

- Severe malnutrition (weight < 75% ideal body weight [IBW])
- Dehydration

- Electrolyte disturbances (hypokalemia, hypophosphatemia, hypomagnesemia most commonly)
- EKG abnormalities
- Sinus bradycardia (HR < 50 bpm)
- Prolonged corrected Q-T interval (>450 if under 18 years, >460 for over 18 years)
- Arrhythmias
- Physiologic instability
- Bradycardia (HR < 50 awake, <40 asleep)
- Hypotension
- Hypothermia
- Orthostatic changes
- Syncope
- Arrested growth and development
- Intractable vomiting, bingeing, or purging
- Acute food refusal
- Acute medical complication of malnutrition
- Seizures
- Cardiac failure, renal failure, other organ failure
- Failure of outpatient management (weight gain 0.5–2 lbs/week)
- Acute psychiatric emergency
- Suicidal ideation
- Acute psychosis
- Comorbid diagnosis interfering with treatment
- Severe depression
- Obsessive-compulsive disorder (OCD)
- Severe family dysfunction

Refeeding Syndrome

Refeeding syndrome is a life-threatening situation of congestive heart failure, liver congestion with elevated liver enzymes, and peripheral edema as a result of total body phosphorus depletion during catabolic starvation followed by increased cellular influx of phosphorus during anabolic refeeding. An initial high glucose load when rapidly increasing caloric intake stimulates insulin secretion, which then increases cellular uptake of phosphorus, potassium, magnesium, and glucose. Within 12–72 hours, the body increases the production of adenosine triphosphate (ATP) from adenosine diphosphate (ADP) and runs out of phosphate, leading to organ failure at the cellular level.

Risk Factors for Refeeding Syndrome

- Degree of malnutrition chronically and/or precipitous weight loss
- Acute malnutrition with little/no energy intake for >10 days
- Prior history of refeeding syndrome
- History of significant alcohol intake
- History of diuretic, laxative, or insulin misuse
- History of electrolyte abnormalities
- History of bariatric surgery with significant weight loss and increased risk of electrolyte losses from malabsorption

Prevention of Refeeding Syndrome

- Correct electrolyte and fluid imbalances WHILE refeeding, not before (can use oral/nasogastric methods
- If no initial electrolyte deficits, carefully monitor while inpatient as electrolyte abnormalities may occur with refeeding
- Monitor vital signs and cardiac/mental status during refeeding
- Underfeeding can lead to further weight loss and has been associated with death in seriously malnourished patients. Start at 2000–2500, follow cmp, mg, phos and increase caloric intake daily to ensure 0.2–1 kg a day gain inpatient, 0.2 kg a week outpatient

Hospitalization

- Can be medical or psychiatric hospital floor, with acute medical stabilization warranted for electrolyte imbalances, prolonged QTc, bradycardia <50 awake and <40 asleep, or high risk of refeeding syndrome.
- For improved outcome need to gain 0.4 lb/day (0.2 kg/day) while inpatient.
- Prevent refeeding syndrome by replenishing phosphorus stores and following cmp, mg, phos regularly and correcting electrolyte imbalances as they occur. Caloric intake can be safely started at 2000–2500 with monitoring of electrolytes and phosphorus, unless there is current evidence of refeeding syndrome, in which case start at lower caloric levels with phosphorus supplementation. Phosphorus can be supplemented using a supplement such as Nutraphos (250 mg phosphorus, 164 mg sodium phosphate, 278 mg potassium phosphate, Willen) with one 250 mg packet mixed in 8 ounces of juice and given orally twice a day for 5 days.
- Thiamine may also need to be repleted in severely malnourished adult patients, and acute change of mental status can be an indication of Wernicke's encephalopathy.
- Monitor fluid intake to prevent fluid overload.
- Nutrition may be given orally from the outset. Closely monitor vital signs, cardiac stability, and mental status. Underfeeding can lead to ongoing weight loss, slower response to treatment, and worse prognosis.

Outpatient Management: "Food is the Medicine That Is Required for Recovery"

Once medically stable, outpatient therapy can occur with multidisciplinary team.

Medical Provider

Validates families' and clinicians' concerns:

- Parents or caregivers are the frontline help-seekers for youth with EDs. Trust their concerns. Even a single consultation about a child's eating behavior, loss of periods, or weight concerns is a strong predictor of the presence or potential development of an ED.
- Helps family understand that they did not cause the illness, nor did their child/family member choose to have it. This awareness facilitates acceptance of the diagnosis, treatment, referral, interventions, while minimizing stigma associated with the diseases.
- Coordinates care team
- Oversees treatment plan

Manages medical issues, interpreting results in context of physiological adaptation to malnutrition and purging

- Weekly to biweekly weigh in (gowned after voiding, backwards on scale for those with undue stress with knowing numbers or without means of processing/managing disordered eating thoughts/behaviors)

- Vital signs lying and standing to assess for orthostatic hypotension by pulse or blood pressure and bradycardia (NOT usually indicative of an athlete's heart in context of starvation)
- Electrolyte/phosphorus abnormalities
- Hydration status and ongoing nutritional monitoring
- Reviews objective physical findings with the patient, gives clear information about growth, menses, osteopenia
- Acknowledge patient's distress: Body image dissatisfaction vs nutritional needs
- Establish alliance with patient to partner in order to work toward health
- Discuss rationale for hospitalization
- Review long-term goals
- Prevent osteopenia; monitor bone density annually if initial amenorrhea
  - Do not use oral contraceptives solely to treat low body weight patient with osteopenia; weight gain alone is the main factor to promote bone gain.
  - Consider the use of physiologic estrogen/progesterone replacement (i.e., transdermal 17β estradiol) in patients with very low bone density (<2 SD below mean)
- Resume/continue menses, contracept as necessary
- Manage medications in patients without suicidal ideation (psychiatrist for latter)
  - Selective Serotonin Reuptake Inhibitors (SSRIs) have a role in anxiety, OCD, with no evidence for weight gain in patients with EDs
  - Antianxiety medications: Short-acting lorazepam (0.5–2 mg usually) may be used before meals or qhs for high anxiety moments
  - Atypical antipsychotics: Olanzapine has some evidence for efficacy to help with patients so anxious that they cannot manage meals
- Pursue life, happiness, and wellness
- Disconnect from electronic media at least 1 hour before bed for restorative sleep
- **Registered dietitian** with experience with EDs
  - Provides nutritional education
  - Six cups fluids a day minimum
  - Five a day fruits and vegetables
  - Four servings of calcium a day
  - Three meals with 3 food groups a day (protein/fat/carb)
  - At least 2 snacks with 2 food groups a day (protein/fat/carb)
  - Zero missed meals or snacks
  - Daily fat intake: 50- to 90-g fat a day for <26-year olds
  - Calcium: 1000 mg daily for patients age 4–8 years, 1200–1500 mg/day for patients age 9–18
  - Vitamin D 600 IU daily
- Help plan appropriate weight goals: 0.5–2 lb/week for patients in need of gain; eating stabilization for patients with binge ED, atypical AN, bulimia nervosa
- Can discuss use of supplements (Nestlé HealthCare Nutrition, 1007 US Highway 202/206, Building JR2, Bridgewater, NJ 08807 for boost and Benecalorie)
  - Boost, Ensure, 250 cal
  - Boost Breeze, 250 cal, fruit flavored, 9-g protein, fat free
  - Boost High Protein, 240 cal, 20-g protein
  - Boost Plus, Ensure Plus, 340 cal
  - Boost VHC (very high calorie) 530 cal
  - Benecalorie, 330 cal, 7-g protein, 33-g fat, lactose free, cholesterol free, kosher (not safe in galactosemis)

Psychologist/Therapist

- Family-based therapist/Maudsley coach for under 18 years old
- Individual therapist for managing comorbid psychiatric illness, to handle anxiety, self-esteem challenges

Psychiatrist

- If suicidal and/or if pharmacotherapy indicated

Long-term Outcomes

- Prognosis for anorexia nervosa variable: 50% of <18 year olds with full recovery using family-based refeeding — Good outcome with return of menses and weight gain
- 25% intermediate outcome: Some weight gain and some relapse
- 25% poor outcome: Associated with later age onset of disorder, longer duration of illness, and lower minimal weight
- Mortality: 0.56% year (increases in mortality rate as duration of illness increases)
  - Patients with AN have a 6- to 10-fold increase in mortality vs unaffected, and 2–3 times higher than all other mental disorders
  - Causes of death include medical complications from disordered eating and suicide

Fertility is preserved in individuals who recover from an ED. Those who persist in restrictive EDs who do conceive may gain less weight have smaller babies with lower 5-minute Apgar scores, experience more complications during pregnancy, have more challenges with breastfeeding, and more difficulties with postpartum adjustment and body image than those without EDs.

Take-Home Messages

- Early intervention and long-term follow-up are essential; if suspect an ED, see the patient back in 2–4 weeks, not longer, to assess weight/growth/menses
- The younger the patient, the greater the need for family therapy/FBT or other interventions
- Have strategies for problematic behaviors (Table 15.1)

Long-term outcomes depend not just on weight restoration and resumption of menses; distorted body image as well as abnormal eating attitudes and behaviors need to be addressed in order to get to full recovery and to decrease risk of relapse.

TABLE 15.1

Problems and Strategies

	Signs/Symptoms	Best Response
Brain starved	Circular thinking, poor memory, indecisive	Provide clear, simple, repetitive explanations
Depressed, anxious	As expected	Set clear expectations Be positive Make comfortable when possible Medications, build team (psychology, psychiatry, dietitian)
Manipulative	Uses one team member against another	Communicate well as a team; If you don't know, ask a colleague

NATIONAL ORGANIZATIONS FOR EATING DISORDERS

1. Academy for Eating Disorders (AED)

   11130 Sunrise Valley Drive, Suite 350

   Reston, VA 20191, USA

   info@aedweb.org

   https://www.aedweb.org/resources/experts-by-experience

2. National Eating Disorders Awareness (NEDA)

   NATIONAL EATING DISORDERS HELPLINE

   Toll-Free Phone Number: 1-800-931-2237

   Hours: 9:00 AM–9:00 PM (ET) Mon–Thurs; and 9:00 AM to 5:00 PM (ET) Fri

   For 24/7 crisis support, text "NEDA" to 741741

   NEDA ADMINISTRATIVE OFFICE

   Business Phone Number: (212) 575-6200

   Fax: (212) 575-1650

   Email: info@NationalEatingDisorders.org

   National Eating Disorders Association

   1500 Broadway, Suite 1101

   New York, NY 10036, USA

3. F.E.A.S.T.: Families Empowered and Supporting Treatment of Eating Disorders

   FEAST is a global support and education community of and for parents of those with eating disorders like anorexia, bulimia, binge eating, and more.

   US: +1 855-50-FEAST

   Canada: +1 647-247-1339

   Australia: +61 731886675

   UK: +44 3308280031

   New Zealand: +64 98875172

   Israel: +972 23748988

   info@feast-ed.org

   www.feast-ed.org

   F. E.A.S.T.

   P.O. Box 1281

   Warrenton VA 20188, USA

4. Gurze Books and Videos on Eating Disorders

   https://www.gurzebooks.com/

BIBLIOGRAPHY

AED Report 2016, 4th Edition. Eating Disorders: A Guide to Medical Care (www.aed.org).

Garber AK, Sawyer SM, Golden NH, Guarda AS, Katzman DK, Kohn MR, Le Grange D, Madden S, Whitelaw M, Redgrave GW. A systematic review of approaches to refeeding in patients with anorexia nervosa. Int J Eat Disord. 2016; 49(3):293–310.

Hornberger LL, Lane MA. Committee on Adolescence. Identification and management of eating disorders in children and adolescents. Pedatrics. 2021; 147(1):E2020040279.

Mond JM, Myers TC, Crosby RD, Hay PJ, Rodgers B, Morgan JF, Lacey JH, Mitchell JE. Screening for eating disorders in primary care: EDE-Q versus SCOFF. Behav Res Ther. 2008; 46:612–622.

Rome ES, Strandjord SE. Eating disorders. Pediatr Rev. 2016 Aug; 37(8):323–336.

Sachs K, Andersen D, Sommer J, Winkelman A, Mehler PS. Avoiding medical complications during the refeeding of patients with anorexia nervosa. Eat Disord. 2015; 23(5):411–421.

Sieke EH, Rome ES. Eating disorders in children and adolescents: what does the gynecologist need to know? Curr Opin Obstet Gynecol. 2016 Oct; 29(5):381–392.

The Society for Adolescent Health and Medicine. Position paper of the Society for Adolescent Health and Medicine: medical management of restrictive eating disorders in adolescents and young adults. J Adolesc Health. 2015; 56(1):121–125.

Statuta S, Asif I, Drezner J. Relative energy deficiency in sport (RED-S). Br J Sports Med. 2017; 51(21):1570–1571.

16

Endometriosis

Jessica Shim and Marc Laufer

Definition

Presence of endometrial glands and stroma outside the normal anatomic location of the lining of the uterus; located primarily in the pelvis in the adolescent (e.g. cul-de-sac, ovarian fossa).

Key Points

- Symptoms of endometriosis commonly start in adolescence
- Adolescents with endometriosis typically have both acyclic and cyclic pelvic pain (dysmenorrhea)
- Endometriomas and infertility are rare presentations in adolescents
- Definitive diagnosis can only be established with laparoscopy with or without histologic confirmation of biopsy specimen

Prevalence

- Not clearly defined in available literature and may be underestimated
- May be present in 50%–70% of adolescents with chronic pelvic pain that is unresponsive to nonsteroidal anti-inflammatory drugs (NSAIDs) or combined oral contraceptive pills (COC)
- Most common after years of menstruation, but symptomatic cases have also been reported prior to menarche or as early as 1 month after menarche

Presentation

- Pelvic pain, dysmenorrhea in combination with acyclic pain
- Pain tends to increase in severity over time and may occur throughout the month
- No correlation between extent of disease and severity of pain
- More than half of patients experience gastrointestinal or bladder symptoms
- Increased risk of migraines and autoimmune comorbidities
- Pain in patients with obstructive Müllerian anomalies (e.g. imperforate hymen, transverse vaginal septum, vaginal agenesis)

Evaluation

History

(See also "Dysmenorrhea" [Chapter 14] and "Pelvic Pain" [Chapter 38].)

DOI: 10.1201/9781003039235-16

Description of Pain

- Location, frequency, and character of pain
- Relation to or association with bowel/bladder function symptoms
  - Up to 50% endometriosis will have at least 1 genitourinary or gastrointestinal symptom (i.e. dysuria, urgency, diarrhea, constipation)
- Relation to menses (cyclic vs. acyclic pain)
- Does the patient miss school/how much?
- Does the patient miss activities of daily living?
- Is pain worse with movement/better with rest?

Family History

- Up to 7-fold increased risk of endometriosis with first degree affected relative

Physical Examination

- (see Chapter 38, "Pelvic Pain")
- Goal is to exclude alternative explanations for the patient's pain such as gastrointestinal, urinary, musculoskeletal, pelvic mass, or reproductive tract anomaly
- Abdominal exam findings vary and can have a nonspecific pattern of tenderness
- Pelvic exam is not always necessary
- Consider Q-tip into the vagina to assess vaginal patency if there is concern for an obstructive anomaly
- Rectal-abdominal exam may also be performed

Laboratory

- No specific blood tests or serum markers identify endometriosis
- Urinalysis to rule out urinary cause of pain
- Sexually transmitted disease and pregnancy testing in the sexually active patient

Imaging

- Not routine but can exclude presence of cyst, pelvic mass, torsion, or an anomaly
- Pelvic ultrasound can be performed trans-abdominally
- MRI if concerned for anomaly

Diagnosis

- Evaluate and consider a trial of NSAIDs, estrogen/progestin therapy, or progestin-only therapy
- Empiric use of gonadotropin-releasing hormone (GnRH) agonist therapy is not recommended due to potential detrimental effects on bone density
- Consider surgery for evaluation and treatment of endometriosis if pain is still present
- Consider surgery even as soon as 3 months into trial if pain interferes with quality of life

Make a definitive diagnosis with laparoscopy

- Red and clear vesicular lesions more common in adolescents than "powder-burn" lesions

- Close tip technique: Move laparoscope close to peritoneum and magnify
- May help to visualize clear lesions by submerging laparoscope in pelvis filled with irrigation fluid (e.g. Normal Saline, Lactated Ringer's)

The American Society for Reproductive Medicine is the accepted staging system standard to assist in comparing response to treatment

- *Stage I*: Minimal disease, 1–5 points
- *Stage II*: Mild disease, 6–15 points
- *Stage III*: Moderate, 16–40 points
- *Stage IV*: Severe, >40 points

Most adolescents have stage I or stage II disease.

Treatment Options

- Endometriosis should be treated with combined surgery and medication (see Figure 16.1)
- Surgery decreases disease burden; medicine can help prevent disease progression
- There is no cure for endometriosis; therefore, staying on medicine is crucial, until desire for fertility

Surgical Therapy

- Remove/destroy all identifiable lesions and restore anatomy
- Techniques include electrocautery, endocoagulation, laser ablation, and excision
- Avoid radical excisional surgery due to risk of adhesion formation
- Consider placement of progesterone-containing intrauterine device at time of surgery for postoperative medical therapy for endometriosis (limited evidence, see below)

Medical Therapy

Treatment should be tailored to the patient with any of the following below.

Combination Estrogen/Progestin Therapy

- Act to suppress the gonadotropic stimulation to the ovary and create a progestin-dominant environment creating an atrophic endometrium
- No data suggests one pill formulation is superior but monophasic regimens preferred
- Cyclic, extended, or continuous regimens are all safe and effective but continuous method may achieve best outcomes through menstrual suppression.
- Continuous method may result in breakthrough bleeding, which may require a hormone-free interval of 3–4 days
- Alternatives for combined oral contraceptive pills (OCPs) include contraceptive patch or vaginal ring

Progestin-Only Therapy

- Commonly used regimens:
  - Norethindrone 0.35 mg by mouth daily

- Norethindrone acetate 5–15 mg by mouth daily
  - Norethindrone acetate dosage can be titrated up to 15 mg but there is small (about 20%) peripheral conversion of norethindrone acetate to ethinyl estradiol, so caution in those with contraindication to estrogen use
- Depot medroxyprogesterone acetate (DMPA) 150 mg intramuscularly or 104 mg subcutaneously every 3 months
  - Used mainly in those who do not respond to combined OCPs or have contraindication to estrogen use
  - Side effects are weight gain, bloating, acne, and irregular bleeding
  - Long-term DMPA use may result in reversible loss of bone density in some patients
- Alternative progestin-only therapies (both with limited evidence in treatment of endometriosis)
  - Etonogestrel implant
  - Levonorgestrel intrauterine device
  - Both may need to be used with an additional hormonal therapy to provide adequate suppression of pain, bleeding, and endometrial implants

GnRH Agonist Therapy

- Induces a reversible hypoestrogenic state that removes the source of stimulation to the endometrial implants
- Available as nasal spray, subcutaneous, or intramuscular injection
- Recommended duration of 12 months by the FDA
- Limit to above the age of 16 years due to potential long-term adverse effects on bone
- Commonly used dosages:
  - Depot leuprolide 3.75 mg IM every 4 weeks or 11.25 mg every 12 weeks
  - Intranasal nafarelin acetate 200 mcg twice daily
- *Side effects*
  - "Flare effect" occurs 21–28 days post-injection due to down-regulation of gonadotrophins, resulting in pain and/or bleeding
  - Osteopenia, hypoestrogenic symptoms like hot flashes, vaginal dryness
- *Add-back therapy:* Use of estrogen and/or progestin to minimize GnRH agonist side effects and osteoporosis
  - Norethindrone acetate 5 mg daily
  - Conjugated equine estrogen 0.625 mg and norethindrone acetate 5 mg daily
  - Add-back should be started once GnRH agonist therapy is started
  - Combination add-back is superior for increasing bone density and quality of life
  - OCPs are not appropriate add-back as it negates GnRH agonist therapy
  - Obtain dual energy X-ray absorptiometry (DXA) scan after at least 12 months use, repeat testing if patient remains on therapy at least every 2 years
- Is not an approved contraceptive

GnRH Antagonist Therapy

- Alternative to GnRH agonist therapy and works immediately without a "flare effect"
- Available in oral or intramuscular forms
  - Elagolix 150 mg daily or 200 mg twice daily
  - Is not approved for use in women under age 18

- May not achieve amenorrhea successfully
- Is not an approved contraceptive

Androgen Therapy

- Inhibits follicular development and induces endometrial atrophy
- Includes Danazol, 400–800 mg daily
- Side effects include acne, hirsutism, weight gain, and possibly deepening of voice, which is irreversible
- May be more desirable for transmasculine adolescents

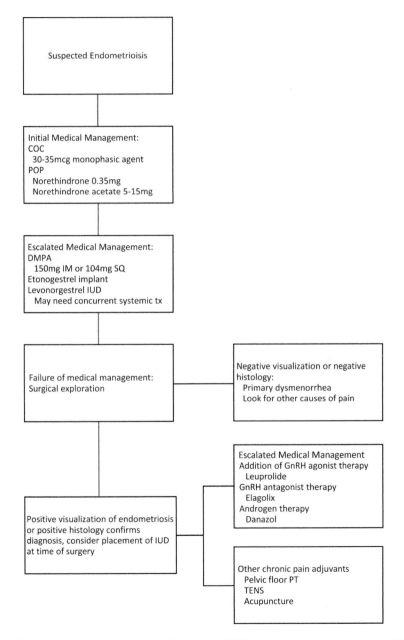

FIGURE 16.1   Treatment options for suspected endometriosis. (COC – continuous oral contraceptives, POP – progesterone only pills, IM – intramuscular, SQ – subcutaneous, IUD – intrauterine device, PT – physical therapy, TENS – Transcutaneous electric nerve stimulation.)

Chronic Pain Therapy

- May need multidisciplinary approach for adolescents with endometriosis and chronic pelvic pain with referral to a pain center or clinic
- Antidepressants may have neuromodulatory/analgesic properties
- Cognitive-behavioral therapy may teach progressive muscle relaxation with pain
- Complementary/alternative therapies
  - Pelvic floor physical therapy
  - Transcutaneous electric nerve stimulation (TENS)
  - Acupuncture

Patient education website: www.youngwomenshealth.org.

BIBLIOGRAPHY

DiVasta AD, Feldman HA, Sadler Gallagher J, et al. Hormonal add-back therapy for females treated with gonadotropin-releasing hormonal agonist for endometriosis: a randomized controlled trial. Obstet Gynecol. 2015; 126(3):617–627.

Laufer MR, Sanfilippo JS, Rose G. Adolescent endometriosis: diagnosis and treatment approaches. J Pediatr Adolesc Gynecol. 2003; 16:S3–S11.

Shim JY, Laufer MR. Adolescent endometriosis: an update. J Pediatr Adolesc Gynecol. 2020; 33:112–119.

17

Female Genital Mutilation (FGM)

Christine Osborne and Sarah K. McQuillan

Definition

The World Health Organization defines female genital mutilation (FGM) as "all procedures involving partial or total removal of the external female genitalia or injury to the female genital organs for non-medical reasons."

In the United States, Federal Law 18 U.S. Code § 116-Female Genital Mutilation, FGM means "any procedure performed for non-medical reasons that involves partial or total removal of, or other injury to, the external female genitalia, and includes:

- A clitoridectomy or the partial or total removal of the clitoris of the prepuce or clitoral hood
- Excision or the partial or total removal (with or without excision of the clitoris) of the labia minora or the labia majora, or both
- Infibulation or the narrowing of the vaginal opening (with or without excision of the clitoris)
- Other procedures that are harmful to the external female genitalia, including pricking, incising, scraping, or cauterizing the genital area"

Key Points

- FMG is internationally recognized as a violation of human rights but is still being reported in 30 countries in Africa and in a few countries in Asia and the Middle East.
- FGM is practiced for a variety of sociocultural reasons with some who believe that FGM is a religious requirement, although it is not mentioned in any major religious text.
- Traditionally performed on children and young adolescents between the ages of 5 and 12, but possibly as young as infants and as old as adults.
- Due to widespread and continued immigration of children, girls, and women into western societies from those countries that continue to practice FGM, providers may see patients who have undergone these procedures.

Important Cultural Background

- In approaching these patients who have had FGM, recognize that the practice of FGM is
  - Deeply entrenched in social, economic, and political structure of the culture in the affected patient
  - Often was supported by the family of the patient without question
  - Anyone who departs from this practice may face condemnation, harassment, and or ostracism

DOI: 10.1201/9781003039235-17

- It is a social convention guided by reward if completed, and punishment if not
    - Extended family often involved in practice (perhaps the accompanying adult with patient)
    - Women family members may have performed the FGM to raise a young woman properly and participate in coming-of-age ritual in their culture
- Therefore, it is difficult for families to abandon this paradigm
- The girl may have felt pressured and/or rewarded to participate and approach the patient with these concepts in mind

Types

- See Abdulcadir et al. (2016) for schematic illustrations and video
- Type I: Partial or total removal of the clitoris and/or the prepuce (clitoridectomy) (Figure 17.1a)
    - Type Ia: Removal of the clitoral hood or prepuce only
    - Type Ib: Removal of the clitoris with the prepuce
- Type II: Partial or total removal of the clitoris and the labia minora, with or without excision of the labia majora (excision) (Figure 17.1b)
    - Type IIa: Removal of the labia minora only
    - Type IIb: Partial or total removal of the clitoris and the labia minora
    - Type IIc: Partial or total removal of the clitoris, the labia minora, and the labia majora
- Type III: Narrowing of the vaginal orifice with creation of a covering seal by cutting and apposing the labia minora and/or the labia majora, with or without excision of the clitoris (infibulation) (Figure 17.1c)
    - Type IIIa: Removal and apposition of the labia minora
    - Type IIIb: Removal and apposition of the labia majora
- Type IV: Unclassified (Figure 17.1d)
- All other harmful procedures to the female genitalia for nonmedical purposes, for example, pricking, piercing, incising (labioplasty), scraping, and cauterization

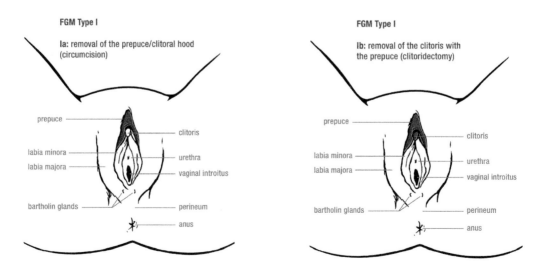

FIGURE 17.1 FGM types: (a) Type I; (From World Health Organization, WHO guidelines on the management of health complications from female genital mutilation. Geneva, Switzerland: World Health Organization; 2016, with permission.)

(Continued)

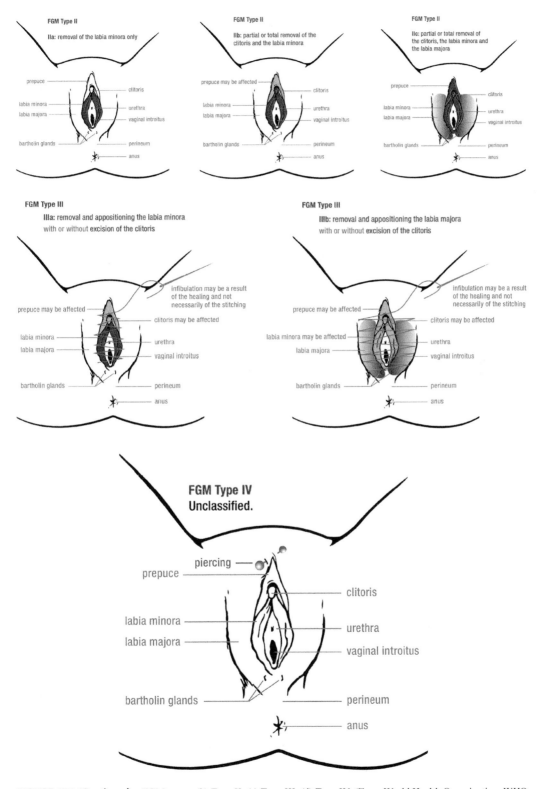

FIGURE 17.1 (*Continued*) FGM types: (b) Type II; (c) Type III; (d) Type IV. (From World Health Organization, WHO guidelines on the management of health complications from female genital mutilation. Geneva, Switzerland: World Health Organization; 2016, with permission.)

Health Complications

FGM Has No Known Health Benefits

- Immediate risks: Hemorrhage, severe pain, genital tissue swelling, infection, wound healing problems, lower urinary tract injuries, shock and death
- Obstetric risks: Requirement for cesarean section, postpartum hemorrhage, episiotomy, prolonged labor, obstetric tears/lacerations, instrumental delivery, difficult labor/dystocia, extended maternal hospital stay, stillbirth and early neonatal death, infant resuscitation at delivery
- Sexual functioning risks: Dyspareunia, decreased sexual satisfaction, reduced sexual desire and arousal, decreased lubrication during sexual intercourse, reduced frequency of orgasm or anorgasmia
- Psychological risks: Post-traumatic stress disorder (PTSD), anxiety, depression
- Long-term risks: Genital tissue damage, vaginal discharge, vaginal itching, menstrual problems, reproductive tract infections, chronic genital infections, urinary tract infections, painful urination
- Violence: FGM is also associated with an increased risk for intimate partner violence (IPV) in the future. Women with previous exposure to violence, particularly physical and sexual trauma during childhood, are more likely to experience violence later in life, leading to a myriad of health complications

Care of the Patient

Communication

Effective sensitive communication with the patient is paramount

- If a translator is needed, have a female interpreter involved
- In some cultures, patients may be accompanied by their father or other family members that are expecting to be involved in the decision-making process
- Health-care providers should explore and assess the decision-making process of the woman and her family and be sure to solicit the patient's views and wishes

Questions

Use of questions may guide you to what care, if any is needed

For example (see further Perron et al., 2020)

- "Do you have any problems passing your urine? Does it take you a long time to urinate?"
- "Do you have any pain with menstruation?"
- "Do you have any itching or burning or discharge from your pelvic area?"
- "(If sexually active) Do you have any pain or difficulty when having relations?"

If changes on genital examination are consistent with FGM be sensitive in how you ask about this.

Consider saying

- "Many women from your country have been circumcised or "closed" as children. If you do not mind telling me, were you circumcised or closed as a child?"
- Or ask similar question to the accompanying parent if that were the case for the patient

Education

Many patients have limited knowledge of female anatomy, use of drawings may be helpful to explain findings.

In many cultures where FGM is practiced, sex, sexuality, and issues related to FGM are considered private matters and not openly discussed.

- Be sensitive to this issue
- Limit providers and staff in the examination room and consider use of female attendants

Interventions

Laws and Reporting

- Performing or assisting in female genital cutting is a criminal offense in Canada.
- In the United States, it is illegal under federal law to perform FGM on anyone under age 18 or to knowingly transport a girl out of the United States to perform FGM under 18 U.S. Code § 116-Female Genital Mutilation.
- The American College of Obstetricians and Gynecologists (ACOG) recommends that a Western provider who encounters a child who has recently been circumcised report to Child Protective Services as per their regional reporting standards.

Culturally Appropriate Care

Every effort should be made to provide culturally appropriate and sensitive care to women with FGM, paying special attention to concerns related to language use and confidentiality.

- Health-care providers must be careful not to stigmatize women who have undergone FGM. As adolescence is a time when feeling normal is of paramount importance, reassuring the young woman is key.
- Health-care providers should use their knowledge and influence to educate and counsel families against having FGM performed on other family members.
- All requests for reinfibulation should be declined.

Deinfibulation

Women experiencing distressing symptoms (including dysmenorrhea, dyspareunia, recurrent urinary tract infections, and voiding dysfunction) or those considering intercourse or pregnancy can be offered deinfibulation.

- Use sedation or general anesthesia
- Incise scar tissue in the midline from the neo-introitus to the level of the urethral orifice using scissors, coagulation/cutting, or laser
- Labial edges may need interrupted sutures (with 4-0 or 5-0 vicryl) to ensure hemostasis.
- Postoperatively, estrogen cream can be applied, as well as topical analgesic gels for pain relief, and frequent sitz baths.

Vaginal dilation postoperatively can also help prevent restenosis of the introitus. In some situations, it can be used alone and instead of surgery.

Clitoral Reconstruction Surgery

Clitorolabial reconstruction using a vaginal graft has been shown to be feasible and associated with improved sexual function in some studies.

Since this is a new technique, the approaches warrant further study and training programs are being developed. This will likely be more widespread in practice in the future.

BIBLIOGRAPHY

Abdulcadir J, Catania L, Hindin MJ, Say L, Petignat P, Abdulcadir O. Female genital mutilation: a visual reference and learning tool for health care professionals. Obstet Gynecol. 2016; 128(5):958–963: https://journals.lww.com/greenjournal/Abstract/2016/11000/Female_Genital_Mutilation__A_Visual_Reference_and.4.aspx

American College of Obstetricians and Gynecologists. *ACOG Statement of Policy on Female Genital Mutilation.* American College of Obstetricians and Gynecologists. *Approved by the Executive Board March 2019. Amended April 2019* Female Genital Mutilation | ACOG. https://www.acog.org/clinical-information/policy-and-position-statements/statements-of-policy/2019/female-genital-mutilation

Center for Reproductive Rights. Legislation on Female Genital Mutilation in the United States. Briefing Papers. 2004. www.reproductiverights.org

Kelly E, Hillard PJA. Female genital mutilation. Curr Opin Obstet Gynecol. 2005; 25(26):1–5.

Mañero I, Labanca T. Clitoral reconstruction using a vaginal graft after female genital mutilation. Obstet Gynecol. 2018; 131(4):701–706.

Perron L, Senikas V, Burnett M, et al. Guideline No. 396-Female genital cutting. J Obstet Gynaecol Can. 2020; 42(2):204–217.

Salihu HM, August EM, Salemi JL, Weldeselasse H, Sarro YS, Alio AP. The association between female genital mutilation and intimate partner violence. *BJOG.* 2012; 119(13):1597–606.

WHO (2008). *Eliminating Female Genital Mutilation. An Interagency Statement.* Geneva: World Health Organization.

WHO (2016). *WHO Guidelines on the Management of Health Complications from Female Genital Mutilation.* Geneva: World Health Organization.

18

Fertility Preservation

Maggie L. Dwiggins

Definition

Preservation of fertility provides options for creating biologic children in those undergoing gonadotoxic therapy or other sterilization procedures due to necessary medical treatment, resulting in iatrogenic infertility.

Key Points

- Fertility preservation is most successful prior to the initiation of gonadotoxic therapy; therefore, prompt referral at the time of diagnosis is optimal
- For females, standard of care includes oocyte, embryo, and ovarian tissue cryopreservation and ovarian transposition
- For postpubertal males, the only standard of care treatment includes sperm banking. Testicular tissue cryopreservation is offered to prepubertal males only under research protocols
- Gonadotropin releasing hormone (GnRH) agonists have not conclusively been identified as a means of fertility preservation in the adolescent patient and should not be offered in lieu of other standard of care options when available
- Iatrogenic infertility has a lasting and significant impact on mental health and relationships; therefore, collaboration with mental health provider should be considered

Evaluation

History: Diagnosis, planned treatment, and pubertal status

- Use of gonadotoxic agents, especially alkylating agents
  - Calculate cyclophosphamide equivalent dose (CED) using the fertility risk calculator at fertilitypreservationpittsburgh.org
- Use of radiation (cranial, pelvic, testicular)
- Determine risk of infertility based on pubertal status and gender (see Table 18.1)
- Understand timeline for planned procedures and start/duration of treatment

Physical exam: Height, weight, and pubertal status

Laboratory

- No necessary lab testing, but consider FSH, LH, and AMH
- If surgery is planned, CBC with ANC and platelets (especially for blood cancers)
- If planning for cryopreservation, infection screening for HIV and hepatitis per protocols

DOI: 10.1201/9781003039235-18

TABLE 18.1

Risk of Gonadotoxicity above Baseline in Females and Males

	Females		Males
Risk	**Pubertal**	**Prepubertal**	
High level of increased risk	• CED > 8 g/m^2 • Hematopoietic stem cell transplant (HSCT) • Ovarian radiation ≥10 Gy • Hypothalamic radiation >40 Gy	• CED > 12 g/m^2 • HSCT • Ovarian radiation ≥15 Gy • Hypothalamic radiation >40 Gy	• CED ≥ 4 g/m^2 • HSCT • Testicular radiation ≥4 Gy • Hypothalamic radiation ≥40 Gy
Significantly increased risk	• CED 4–8 g/m^2 • Ovarian radiation <10 Gy • Hypothalamic radiation 30–39.9 Gy	• CED 8–12 g/m^2 • Ovarian radiation <15 Gy • Hypothalamic radiation 30–39.9 Gy	• Cisplatin >500 mg/m^2 • Testicular radiation 0.7–3.9 Gy • Hypothalamic radiation >30–39.9 Gy
Minimally increased risk	• CED < 4 g/m^2 • Heavy metals • Hypothalamic radiation 22–29.9 Gy	• CED < 8 g/m^2 • Heavy metals • Hypothalamic radiation 22–29.9 Gy	• CED < 4 g/m^2 • Heavy metals • Testicular radiation 0.2–0.6 Gy • Hypothalamic radiation 26–29.99 Gy

Abbreviation: CED = cyclophosphamide equivalent dose of alkylators.

Source: Adapted from Meacham LR, Burns K, Orwig KE, Levine J. Standardizing risk assessment for treatment-related gonadal insufficiency and infertility in childhood adolescent and young adult cancer: the Pediatric Initiative Network risk stratification system. J Adolesc Young Adult Oncol. 2020; 9(6):662–666.

Management

Oocyte/Embryo Cryopreservation

- Can be offered to any postpubertal patient with understanding of procedure and assent to treatment with frequent blood testing, transvaginal ultrasonography, and transvaginal oocyte retrieval
- Refer to reproductive endocrinology (REI) specialist with understanding of random-start stimulation
- Requires delay of cytotoxic cancer treatment by 10–21 days
- Counseling difficult as results may not be generalizable, response to stimulation may be impaired, and patients typically only have time for single cycle
- *Risks*: Ovarian hyperstimulation syndrome (OHSS), delay in cancer therapy, theoretic stimulation of estrogen sensitive cancers, increased thromboembolic events, intra-abdominal hemorrhage, pain, inadequate number of mature oocytes retrieved
- Live birth rates are the same or slightly decreased compared to age-matched cohorts undergoing single cycle

Ovarian Tissue Cryopreservation (OTC)

- Only method of fertility preservation for prepubertal girls
  - Although standard of care, should counsel regarding limited data on live birth rates and success in the prepubertal patient
- Surgically obtain ovarian cortical tissue, typically by laparoscopy
  - Can be done at the time of other planned procedures
  - Whole ovary yields better outcomes versus wedge biopsy
  - Contraindicated in ovarian cancer or if results in complete removal of both ovaries

- Tissue is cryopreserved until pregnancy attempt is desired
  - Tissue can only be used by patient
  - Requires second surgery for grafting of tissue orthotopically into remaining ovary, ovarian fossa, or posterior uterus (heterotopic transplantation unsuccessful)
- *Risks*: Risk of surgery and anesthesia, reintroduction of malignancy (especially for blood cancers or in hereditary cancers involving the ovaries)
- Live birth rates suggested to be around 30%; however, exact rates are poorly documented due to unknown number of pregnancy attempts in the available literature

Ovarian Transposition

- Surgical removal of ovaries from radiation field in those undergoing pelvic radiation
- Widely available conservative method of treatment
- *Risks*: Risks of surgery and anesthesia, may remove ovary from anatomic position for spontaneous pregnancy and transvaginal oocyte retrieval

GnRH Analog

- Data inconclusive regarding efficacy in the adolescent, not FDA approved for fertility preservation
- Should not be used in place of other fertility preservation alternatives
- Theoretic ovarian protection due to ovarian suppression
- Can be used for menstrual suppression (see Chapter 30, "Oncology")
- *Risks*: Decreased bone mineral density — For prevention use in conjunction with norethindrone acetate and calcium supplementation

Sperm Banking

- Only available to postpubertal males with ability to masturbate
  - In those with sperm production but unable to masturbate, vibratory stimulation or electro-ejaculation may be an option
  - In those without ability to ejaculate or with azoospermia/insufficient sperm, surgical sperm extraction can be performed for use with IVF/intracytoplasmic sperm injection (ICSI) at a later time, requires a specialist in male infertility
- *Risks*: Poor collection prior to treatment start

Testicular Tissue Cryopreservation

- Only option for prepubertal boys, should be performed under research protocol
- Removal of testicular tissue via wedge biopsy
- Theoretic reactivation of spermatogenesis with autologous transplantation of spermatogonial stem cells; no sperm have been recovered, and no pregnancies to date
- *Risks*: Risk of surgery and anesthesia, reintroduction of malignancy (especially for blood cancers or cancers involving the testicles)

Special Considerations

Adoption
- Studies have shown adoptions agencies may discriminate against cancer survivors, making adoption more difficult

Fertility Preservation for Special Populations

- Turner syndrome
  - OTC best option for fertility preservation
  - Mechanism of oocyte destruction is rapid and often significantly decreased by birth, therefore, may not have success at establishing endocrine function or oocyte creation
  - Performed under research protocol, must carefully weigh the risks of surgery and potential loss of endocrine function with the removal of ovary versus benefits regarding small possibility of live birth in this population
  - Turner syndrome is a relative contraindication to pregnancy due to increased risk cardiovascular mortality
  - Use of a surrogate may be a better option
- Transgender patients
  - May be especially important in those treated with puberty blockers followed immediately by gender-affirming hormone therapy who never undergo natal pubertal development and are unable to proceed with standard fertility preservation techniques
  - Oocyte/embryo cryopreservation and sperm banking should be performed prior to hormone treatment due to risk of infertility (see Chapter 51, "Transgender Care")
  - Gonadal tissue cryopreservation performed under research protocols at most institutions due to insufficiency of data regarding pregnancy outcomes versus risk of surgery and possible endocrine dysfunction

BIBLIOGRAPHY

Gynecologic issues in children and adolescent cancer patients and survivors. American College of Obstetricians and Gynecologists Committee Opinion no 747. Obstet Gynecol. 2018; 132(2):e67–e77.

Meacham LR, Burns K, Orwig KE, Levine J. Standardizing risk assessment for treatment-related gonadal insufficiency and infertility in childhood adolescent and young adult cancer: the Pediatric Initiative Network risk stratification system. J Adolesc Young Adult Oncol. 2020; 9(6):662–666.

Practice Committee of the American Society for Reproductive Medicine. Fertility preservation in patients undergoing gonadotoxic therapy or gonadectomy: a committee opinion. Fertil Steril. 2019; 112(6):1022–1033.

Practice Committee of the American Society for Reproductive Medicine Increased maternal cardiovascular mortality associated with pregnancy in women with Turner Syndrome. Fertil Steril 2012; 97(2): 282–284.

19

Genital Trauma

Diane F. Merritt

Definition

Genital injuries that involve the mons, vulva, labia, clitoris, vagina, and adjacent urogenital and anogenital structures.

The trauma may occur accidently or as a result of sexual assault.

Key Points

- Accidental genital trauma is the most common cause of prepubertal vaginal bleeding in an emergency setting
- Must ensure the history matches the physical exam findings

Evaluation

History

Determine "How did this happen" (accidental vs non-accidental)

- Were any eyewitnesses present?
- Is the child preverbal or able to tell her story?
- Is the history given compatible with the injuries found?
  - *Accidental*: History given by patient or reliable witness is compatible with injury.
  - *Non-accidental*: History by patient not compatible with injury, unwitnessed event, delay in presentation

Inconsistencies in the history raise concern for sexual abuse or assault

If sexual abuse is suspected or the injury does not fit the history, consult with child protection services at your institution

- If the injury occurred within 72 hours of the visit, a rape kit, forensic material collection, and cultures/serologies for sexually transmitted infections (STIs) should be obtained
- Report to the appropriate law enforcement officials (see Chapter 46, "Sexual Abuse")

Physical Exam

- Maintain calm and reassuring "demeanor throughout the examination.
- Vital signs, airway, breathing, site of trauma, and hemodynamic stability

Genitourinary Exam (GU): Adequate visualization and good light source are paramount; reassurances and cooperation of the child is key (see Chapter 20, "Gynecologic Examination")

DOI: 10.1201/9781003039235-19

- Straddle injuries usually affect the mons, labia, and/or posterior fourchette
- Penetrative injuries usually affect the hymen, vagina, and rectum
- Assess ability to void
- *GI*: Assess for signs of concomitant or intra-abdominal injury

Determine need for repair: Active bleeding, large laceration, penetrative injury, rectal/intra-abdominal injury, and rapidly expanding hematoma

Management

Superficial genital lacerations and abrasions not actively bleeding

- Rinse blood and debris with warm tap water and syringe (without needle) or IV tubing and saline
- Cover the injury with 2% lidocaine jelly (before and after rinsing)
- If injury is well visualized with no active bleeding, observation
- *Home care*: Topical petroleum jelly, warm water sitz baths, two to three times daily, minimal activity

Small vulvar hematomas that do not distort the anatomy or affect voiding

- Ensure hematoma not expanding and no evidence of necrosis to surrounding tissue
- Document that patient can urinate spontaneously prior to discharge
- *Home care*: Ice pack to area for 20–30 min QID for 48 hours (wear two pairs of underwear, place ice pack in between to also apply pressure); maintain hygiene with warm water sitz baths, two to three times daily until resolves; minimal activity; supine position preferred

Bite wounds to genitals

- Irrigate copiously, clean with soap (or antiseptic solution) and water
- Provide local anesthesia (if needed) and debride necrotic tissue cautiously
- Option of primary closure (if simple laceration, clinically uninfected, <12 hours old) versus allow to heal by secondary intention
- Antibiotic prophylaxis suggested after primary closure (see Stevens et al. 2014)
- Preemptive early antimicrobial therapy (both aerobic and anaerobic bacteria coverage such as amoxicillin-clavulanate) for three to five days is recommended for:
  - Immunocompromised patients
  - Asplenic patients
  - Those with advanced liver disease
  - Those with preexisting or resultant edema of affected area
  - Moderate or severe injuries
- Tetanus booster should be provided if none within 10 years
- Reevaluate in 24–48 hours to assess for signs of infection; tetanus prophylaxis is indicated
- *Home care*: Topical petroleum jelly to site. Maintain hygiene with warm water sitz baths, 2–3× daily until healed

SEVERE INJURY seek expertise from gynecology or trauma service

- If injury more than described above (i.e. active bleeding despite compression, unable to assess full extend of injury, involves a hematoma that is affecting voiding or anatomy or overlying tissue is necrotic)
  - Evaluate and treat under anesthesia
  - May need Foley catheter for voiding assistance immediately postoperatively

- Use absorbable sutures
- Caution closing a wound over 24 hours old, consider packing until hemostatic and/or begins to granulate

- If injury extends through or above the hymen or was caused by a penetrating object long enough to extend into the peritoneal cavity:
  - Perform CT or abdominal plain films to rule out intra-abdominal and/or bony pelvis injury
  - Complete comprehensive examination under anesthesia
  - Once anesthesia induced and prior to sterile prep, obtain forensic and STD specimens if indicated
  - Make a careful anatomic description of the injury with photo documentation if possible
  - *Perform vaginoscopy*: See Chapter 31, "Operative Care"
  - Perform cystoscopy and sigmoidoscopy by appropriate specialist if extensive injury warrants
  - If severe rectal injuries are noted, determine if a diverting colostomy is indicated
  - If visualization is still compromised, use small ribbon retractors and headlight to visualize deep vaginal penetrative injuries
  - Ensure hemostasis
  - Repair with fine absorbable suture material in layered fashion

Additional Therapy

- Tetanus booster should be provided if none within ten years
- Broad-spectrum antibiotics should be used therapeutically not prophylactically (see Stevens et al. 2014)
- Postoperative visit
  - Repetitive reassurance that injuries will not affect the ability to have healthy sexual relations and bear children in the future
  - With proper care and support, long-term morbidity rare, even when there is an impalement injury with severe anogenital trauma.

BIBLIOGRAPHY

Lopez HN, Focseneanu MA, Merritt DF. Genital injuries acute evaluation and management. Best Pract Res Clin Obstet Gynaecol. 2018; 48:28–39.

Patel BN, Hoefgen HR, Nour N, Merritt DF (2020). Genital Trauma. In Emans SJ, Laufer MR, DiVasta AD, eds., *Emans, Laufer, Goldstein's Pediatric and Adolescent Gynecology* (7th ed., pp. 237–250). Philadelphia, PA: Wolters Kluwer.

Stevens DL, Bisno AL, Chambers HF, et al. Practice guidelines for the diagnosis and management of skin and soft tissue infections: 2014 update by the Infectious Diseases Society of America. Clin Infect Dis. 2014; 59(2):e10–e52. Date accessed 5/13/2020 https://doi.org/10.1093/cid/ciu296

20

Gynecologic Examination

S. Paige Hertweck

Key Points

- A detailed gynecologic exam is not routinely part of all office visits but may be warranted even in the young patient
- Consent and assent, when able to be obtained, should be provided by both patient and parent
- Gentle exam techniques are needed in the prepubertal patient, never force an exam on an unco-operative child due to risk of trauma to the unestrogenized tissue
- Confidentiality is an important component to the gynecologic exam

Newborn/Infant

Examination of the genitalia of a newborn should be routine in the delivery room:

Location:	Isolette/exam table
Position:	Frog-leg position
Technique:	Labial separation/traction
	Perform gentle abdominal exam to palpate any masses
	(Pelvic masses i.e. ovarian cysts tend to be abdominal in infants due to their small bony pelvises)
Common findings:	
Newborn:	Maternal estrogenization (see Figure 20.1)
	Plump/full labia majora
	Mucous vaginal discharge
	Thick pale pink hymen
	Signs of estrogenization diminish after 2–3 weeks
Older infant:	Hypoestrogenic vulvar tissue (see Figure 20.1)
	Less prominent labia majora/minora
	Hymen recessed into vestibule appears thin/red

Prepubertal Female

Most gynecologic concerns at this age are

- Concerns about anatomical development
- External epithelial conditions
- Vulvovaginitis

DOI: 10.1201/9781003039235-20

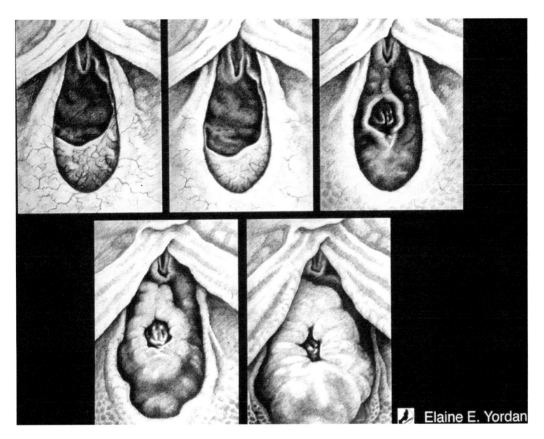

FIGURE 20.1 Progressive effects of estrogen on hymenal appearance: (upper three images) unestrogenized prepubertal appearance and (lower two images) estrogenized (neonatal/pubertal) appearance. (From Yordan EM (ed), The PediGYN Teaching Slide Set. North American Society for Pediatric and Adolescent Gynecology, with permission.)

History

- Spend time during the history establishing a rapport with the young patient by including questions about family, best friends, favorite activities before performing exam
- Elicit concerns from both patient and guardian
- Explain the concept of the exam after obtaining history

Physical Examination

Involve the patient in the exam to emphasize that they have some control
- Would you like to wear a blue gown or a green gown?
- Would you like to sit on your mom/dad's lap or on the table?

Perform a thorough exam
- Start by listening to heart and lungs while assessing body habitus/hygiene/skin disorders or discoloration and allow patient to feel comfortable

Position the child appropriately for genitalia examination
- Most children over age 2 are able to use the stirrups or parent's lap for dorsolithotomy (see Figure 20.2)
- Other positions include
  - Frog leg (see Figure 20.3)

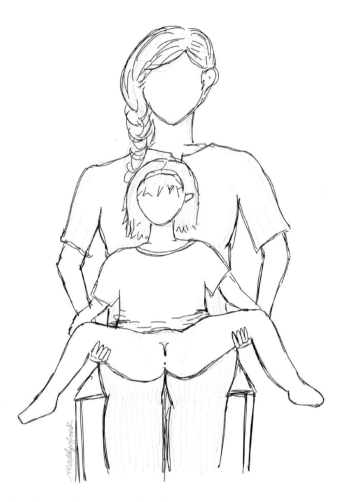

FIGURE 20.2   Child in supine dorsolithotomy position while in mother's lap. (By courtesy of Madelyn Frank.)

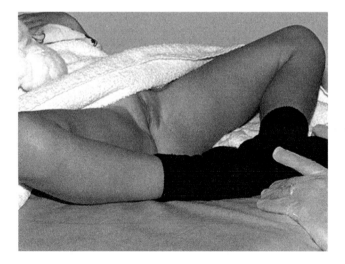

FIGURE 20.3   A 5-year-old demonstrating the supine 'frog-leg' position. (Reproduced with permission from McCann JJ, Kerns DL. "Visualization Techniques" The Child Abuse Atlas, Evidentia Learning, 2017, www.childabuseatlas.com.)

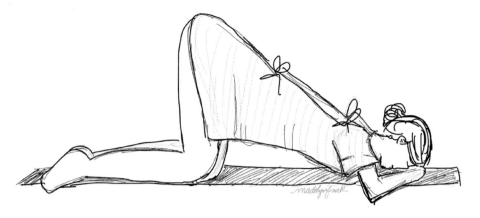

FIGURE 20.4   Child in prone knee-chest position for genital examination. (By courtesy of Madelyn Frank.)

- Knee-chest position (see Figures 20.4 and 20.5)
    - Helpful adjunctive position
    - May allow visualization of the lower and even upper vagina with use of otoscope or ophthalmoscope

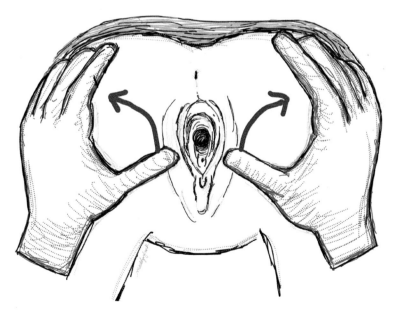

FIGURE 20.5   Technique for examination of female genitalia in prone knee-chest position. (By courtesy of Madelyn Frank.)

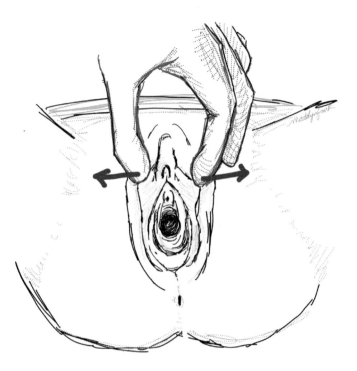

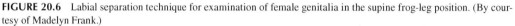

FIGURE 20.6   Labial separation technique for examination of female genitalia in the supine frog-leg position. (By courtesy of Madelyn Frank.)

Visualize the Vestibule

- Labial separation (see Figure 20.6)
- Labial traction (see Figure 20.7)

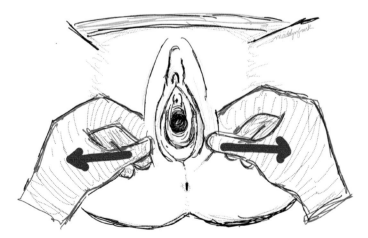

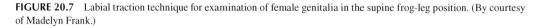

FIGURE 20.7   Labial traction technique for examination of female genitalia in the supine frog-leg position. (By courtesy of Madelyn Frank.)

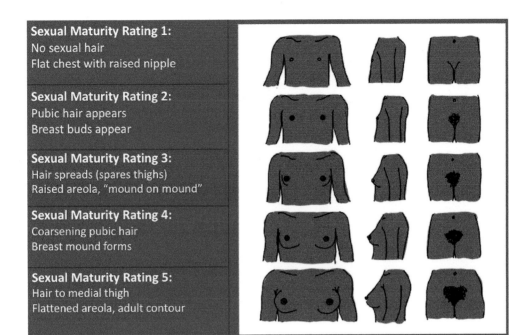

| Sexual Maturity Rating 1:
No sexual hair
Flat chest with raised nipple |
| Sexual Maturity Rating 2:
Pubic hair appears
Breast buds appear |
| Sexual Maturity Rating 3:
Hair spreads (spares thighs)
Raised areola, "mound on mound" |
| Sexual Maturity Rating 4:
Coarsening pubic hair
Breast mound forms |
| Sexual Maturity Rating 5:
Hair to medial thigh
Flattened areola, adult contour |

FIGURE 20.8 Tanner stages: female pubic hair. (By courtesy of Meredithe McNamara, MD MS, Associate Professor of Pediatrics, Yale University School of Medicine.)

Assess

- Presence of pubic hair (Tanner staging, see Figure 20.8)
- Clitoral size
- Hymenal shape (see figures showing hymenal shapes in "Hymenal Anatomy", Chapter 24)
- Signs of estrogenization (pale pink hymenal tissue vs reddened tissue), presence or absence of vaginal discharge
- Perianal hygiene

Obtain Specimens

- Use small Dacron swabs (male urethral size) to obtain vaginal swabs when necessary (see Figure 20.9)
- The prepubertal hymen is hypoestrogenic and sensitive to touch; therefore, consider using a 'catheter-within-a-catheter' technique by cutting a 4.5" butterfly catheter and putting it inside a #12 red rubber catheter attached to a 1–3-ml syringe to first instill 1 ml of fluid and then aspirate for use (Figure 20.10)

Document and Describe Findings

- In prepubertal girls, it is preferable to list each genital structure examined because future examiners will use the previous exams for the basis of their findings. This is particularly helpful in suspected abuse cases where a structure may have been altered by trauma, like a hymen

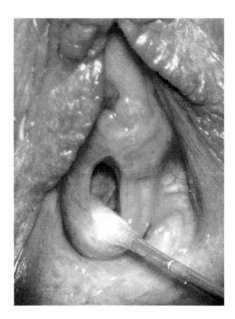

FIGURE 20.9   Use of small Dacron swabs to obtain vaginal swabs. (Reproduced with permission from McCann JJ, Kerns DL. "Visualization Techniques" The Child Abuse Atlas, Evidentia Learning, 2017, www.childabuseatlas.com.)

- List includes labia majora, labia minora, hymenal shape or variations (bumps, clefts in hymen), urethra, vagina, rectal findings even if normal (see Figure 20.11)
- It is helpful to use a clockface method to delineate location of any abnormal findings (see Figure 20.12)

Remember

- Avoid iatrogenic trauma, do not force exams on noncooperative children
- Allow child to have sense of control by participating in exam (choosing gown, position for exam, putting on gloves)
- Tell the truth to children: If something will hurt, tell them it will hurt
- An examination under anesthesia may sometimes be necessary for patients who are non-compliant with exam

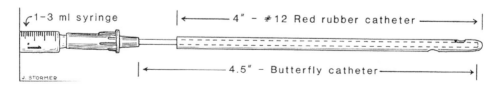

FIGURE 20.10   Assembled catheter-within-a-catheter, as used to obtain samples of vaginal secretions from prepubertal patients. (From Pokorny SF, Stormer J. A traumatic removal of secretions from the prepubertal vagina. Am J Obstet Gynecol 1987;156:581–2, with permission.)

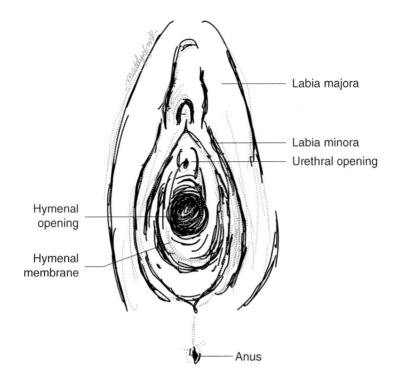

FIGURE 20.11 External structures of the female genitalia. (By courtesy of Madelyn Frank.)

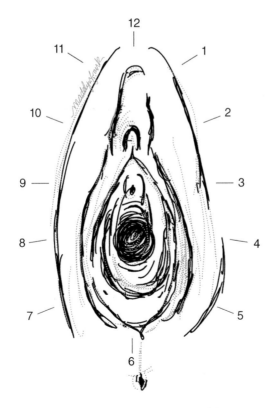

FIGURE 20.12 Face of clock orientation with patient in frog-leg supine position. (By courtesy of Madelyn Frank.)

Adolescent Patient

Indications for Adolescent Gyn Exam

Preventative visits

- Age 13–15: Initial visit; does not necessarily include pelvic exam
- Yearly visits thereafter; pelvic when indicated

Annual/semi-annual for sexually active teens

- Need sexually transmitted disease (STD) screening with each new partner
- Annual if regular partner

Indications for pelvic examination

- Pubertal aberrancy
- Abnormal bleeding
- Abdominal or pelvic pain
- Vulvovaginal concerns

History

Confidentiality

- Confidentiality is key to provision of care to adolescent patients
- Consider use of the American College of Obstetricians and Gynecologists (ACOG) adolescent spe-
  cific information regarding the first reproductive visit and confidentiality listed in reference section
- Consider use of a confidential questionnaire (ideally completed online but could be written in
  private location away from parent/guardian) to assist patients in expressing their concerns (see
  Figures 20.13 and 20.14 for examples)

History Hints

Start history by building trust with a friendly, respectful greeting:
   'How may I help you today?'
   Avoid: 'What's your problem/complaint today?'
Initially meet with teen and her parent(s) or guardian(s) if possible to explain the course of the visit
   Explain concept of confidentiality and privacy to both parents and teen (ACOG has a helpful docu-
      ment on confidentiality and promotion of healthy relationships in adolescence). For example,
      "We will spend some time talking together about your teen's health history and any concerns that
      you or they might have, and then I will also spend some time alone with your teen. At the end
      of the visit, we will all meet together again to clarify any tests, treatments or follow-up plans".

Acknowledge that the youth is a minor and, therefore, has specific legal rights related to consent and
confidentiality.

   INTRODUCE the concept of fostering adolescent self-responsibility and self-reliance.
   REINFORCE that this policy applies to all adolescents in your practice or clinic (in other words,
      this is not specific to YOUR child).

   Validate the parental role in their child's health and well-being. Elicit any specific questions or
   concerns from the parent. Direct questions and discussion to the youth while attending to and
   validating parental input.

REMOVE Invite the parents to have a seat in the waiting area, assuring them that you will call them prior to closing the visit.

REVISIT Once the parent is out of the room,

Revisit issues of consent and confidentiality with the youth, including situations when confidentiality has to be breached (suicidality, abuse).

Revisit areas of parental concern with the youth and obtain the youth's perspective.

Conduct the psychosocial interview and physical exam (ascertain whether youth desires parent's presence during PE and accommodate youth's preference).

If you do not have the ability to have a written psychosocial sexual history from the patient, use the quick **HEADSSS/Body** screen (see Chapter 21, "High-Risk Behaviors").

Clarify what information from the psychosocial interview and PE the youth is comfortable sharing with the parent.

REUNITE Invite the parent back to close the visit with both parent and youth.

Tips

When asking questions of teens

Give a range of acceptable answers

- 'Some teens can talk about sex with their parents; others can't. How do you feel?'

Create a context for questions

- 'A lot of people your age … how do you feel about that?'

When screening, begin discussions/questions with less-sensitive issues

- Ask about home and education before affect and sexuality

Obtain

- *Routine history*: Chief complaint, history of present illness, past medical history, family and social history
- *Gynecologic history*: Menarche, flow duration, cycle interval, pad/tampon saturation, dysmenorrhea (see Chapter 27, "Menstruation" and Chapter 14, "Dysmenorrhea" for what is normal)
- *Sexual*: Coitarche, number of partners (total and recent), condom use, sexual attraction, body parts used for intimacy, history of STI or pregnancy, parental knowledge

Examination

Start by completing thorough routine head-to-toe assessment prior to pelvic

- Allows for complete assessment while patient is comfortable
- May observe somatic signs that affect gyn complaints: Café au lait spots, hirsutism/acne, very low body weight, obesity, other skin conditions (atopic dermatitis or psoriasis), abdominal trigger points/musculoskeletal pain

Pelvic examination

- Explain process of exam before performing
- Position
  - Use semi-sitting dorsal lithotomy (lift back of exam table to allow better eye contact with provider giving better sense of control)
  - Consider using mirror to show genital anatomy to patient

Please answer the following questions to help your healthcare provider take better care of you. This document will not be shared with your parent/guardian, and the information you provide will be kept confidential unless we feel that you or someone else may be in danger.

Gender you identify with: Female   Male   Non-binary   Transgender male   Transgender female

Preferred pronoun: she/her   he/him   they/them   other:_____

Is there anything you would like to discuss with your provider today:_____

_____

_____

Do you have concerns that you would like to discuss in private with your provider?   Yes   No

FRIENDS AND FAMILY

1. Who lives at home with you? Circle all that apply.

    Mother   Father   Stepparent   Guardian(s)   Foster parent(s)   Sibling(s)   Other:_____

2. Do you feel safe at home?   Yes   No
3. Do you have one or more friends that you feel comfortable talking to?   Yes   No

SCHOOL AND WORK

4. What school do you go to?_____
5. What grade are you in?_____
6. Do you participate in any after school sports or clubs?_____
7. Do you have a job? If so, where at?_____

HEALTH HABITS

8. Do you exercise or participate in a sport at least 5 times/week that makes you sweat or breathe hard for at least 30 minutes at a time? If yes, what?_____
9. Are you happy with your current weight?   Yes   No   If no, why not?_____
    _____
10. Have you ever used diet pills or laxatives, made yourself throw-up, or starved yourself to lose weight? Yes   No

SAFETY

11. Have you ever been forced or pressured to do something sexual that you didn't want to do?   Yes   No
12. Have you ever been in a relationship with someone who threatened or hurt you?   Yes   N

TOBACCO, ALCOHOL, AND DRUGS

13. Have you ever used alcohol?   Yes   No

FIGURE 20.13   Adolescent confidential questionnaire. (*Continued*)

14. Have you ever used drugs? Yes No If yes, circle all that apply.
   Marijuana Meth Ecstasy Cocaine Heroin Inhalants Prescription pills
15. Do you ever forget things that you did while using drugs or alcohol? Yes No
16. Do you use tobacco products including cigarettes, e-cigarettes, or Juul? Yes No

RELATIONSHIPS

17. Are you dating anyone? Yes No
18. Who are you attracted to? Males Females Both Other:_____
19. Have you ever had any type of sex? Yes No No, but considering
   If yes, circle all that apply. Vaginal Anal Oral

**IF YOU ANSWERED "NO" TO QUESTION 19, YOU CAN SKIP QUESTIONS 20-30. IF YOU ANSWERED "YES" TO QUESTION 19, PLEASE ANSWER THE QUESTIONS BELOW.

20. How old were you when you first had sex?_____
21. How many partners have you had in the past 3 months?_____
22. How many partners have you had in total?_____
23. When was the last time that you had sex?_____
24. How often do you use a condom? Never Sometimes Always
25. Have you ever had sex for drugs or money? Yes No
26. Are your parents aware that you are sexually active? Yes No
27. Have you ever been pregnant? Yes No If yes, when?_____
28. Have you ever had a sexually transmitted infection (STI)? Yes No
29. Would you like to be tested for sexually transmitted infections (STIs)? Yes No
30. Can we discuss your test results with your parents? Yes No
   ** ALL STI RESULTS ARE CONFIDENTIAL. PLEASE PROVIDE US WITH YOUR CELL PHONE NUMBER SO WE CAN CONTACT YOU WITH RESULTS:_____

FIGURE 20.13 (*Continued*)

- Inspect
  - External genitalia (Tanner staging)
  - Vaginal/cervical exam (when indicated)
- Use appropriate size speculum
- Virginal/nulliparous patients – Huffman specula ($1/2 \times 4$ inches long) (see Figure 20.15)
- Sexually active teens – Huffman or Pederson specula ($7/8 \times 4$ inches long)
- Vaginal testing for chlamydia and gonorrhea, if sexually active
- If no pelvic exam completed, may do urine screening for chlamydia/gonorrhoea or patient performed self-swab
- Bimanual exam (when indicated)
  - Put single finger in the vagina
  - Assess for vaginal levator pain by assessing for pain at 5 and 7 o'clock in vaginal side wall
  - Palpate cervix evaluating for cervical motion tenderness
  - Assess uterine size and position (ante- or retroverted)
  - Assess adnexa for tenderness, masses, and ovarian enlargement
  - Perform rectovaginal bimanual exam only if need additional clarification for exam (e.g. pelvic mass, pain, cul-de-sac nodularity)
- For patients with abdominal pain or severe dysmenorrhea
- Assess cul-de-sac area for nodularity indicating endometriosis
- Assess for adnexal masses, uterine anomalies

Name: _____   Date: _____

Instructions: *How often have you been bothered by each of the following symptoms during the past two weeks? For each symptom put an "X" in the box beneath the answer that best describes how you have been feeling.*

Questions	Not At All (0)	Several Days (1)	More Than Half the Days (2)	Nearly Every Day (3)
1. Feeling down, depressed, irritable or hopeless?				
2. Little interest or pleasure in doing things?				
3. Trouble falling asleep, staying asleep, or sleeping too much?				
4. Poor appetite, weight loss, or overeating?				
5. Feeling tired, or having little energy?				
6. Feeling bad about yourself – or feeling that you are a failure, or that you have let yourself or your family down?				
7. Trouble concentrating on things like school work, reading, or watching TV?				
8. Moving or speaking so slowly that other people could have noticed? Or the opposite – being so fidgety or restless that you were moving around a lot more than usual?				
9. Thoughts that you would be better off dead, or of hurting yourself in some way?				

In the **PAST YEAR** have you felt depressed or sad most days, even if you felt okay sometimes?	☐YES ☐NO
If you are experiencing any of the problems on this form, how difficult have these problems made it for you to do your work, take care of things at home or get along with other people?	

☐Not Difficult At All   ☐ Somewhat Difficult   ☐Very Difficult   ☐Extremely Difficult

Has there been a time in the past month when you have had serious thoughts about ending your life?	☐YES ☐NO
Have you **EVER**, in your **WHOLE LIFE**, tried to kill yourself or made a suicide attempt?	☐YES ☐NO

For Office Use Only   Score _____

FIGURE 20.14   Patient Health Questionnaire modified for teens.

Assessment/Plan

Hints on conveying information
  After the exam

- In the non-sexually active teen – Meet with family member and patient together to review findings and make plan.
- In the sexually active teen, if confidentiality is a concern – First discuss findings with patient alone while in the examination room. Make a plan together about how to discuss with parent/guardian. Encourage the teen to allow you to be the liaison between her and her family stressing the benefits of informing everyone of contraception use and her situation. Then meet together with family.

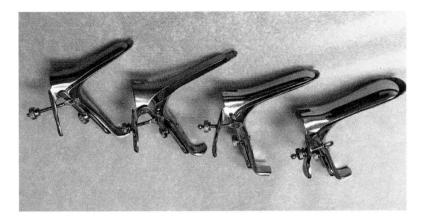

FIGURE 20.15 Types of specula (from left to right): infant. (Huffman, Pederson, and Graves reproduced with permission from Lara-Torre E. In Sanfilippo JS, Lara-Torre E, Gomez-Lobo V. *Sanfilippo's Textbook of Pediatric and Adolescent Gynecology*, 2nd edn. Boca Raton, FL: CRC Press, Taylor & Francis, 2020.)

After discussions about outcome of the exam and findings, when it is time to make a decision between medical therapies, make it clear that a decision is needed and that the decision belongs to the patient not to the parent

Ask: 'What have you decided to do?'

If any indecision indicates need for further discussion, reflecting patient's decision back can often clarify situation

- 'So, you have decided to …' then allow patient to agree or disagree

When providing instructions

- Give, short, simple, repetitive instructions
- Make links for taking medicine 'When brush teeth, take pill'
- Check understanding by having teen repeat back to you
- Send printed instructions home

Encourage follow up by anchoring experience to external events

- 'Come back during week of Thanksgiving' instead of 'end of November'

BIBLIOGRAPHY

Confidentiality in Adolescent Health Care. American College of Obstetricians and Gynecologists Committee Opinion 803. Obstet Gynecol. 2020; 135:e171–e177.

The initial reproductive health care visit. American College of Obstetricians and Gynecologists Committee Opinion 811. Obstet Gynecol. 2020; 136:e70–e80.

Lara-Torre E (2020). The Physical Exam in the Pediatric and Adolescent Patient. In Sanfilippo JS, Lara-Torre E, Gomez-Lobo V, eds., *Sanfilippo's Textbook of Pediatric and Adolescent Gynecology* (2nd ed.). Boca Raton, FL: CRC, Taylor & Francis Group.

Promoting healthy relationships in adolescents. American College of Obstetricians and Gynecologists Committee Opinion 758. Obstet Gynecol. 2018; 132:e213–e220.

21

High-Risk Behaviors (HRB)

How to Assess for and Help Patients become Resilient and Not Engage in HRB

Ellen Rome

Key Points

- Appropriate preventative care for the adolescent includes annual assessment of both protective factors and risk factors that lead to wellness or illness, including risks at home, school, and in the community.
- High-risk behaviors include vaping and other substance use, alcohol abuse, unprotected sexual activity, intimate partner violence and nonconsensual sex, self-harm, and other challenges to mental and physical health.
- Protective factors develop from connection at home and at school, internal and external factors, mediated by genetic risk and the effects of toxic stress in a vulnerable individual.

Evaluation

Taking a History

Meet with parent and patient initially to identify reason for the visit, then excuse the parent for the duration of the interview

Confidentiality and its limits should be defined and discussed with both parent and child

- In all 50 states, adolescents have the right to seek help and intervention for diagnosis and treatment of sexually transmitted infections without parental involvement. Many states also allow provision for youth to seek care for substance abuse, as well.
- If the clinician feels the adolescent is at high risk of harm that confidentiality may be relinquished.

Confidential interview: Relaxed; listening actively; nonjudgmental in responses; straightforward and respectful

Screening tool can be filled out by the adolescent (see Figure 20.14: The self-administered confidential adolescent visit questionnaire) or by the practitioner (HEADSFIRST Screening Tool)

H: Home – Relationships, space, freedom and restrictions, support

Who lives at home? What happens when there is an argument at home?

DOI: 10.1201/9781003039235-21

E: Education/employment – Expectations, study habits, future, achievement, jobs

What grade are you in school?
How were your grades last year? This year?
How connected do you feel to your school/community?
For those out of school: Where are you working now? How is that going?

A: Activities – Abuse – physical, sexual, emotional, verbal neglect

Has anyone ever done anything to you that made you uncomfortable? Activities: How do you
spend your time?

D: Drugs – Vaping, marijuana, tobacco/nicotine, alcohol, illicit drugs

Do your friends vape/smoke? Do you vape/smoke? What form, how much, how often? Have
you ever tried to quit or cut back?
Any marijuana/CBD? In what form, how much, how often? Have you ever tried to quit or cut back?
Same questions for alcohol, other drugs, over-the-counter drugs misused. If YES, ask the
CRAFFT questions (see Chapter 49, "Substance Abuse")
*Have you ever ridden in a **C**ar driven by someone/yourself who was high or had been*
using alcohol or drugs?
*Do you ever use alcohol/drugs to **R**elax, feel better about yourself, or fit in?*
*Do you ever drink/use drugs **A**lone?*
*Do you ever **F**orget things you did while using alcohol/drugs?*
*Do your **F**amily or **F**riends ever tell you that you should cut down on your drinking or*
drug use?
*Have you ever got in **T**rouble from drinking/using drugs?*

S: Sexuality – Sexual identity and gender identity, relationships, activity, safety, body changes

Are you attracted to guys, girls, or both?
Do you see yourself as male, female, nonbinary, or other?
Have you ever had sex? Oral, vaginal, anal?
Use condoms all/most/some/none of the time? Second method of protection for heterosexual
sexual activity?
Have you ever had STIs or pregnancy? If yes – Do you want to be pregnant/parenting this year?
Has anyone ever asked you to have sex in exchange for something you wanted or needed?
(food, clothing, money, shelter, other items?)
Has anyone ever asked you to have sex with another person?
Has anyone ever taken sexual pictures of you, asked you to send pictures of your private parts,
or posted such pictures on the internet?

F: Friends – Peer pressure, positive and negative interactions

I: Image – Self-esteem, appearance, body image, nutrition

R: Recreation – Exercise, relaxation and sleep, media use, sports

S: Safety – Hazardous activities, seatbelts, bike/motorcycle helmets, driving

T: Threats – Harm to self or others, running away/getting "thrown away," homelessness

Other Red Flags for Risk Behaviors

- Low self-esteem
- Need for peer approval
- Poor relationship with family
- Substance abusing friends or family
- Early alcohol/substance abuse
- Easy availability of alcohol or drugs
- ADHD, impulsivity
- Poor academic achievement, marginalized at school
- Depression, anxiety
- Loss of a parent or loved one

Red Flags for Substance Use, Intimate Partner Violence, Sex Trafficking, and Other Unsafe Situations (See Chapter 46, "Sexual Abuse" and Chapter 49, "Substance Abuse")

- Suspicious trauma or injury without plausible explanation
- Altered level of consciousness (substance use? Head trauma?)
- Excessive fatigue, abnormal sleep habits
- Red eyes, track marks, and suspicious odors
- Change in weight or general appearance
- Tattoos without a story, especially bar codes or other branding as property
- Change in friends to known troublemakers
- Change in music, clothes
- Pushing the limits at home, school
- Drug paraphernalia found in house or in purse/backpack
- Incomplete homework assignments or not turned in
- Inattentiveness in class, laughs inappropriately
- Irritability
- Memory problems
- Law enforcement involvement
- High-risk sexual behaviors

Red Flags for Depression (see Chapter 13, "Depression")

- Anger
- Anxiety
- Changes in appetite, weight, and/or eating habits
- Depression, low self-esteem, feelings of sadness/helplessness/emptiness
- Insomnia, disturbed sleep, excessive sleep, and fatigue
- Guilt and shame
- Self-harm

Management

Plan is dependent on the level of risk assessed

- Reinforce and commend abstinence/healthy choice; include age-appropriate anticipatory guidance
OR

Assess for immediate risk

- Survival mode: *What will make things better for you at this moment?*
- Layers of problems to unravel: *What other problems exist in your life beyond the physical stuff?*

Motivational interviewing to decrease the risk behavior

- Praise changes made
- Reflect what you have heard
- Roll with resistance: "I am sensing you do not want to talk about XXX. Tell me more about that and concerns you may have."
- Encourage the patient to set her/his/their own goals
- Ask permission before giving advice (unwelcome advice is not likely to be heeded)
- Accept patient's motivation (or lack thereof) to change without confronting or judging
- Work collaboratively while supporting patient autonomy while moving towards positive change
- And, as needed, refer for appropriate treatment

Accentuate the Positive: What Works to Transform Teen Lives?

- Help youth moved from fixed mindset to growth mindset: Praise effort, not the results
- Create connections:
  - Connections to both family and school are HIGHLY protective
  - Connections to community: Volunteering, service
  - Connections to caring adults, including health-care provider, coaches, and teachers
- Explore the role of social media in the young person's life: Is it time for a social media time-out?
- See the youth as an asset and positive solution-generator, not a problem to be solved
- Ask (questions), reflect (back your understanding to patient), and encourage change

BIBLIOGRAPHY

Do KT, Guassi Moreira JF, Telzer EH. But is helping you worth the risk? Defining prosocial risk taking in adolescence. Dev Cogn Neurosci. 2017; 25:260–271.

Dweck C. *Mindset: the New Psychology of Success*, 2008.

Ginsberg K. *Raise Kids to Thrive*, 2015.

Greenbaum VJ, Dodd M, McCracken C. A short screening tool to identify victims of child sex trafficking in the health care setting. Pediatric Emer Care. 2018; 34:33–37.

Jankowski MK, Rosenberg HJ, Sengupta A, Rosenberg S, Wolford G. Development of a screening tool to identify adolescents engaged in multiple problem behaviors: the Adolescent Risk Behavior Screen (ARBS). J Adol Health. 2007; 40(2):180.e19–180.e26.

Levy S, Sherritt L, Gabriellie J, Shrier L, Knight JR. Screening adolescents for substance use-related high-risk sexual behaviors. J Adol Helath. 2009; 45(5):473–477.

Maslyanskaya S, Alderman EM. Confidentiality and consent in the care of the adolescent patient. Pediatr Rev. 2019; 40(10)508–516.

Nesi J, Prinstein MJ. In search of likes: longitudinal associations between adolescents' digital status seeking and health-risk behaviors. J Clin Child Adolesc Psychol. 2019; 48(5):740–748.

Pollak KI. Incorporating MI techniques into physician counselling. Patient Educ Couns. 2011; 84:1–2.

Rome ES, Miller E. Intimate partner violence in the adolescent. Pediatr Rev. 2020; 41(2):73–80.

22

Hirsutism

Benjamin L. Palmer and Lauren A. Kanner

Definition

Appearance of excessive coarse (terminal) hair in androgen-sensitive sites (upper lip, chin, mid-sternum, abdomen, back – i.e. male pattern) in women; increase in distribution and quantity of terminal hair.

Key Points

- In most cases, it is due to excess androgen production
- In children, may be the first sign of central precocious puberty
- In adolescents, may be idiopathic or an early sign of a tumor or pathologic condition of ovary or adrenal gland
- Can be the first sign of impending virilization (clitoromegaly, temporal hair recession, deepening of the voice, changes in muscle pattern, breast atrophy)
- Tends to be terminal coarse, long curly hair compared to vellus, soft body hair
- Must be distinguished from hypertrichosis, which refers to generalized growth of hair in excess of normal limited to normal distribution

Differential Diagnosis

Pediatric

- Premature adrenarche: Most common etiology
- Congenital adrenal hyperplasia (CAH)
- Adrenocortical tumor
- Idiopathic/genetic predisposition

Adolescent

Idiopathic/genetic predisposition

Ovarian causes

- Anovulation/polycystic ovary syndrome (PCOS): Most common pathologic etiology (see Chapter 39, "Polycystic Ovary Syndrome")
- Stromal hyperthecosis
- Ovarian tumors
- Enzyme deficiency (17-ketosteroid reductase)

DOI: 10.1201/9781003039235-22

Adrenal causes

- CAH (21-hydroxylase/11-beta-hydroxylase/3-beta-hydroxysteroid dehydrogenase deficiencies) – (see Chapter 3, "Ambiguous Genitalia")
  - Can be from early childhood or into adolescence
- Cushing's syndrome: 2–5% of cases
- Adrenocortical tumors
- Macronodular hyperplasia
- Hypothalamic-pituitary tumors causing Cushing's disease

Disorders of Sexual Differentiation (see Chapter 3)

Drug-induced

- Cyclosporin, androgens, danazol, diazoxide, glucocorticoids, minoxidil, phenytoin, testosterone, and valproic acid

Other causes

- Hypothyroidism/hyperprolactinemia
- Stress/anorexia
- Central nervous system disorders (mental and motor retardation)

Diagnosis

- Distinguish between idiopathic hirsutism and a pathologic condition

History

- *General*: Age, focus on growth parameters, any recent change in height/weight and ethnicity
- *Hair growth*: Onset and timing, location/distribution, progression, relation to other secondary sexual characteristics and/or menses
  - Gradual and isolated onset and progression suggest idiopathic condition, medications, CAH, or chronic anovulation
  - Rapid progression with other signs of virilization like deepening of the voice and severe acne may indicate acute pathology, like a tumor
- *Puberty and menstruation history*: Adrenarche, thelarche, menarche, frequency, regularity of periods
- *Assess family history*: PCOS, CAH, pubertal tempo, hirsutism, and hypertrichosis
- Medication use: In particular, use of testosterone and valproic acid
- Assess for use of prior hair-control methods (shaving, waxing, cream, electrolysis, laser)

Physical Examination

- *NOTE*: Look for signs of thyroid disorder, galactorrhea, acne, signs of Cushing's, and presence of abdominal/pelvic masses
- Check weight, height, growth velocity
- Evaluate hair pattern
  - Determine terminal vs vellus hair
  - Quantify extent of hirsutism objectively with a Ferriman and Gallwey score (a score of >8 indicates hirsutism but does depend on race and ethnicity, see Figure 22.1) – ask if patient has removed hair recently

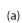
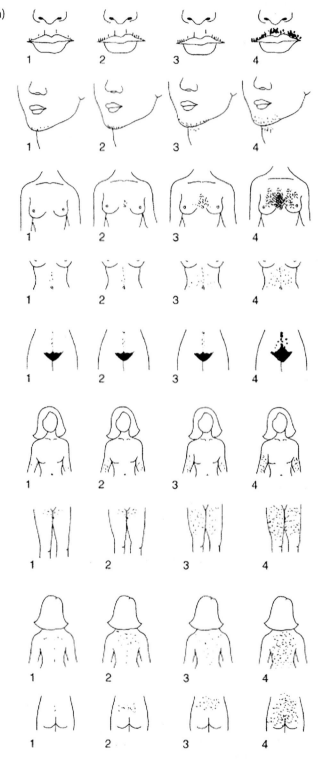

FIGURE 22.1 Hirsutism scoring sheets. (a) The original Ferriman-Gallwey scoring graded 9 body areas with score 0–4, with an overall score of 8 or more indicating hirsutism. (Reproduced with permission from Ferriman D, Gallwey JD. Clinical assessment of body hair growth in women. J Clin Endocrinol Metab 1961;21:1440.) (*Continued*)

(b) *(Grade 0 at all sites indicates absence of terminal hair).*

Site	Grade	Definition
1. Upper lip	1	A few hairs at outer margin.
	2	A small moustache at outer margin.
	3	A moustache extending halfway from outer margin.
	4	A moustache extending to midline.
2. Chin	1	A few scattered hairs.
	2	Scattered hairs with small concentrations.
	3 & 4	Complete cover, light and heavy.
3. Chest	1	Circumareolar hairs.
	2	With mid-line hair in addition.
	3	Fusion of these areas, with three-quarter cover.
	4	Complete cover.
4. Upper back	1	A few scattered hairs.
	2	Rather more, still scattered.
	3 & 4	Complete cover, light and heavy.
5. Lower back	1	A sacral tuft of hair.
	2	With some lateral extension.
	3	Three-quarter cover.
	4	Complete cover
6. Upper abdomen	1	A few mid-line hairs
	2	Rather more, still mid-line.
	3 & 4	Half and full cover.
7. Lower abdomen	1	A few mid-line hairs
	2	A mid-line streak of hair.
	3	A mid-line band of hair.
	4	An inverted V-shaped growth.
8. Arm	1	Sparse growth affecting not more than a quarter of the limb surface.
	2	More than this; cover still incomplete.
	3 & 4	Complete cover, light and heavy.
9. Foream	1, 2, 3, 4	Complete cover of dorsal surface; 2 grades of light and 2 of heavy growth.
10. Thigh	1, 2, 3, 4	As for arm.
11. Leg	1, 2, 3, 4	As for arm.

FIGURE 22.1 (*Continued*)   Hirsutism scoring sheets. (b) The modified Ferriman-Gallwey scoring shown here graded 11 body areas minus the forearm, whereby a score of 8 or more indicates hirsutism but can be varied or overlaid in various racial/ethnic groups. (Reproduced with permission from Hatch R, Rosenfield RL, Kim MH, et al. Hirsutism: implications, etiology, and management. Am J Obstet Gynecol 1981;149:815.)

- Identify location and distribution of hair growth (androgen-sensitive sites vs diffuse growth)
- Evaluate for temporal or vertex alopecia (male-patterned hair loss)
- Look at skin for acne and/or acanthosis nigricans (darkly pigmented skin at the nape of the neck, axilla, waist – associated with hyperinsulinemia/PCOS)
- Look for stigmata of Cushing's disease (striae, moon facies)

- Palpate for thyroid enlargement
- Puberty
  - Sexual Maturity Rating/Tanner staging
  - Examine breasts for galactorrhea/atrophy
  - Monitor for signs of virilization
- Evaluate for abdominal or pelvic masses on palpation

Laboratory Evaluation

Determine presence of adrenal and ovarian hyperandrogenism

- Free/total testosterone
  - Elevation reflects ovarian androgen production (ideally done via quantitative high-performance liquid chromatography-tandem mass spectrometry)
  - If checking free testosterone, also obtain a sex hormone binding globulin (SHBG) for PCOS screening
- Dehydroepiandrosterone sulfate (DHEAS)
  - Elevation reflects adrenal androgen production

If patient not virilized, rule out other causes of androgen excess

- First screen for causes of anovulation:
  - Prolactin, thyroid-stimulating hormone (TSH), human chorionic gonadotropin (hCG) level
- Then check serum testosterone, DHEAS level
- Screen for nonclassical CAH
  - Obtain 7 a.m. 17-hydroxyprogesterone level (17-OHP)
    - Level > 300 ng/dl confirms CAH
    - Level > 100 ng/dl needs adrenocorticotropic hormone (ACTH) stimulation test to clarify the diagnosis

If cushingoid symptoms, screen for Cushing's syndrome

- Obtain overnight low-dose dexamethasone suppression test
  - Give patient 1-mg dexamethasone at 11 p.m.
  - Draw fasting serum cortisol at 8 a.m.
  - Normal is <5 ng/dl

If patient virilized or rapid progression of hair growth and other features of hyperandrogenism (raises concern for tumor)

Pediatric

Obtain DHEAS level

- Usually between 40 µg/dL (above range for 1–9 years olds) and 130 µg/dL (average for early puberty) if isolated adrenarche
- If elevated above this, look for adrenal tumor or CAH

Obtain serum testosterone

- If above 100 mg/dL, look for ovarian or adrenal androgen-secreting tumor

Obtain ultrasound

Obtain 7 a.m. 17-OHP level

- If >100 ng/dl, need ACTH stimulation test
  - Draw baseline 17-OHP, 17-OH pregnenolone, aldosterone, androstenedione, 11-deoxycorticosterone, corticosterone level
  - Then give 250-µg cosyntropin IV

- Redraw 17-OHP, 17-OH pregnenolone, aldosterone, androstenedione, 11-deoxycorticosterone, corticosterone level at 60 minutes (see Chapter 3, "Ambiguous genitalia and Differences in Sexual Development")
- If >300 ng/dL, diagnostic of CAH but can obtain an ACTH stimulation test to confirm enzyme defect

Adolescent

Obtain serum testosterone

- If above lab reference range (generally 45–60 ng/dL) and below 150 ng/dL, suggests ovarian hyperandrogenism and PCOS
- Abnormal >150 ng/dL suggests an ovarian or adrenal androgen-secreting tumor, so check pelvic ultrasound

Obtain a serum (DHEAS)

- Abnormal >700 µg/dL suggests adrenal tumor
- Check CT or MRI of adrenals
- If negative, may need to do adrenocorticotropic hormone (ACTH) stimulation test to rule out CAH, (see Chapter 3, "Ambiguous genitalia and Differences in Sexual Development")

Management

- Treatment is targeted at the underlying cause
- Eliminate causative factors
- Optimize weight
  - Obesity is linked to anovulation, insulin resistance, lowered sex-hormone-binding globulin levels and PCOS
- Further treatment can be divided into cosmetic/physical and pharmacologic
  - *Cosmetic/physical treatment*-manages hair:
    - Bleaching
    - Cutting or shaving
    - Depilatory creams
    - Electrolysis
    - Laser depilation
    - Plucking
    - Waxing
  - *Pharmacologic treatment* (may take up to 6–12 months for improvement due to length of hair growth cycle)
  - *Management of excess ovarian androgen production, most commonly PCOS:*
    - Combination estrogen/progestin treatment:
      - Oral contraceptive pills may be better than transdermal contraceptive patch or vaginal ring
      - Estrogen component increases sex-hormone-binding globulin, which binds circulating androgen, thus decreasing androgen action at hair follicle
      - Progestin component inhibits luteinizing hormone (LH) secretion, creating less ovarian androgen output
    - Gonadotropin-releasing hormone (GnRH) agonists in severe cases:
      - Depot leuprolide (Lupron Depot®, TAP Pharmaceuticals, Inc., Lake Forest, IL) 3.75-mg IM monthly
      - Will result in hypoestrogenism, may need to combine with estrogen or estrogen/progestin add-back (see Chapter 16, "Endometriosis")

- If associated with insulin resistance, consider use of metformin (see "Polycystic Ovarian Syndrome", Chapter 39)
- May need endocrinology consult

- *Management directed at hair follicle*
  - Spironolactone
    - Aldosterone antagonist with antiandrogenic effects
    - Decreases androgen production by inhibiting 5-alpha-reductase activity and blocks the androgen receptor at hair follicle. May also help with acne
    - May use in combination with oral contraceptives or alone but recommended that patients are required to have concurrent use of birth control if sexually active due to a risk of teratogenicity in a male fetus
    - Dose 50 mg po daily, which can be increased up to 100 mg po twice daily
    - Does not alter hair distribution already present but will decrease new growth
    - May take up to 6–12 months to see response
  - Eflornithine hydrochloride 13.9% cream (Vaniqa®)
    - Topical antiandrogen that inhibits ornithine decarboxylase
    - Approved by US FDA for treatment of female hirsutism
    - Apply 2× per day to face and chin
    - May be used alone or in combination with other pharmacotherapies
    - *Side effects*: Burning, folliculitis
    - Allow 4–8 weeks for clinical improvement

- *Management of excess adrenal androgen production*
  - Little role for corticosteroid treatment unless adrenal enzyme deficiency
  - If CAH, (see Chapter 3, "Ambiguous genitalia and Differences in Sexual Development") for workup/management
  - If ovarian or adrenal tumor (see Chapter 35, "Ovarian Masses"): Needs surgical excision

BIBLIOGRAPHY

American Academy of Pediatrics (2017). Hirsutism, Hypertrichosis, and Precocious Sexual Hair Development. In McInerny TK, Adam HM, Campbell DE, DeWitt TG, Foy JM, Kamat DM, eds., *American Academy of Pediatrics Textbook of Pediatric Care* (2nd ed.). Elk Grove, IL: American Academy of Pediatrics.

Divasta AD, Barbieri RL, Emans SJ (2020). Polycystic Ovarian Syndrome in the Adolescent. In Emans SJ, Laufer MR, DiVasta AD, eds., *Emans, Laufer, Goldstein's Pediatric and Adolescent Gynecology* (7th ed., pp. 443–451). Philadelphia, PA: Wolters Kluwer.

Martin KA, Anderson RR, Chang RJ, Ehrmann DA, Lobo RA, Murad MH, Pugeat MM, Rosenfield RL. Evaluation and treatment of hirsutism in premenopausal women: an endocrine society clinical practice guideline. J Clin Endocrinol Metab. April 2018; 103(4):1233–1257.

23

Human Immunodeficiency Virus (HIV)

Prevention and Management in Adolescents and Young Adults

Kimberly Huhmann and Andrea Zuckerman

Definition

Human immunodeficiency virus (HIV) is a virus that attacks the body's immune system, so the body is unable to adequately fight off infections.

This virus is transmitted through sex and body fluids.

Key Points

There is no cure for HIV

Of yearly new diagnoses of HIV, youth aged 13–24 made up 21% of cases.

- 87% males: The most common mode of transmission was male-to-male sexual contact (93%).
- 13% females: Heterosexual contact was the most common mode of transmission (86%).

There is increased risk in the transgender population

- About one in seven transgender women are HIV positive.
  - Higher prevalence among Black/African American and Hispanic/Latina.
- Nearly 3% of transgender men are HIV positive.
- Those with an STI are 2–5 times more likely to become infected with HIV if exposed.
  - Syphilitic and herpetic ulcers increase sexual transmission by increasing blood-mucosal contact.
  - Gonorrhea and chlamydia facilitate transmission by increasing amount of viral shedding in genital secretions.
- Preexposure prophylaxis (PrEP) is a daily medication that helps protect against HIV transmission in those who are high risk and, when taken every day, can reduce the risk of transmission through sex by approximately 99% and through intravenous drug use by 74–84%.
- Postexposure prophylaxis (nPEP) is medication taken after a nonoccupational HIV exposure to prevent an HIV infection.
- Vigilant STI screening and pap testing should be performed.

DOI: 10.1201/9781003039235-23

Evaluation

Screening

Offer screening to

- All adolescents and adults aged 13–64 at least once
- Anyone seeking evaluation/testing for STIs
- Heterosexual persons who themselves or whose sex partners have had more than one sex partner since their most recent HIV test
- Occupational exposure (e.g., needle stick)
- Those individuals initiating treatment for tuberculosis (TB)
- Prior to beginning a new sexual relationship
- Medical/gynecologic conditions consistent with HIV-related illness
- History of substance abuse associated with unprotected sex
- Persons who exchange sex for money or drugs
- Partner known to be HIV-infected or at high risk
- Victims of rape/sexual abuse (baseline and 3–9 months later)
- History of STDs
- Pregnancy
- History of unprotected sex with multiple partners, older men, or partner from area where HIV is prevalent
- Anyone with acute retroviral syndrome: Fever, malaise, lymphadenopathy, sore throat, myalgia, and skin rash within first few weeks of HIV infection before antibody test positive

Diagnosis

- Informed consent must be obtained before HIV testing
- Opt-out screening is recommended (notify patient the testing will be performed unless they decline)

Ideal testing algorithm

- HIV-1/HIV-2 antigen/antibody (Ag/Ab) immunoassay

If positive

- Obtain HIV-1/HIV-2 supplemental testing (HIV-1/HIV-2 antibody differentiation assay, Western Blot, or indirect immunofluorescence assay)
- If the immunoassay is positive and supplemental testing is negative or indeterminate, obtain serum HIV RNA testing to identify acute infection

Alternative testing strategies exist

- Rapid testing if positive requires HIV-1/HIV-2 Ag/Ab immunoassay confirmation
- Enzyme-linked immunosorbent assay (ELISA) and if positive followed by confirmatory Western Blot (may not identify acute infections)

Retest: Persons with an exposure within the past 3 months
NOTE: When delivering test results, always ensure that

- The correct test result is being discussed
- Results are being delivered confidentially

- The patient has consented to testing and hearing results at this time
- You are prepared to counsel the patient on results and provide resources necessary

---

Management

- Refer patient immediately for initial counseling and behavioral, psychosocial and medical evaluation, and treatment services
- Evaluate patient for symptoms or signs that suggest advance HIV infection (e.g. fever, weight loss, diarrhea, cough, shortness of breath, and oral candidiasis) – this should prompt urgent referral for medical care
- Encourage HIV-positive patients to notify partners. Refer patient to health department partner-notification programs. If patient is unwilling to notify their partners, the health department should be informed to use confidential procedures to notify partners
- Draw hCG, ensure patient is not pregnant

PrEP

Should be offered to HIV-negative individuals at substantial risk of acquiring HIV

- Multiple sexual partners
- Anal and/or vaginal sex with inconsistent or no condom use
- Needle sharing (e.g. drugs or gender affirming hormones)
- Commercial sex worker
- HIV-positive sexual partner
- High-prevalence network
- Recent bacterial sexually transmitted infection
- Recent drug treatment and currently injecting

Testing prior to initiation

- HIV-negative test
- Hepatitis B surface antigen
- Serum creatinine
- Urine pregnancy test (for female sex assigned at birth patients)

Dosing

- *Truvada*®: Emtricitabine 200 mg and tenofovir disoproxil fumarate 300 mg taken by mouth daily.
  - Protects against transmission of HIV during sexual and intravenous drug exposures
  - At-risk adult and adolescents ($\geq$35 kg)
- *Descovy*®: Emtricitabine 200 mg and tenofovir alafenamide 25 mg taken by mouth daily.
  - Protects against sexual transmission of HIV infection (excluding receptive vaginal sex)
  - At-risk adult and adolescents ($\geq$35 kg)
- *Common side effects*: Transient nausea
- If creatinine clearance (GFR) <30 mL/min, PrEP should be stopped
- Individuals without hepatitis B immunity should be vaccinated. Hepatitis B positive individuals can have disease flares with discontinuation of PrEP

Follow-up

- *Every 3 months*: HIV testing
- *Every 6 months*: Sexually transmitted infection testing

Adequate protection

- *Receptive anal sex*: 7 days after initiating
- *Receptive vaginal sex and intravenous drug use*: 21 days after initiating
- There is no insufficient data regarding time to protection for receptive anal or vaginal sex

Sero-different couples (one partner is HIV positive, one partner is HIV negative)

- Most patients do get PrEP because it has been shown to be safe and well tolerated. However, there is support for and against PrEP use in this population
- Support for *not* using
  - Optimally treating HIV with antiretroviral therapies also prevents transmission
  - PrEP is an additional medication and has cost associated with its use
- Support for using
  - Viral counts can rebound during antiretroviral treatments
  - Not all relationships are monogamous
  - Use of PrEP gives the HIV-negative user control of their infection risk

Reproductive effects

- Studies have not shown decreased efficacy of hormonal contraceptives associated with PrEP use
  - Advocate for reliable contraception that avoids first-pass metabolism, such as LARC
  - When pregnancy is not desired, counsel on importance of back up method (such as barrier methods)
- PrEP does not affect rates of birth defects or birth outcomes
- If the HIV-positive partner is taking antiretroviral therapy, PrEP is not offering much additional protection. The HIV-negative partner may not need to take PrEP during pregnancy (see information about sero-different couples above)
- No decreased efficacy of gender affirming hormones

nPEP

Should be offered to individuals who are at risk of contracting HIV *after* being exposed to HIV-positive person (e.g. sexual exposure, needle sharing, sexual assault, etc.)
  Type of contact that would warrant nPEP

- Contact to a mucosal surface (vaginal, rectal, eye, mouth, etc.), non-intact skin, or percutaneous
- One of those surfaces had blood/blood contaminated fluid, semen, vaginal/rectal secretions, or breast milk present
- By a known HIV-positive individual

In situations with exposure to an individual with unknown HIV status, the provider should assess risk and determine whether to prescribe nPEP.
  Testing prior to starting medication

- HIV testing
- Creatinine and liver function tests

- Hepatitis B and C antibodies
- Syphilis, gonorrhea, and chlamydia

Dosing

- Typically involves a 3-drug regimen
- No evidence that one combination is superior to another. There are multiple available regimens with different side effects and dosing schedules. See CDC nPEP guideline for options (Table 23.1)
- Must be started within 72 hours of exposure. Taken once or twice a daily for 28 days
- *Side effects*: Transient nausea

Follow-up

- *At 12 weeks postexposure*: Repeat HIV testing
- *At 24 weeks postexposure*: Repeat HIV testing (only if HCV contracted), Hepatitis B and C antibodies, syphilis

Insurance Coverage

Most insurance providers (including state Medicaid) cover PrEP. However, some carriers may require a prior authorization to be completed.

- For access to free medications, visit getyourprep.com
- For assistance with co-payments, visit gileadvancingaccess.com
- For state assistance programs, visit nastad.org/prepcost-resources/prep-assistance-programs

Sexually Transmitted Infection Screening

- *Gonorrhea, chlamydia, trichomonas, and syphilis*: Screen at entry of care and at least annually.
- *Hepatitis B and C*: Screen at entry of care and as needed based on risk thereafter.
  - Hepatitis B vaccine recommended if patient does *not* have chronic hepatitis B and/or is *not* immune.
- Recommend barrier precautions for infection prevention.

Pap Smear Recommendations for HIV-Positive Women

- HPV vaccine recommendations are the same as non-HIV-positive patients.
- Start screening with cytology alone:
  - Within 1 year of coitarche
  - If HIV diagnosis occurs after coitarche, start screening with cytology alone within 1 year of HIV diagnosis
  - If no coitarche by 21 years old, start screening with cytology alone at 21 years old
- Screen with cytology alone annually until three consecutive negative results. Then, screen with cytology alone every 3 years
- At age 30, screening can be with cytology alone or co-testing (cytology with HPV testing)
  - *Cytology alone*: Annual until three consecutive negative results. Then, screen every 3 years
  - *Co-testing*: After one negative result, repeat screening every 3 years
- Screening continues for complete lifespan. Do *not* stop screening at age 65 regardless of Pap smear history.

TABLE 23.1

Preferred and Alternative Antiretroviral Medication 28-Day Regimens for nPEP[a,b]

Age Group	Preferred/ Alternative	Medication
Adults and adolescents aged ≥ 13 years, including pregnant women, with normal renal function (creatinine clearance ≥ 60 mL/min)	Preferred	A 3-drug regimen consisting of tenofovir DF 300 mg and fixed dose combination emtricitabine 200 mg (Truvada[c]) once daily with raltegravir 400 mg twice daily or dolutegravir 50 mg once daily
	Alternative	A 3-drug regimen consisting of tenofovir DF 300 mg and fixed dose combination emtricitabine 200 mg (Truvada) once daily with darunavir 800 mg (as two 400-mg tablets) once daily and ritonavir[b] 100 mg once daily
Adults and adolescents aged ≥ 13 years with renal dysfunction (creatinine clearance ≤59 mL/min)	Preferred	A 3-drug regimen consisting of zidovudine and lamivudine, with both doses adjusted to degree of renal function with raltegravir 400 mg twice daily or dolutegravir 50 mg once daily
	Alternative	A 3-drug regimen consisting of zidovudine and lamivudine, with both doses adjusted to degree of renal function with darunavir 800 mg (as two 400-mg tablets) once daily and ritonavir[b] 100 mg once daily
Children aged 2–12 years	Preferred	A 3-drug regimen consisting of tenofovir DF, emtricitabine, and raltegravir, with each drug dosed to age and weight
	Alternative	A 3-drug regimen consisting of zidovudine and lamivudine with raltegravir or lopinavir/ritonavir[b], with raltegravir and lopinavir/ritonavir dosed to age and weight
	Alternative	A 3-drug regimen consisting of tenofovir DF and emtricitabine and lopinavir/ritonavir[b], with each drug dosed to age and weight
Children aged 3–12 years	Alternative	A 3-drug regimen consisting of tenofovir DF and emtricitabine and darunavir[d]/ritonavir[b], with each drug dosed to age and weight
Children aged 4 weeks[e] –<2 years	Preferred	A 3-drug regimen consisting of zidovudine oral solution and lamivudine oral solution with raltegravir or lopinavir/ritonavir[b] oral solution (Kaletra[f]), with each drug dosed to age and weight
Children aged 4 weeks[e] –<2 years	Alternative	A 3-drug regimen consisting of zidovudine oral solution and emtricitabine oral solution with raltegravir or lopinavir/ritonavir[b] oral solution (Kaletra), with each drug adjusted to age and weight
Children aged birth–27 days	Consult a pediatric HIV specialist	

Abbreviations: HIV, human immunodeficiency virus; nPEP, nonoccupational postexposure prophylaxis; tenofovir DF, tenofovir disoproxil fumarate.

Source: From CDC, Updated Guidelines for Antiretroviral Postexposure Prophylaxis After Sexual, Injection Drug Use, or Other Nonoccupational Exposure to HIV, CDC 2016, with permission; https://www.cdc.gov/hiv/pdf/ programresources/cdc-hiv-npep-guidelines.pdf

[a]   These recommendations do not reflect current Food and Drug Administration-approved labeling for antiretroviral medications listed in this table.

[b]   Ritonavir is used in clinical practice as a pharmacokinetic enhancer to increase the trough concentration and prolong the half-life of darunavir, lopinavir, and other protease inhibitors. Ritonavir is not counted as a drug directly active against HIV in the above "3-drug" regimens.

[c]   Gilead Sciences, Inc., Foster City, California.

[d]   Darunavir only FDA-approved for use among children aged ≥3 years.

[e]   Children should have attained a postnatal age of ≥28 days and a postmenstrual age (i.e., first day of the mother's last menstrual period to birth plus the time elapsed after birth) of ≥42 weeks.

[f]   AbbVie, Inc., North Chicago, Illinois.

BIBLIOGRAPHY

Antiretroviral Postexposure Prophylaxis after Sexual, Injection-Drug Use, or Other Nonoccupational Exposure to HIV in the United States: Recommendations from the U.S. Department of Health and Human Services [Internet]. [cited 2020 May 4]. Available from: https://www.cdc.gov/mmwr/preview/mmwrhtml/rr5402a1.htm

Transgender Health Archives » LGBT Health Education Center [Internet]. [cited 2020 May 4]. Available from: https://www.lgbthealtheducation.org/category/transgender-health/

Learn About PrEP | Preventing New HIV Infections | Clinicians | HIV | CDC [Internet]. [cited 2020 May 4]. Available from: https://www.cdc.gov/hiv/clinicians/prevention/prep.html

Gynecologic Care for Women and Adolescents with Human Immunodeficiency Virus | ACOG [Internet]. [cited 2020 Sep 11]. Available from: https://www.acog.org/clinical/clinical-guidance/practice-bulletin/articles/2016/10/gynecologic-care-for-women-and-adolescents-with-human-immunodeficiency-virus

24

Hymenal Anatomy (Normal and Abnormal)

Kate McCracken

Key Points

- Hymenal anatomy may vary; however, absence of the hymen has not been reported in the literature; if absent, look for a reason.
- Typically, hymen anomalies are isolated findings and do not have long-term implications on sexual function, fertility, or obstetric outcomes.
- Menstrual outflow obstructions – i.e. imperforate hymen – increase the risk of endometriosis. Women with a history of an imperforate hymen should be evaluated if they have ongoing dysmenorrhea.
- Virginity is a sociocultural construct, rather than a medical diagnosis, and is not affected by a hymenectomy (removal of excess hymen tissue) nor can virginity be determined based on a hymenal/physical examination.

Examination

- Please refer to the chapter on gynecologic examination in the pediatric patient (Chapter 20) for a description on how to visualize the hymen.
- Gentle labial traction as well as asking the patient to Valsalva are helpful maneuvers to aid in visualization of the hymen.
- Prepubertal patients: Use a moistened Dacron swab or lubricated 5-mm pediatric feeding tube to best evaluate the perimeter of the hymen.
- Pubertal non-sexually active patients: Run the hymen's perimeter using a moistened Q-tip to assess confluence
  - Hormonal stimulation can heal hymenal lacerations, making the perimeter appear uninterrupted.
  - Examination of the hymen cannot be used to prove or disprove penetration.

Prepubertal Morphology

- Annular (circumferential) (Figure 24.1): Hymen extends completely around the circumference of the vaginal orifice
- Crescentic (posterior rim) (Figure 24.2): Hymen with anterior attachments at approximately the 11 o'clock and 1 o'clock positions with no hymenal tissue visible between the two attachments

DOI: 10.1201/9781003039235-24

- Redundant (Figure 24.3): Abundant hymenal tissue that tends to fold back upon itself or protrude
- Fimbriated (Figure 24.4): Hymen with multiple projections or indentations along the edge

There are reports of several nonspecific prepubertal hymenal findings – including periurethral/ perihymenal bands, hymenal tags, hymenal bumps/mounds.

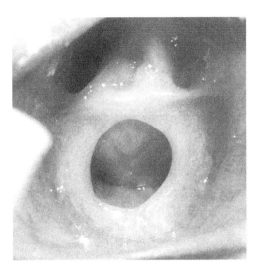

FIGURE 24.1 Four year old African American female, normal annular hymen. (From Kerns D, McCann D, Child Abuse Atlas, EvidentiaLearning.com, with permission.)

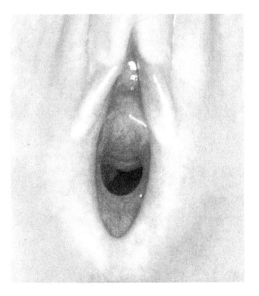

FIGURE 24.2 Three year old Anglo female with crescentic hymen. Non-abuse study. Intravaginal longitudinal ridges. Labial separation, traction and prone knee-chest position. (From Kerns D, McCann D, Child Abuse Atlas, EvidentiaLearning.com, with permission.)

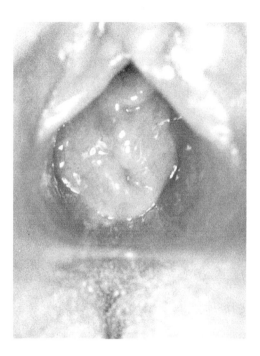

FIGURE 24.3 Two year old Anglo female with a redundant hymen. Non-abuse study. Labial separation, traction and prone knee-chest position. (From Kerns D, McCann D, Child Abuse Atlas, EvidentiaLearning.com, with permission.)

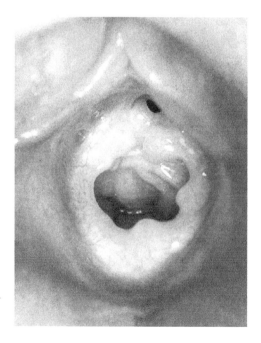

FIGURE 24.4 Two year old Anglo female with a fimbriated hymen, a normal variation. (From Kerns D, McCann D, Child Abuse Atlas, EvidentiaLearning.com, with permission.)

Morphology Changes with Aging toward Puberty

- With advancing age, there is an increase in the number of children with a crescentic configuration and increasing transverse and vertical diameters.
- The number of mounds and intravaginal ridges increases with age but frequently is associated with preexisting ridges.
- There is no significant change in the number of tags, vestibular bands, notches, periurethral bands, or external ridges.
- At menarche, the hymen typically has progressed from crescentic to fimbriated and thickened due to increased exposure to endogenous estrogen.

Indications of Sexual Abuse

Penetrative abuse may lead to hymenal changes – including

- Acute laceration or ecchymosis of the hymen
- Absence of hymenal tissue in the posterior half
- Healed hymenal transection or complete cleft

Remember, the hymen heals quickly, and a normal appearing hymen cannot prove or disprove penetration.

Congenital Abnormalities

Imperforate Hymen

Newborn

With mucocolpos (Figure 24.5)

- Presents as a bulging yellow or translucent mass at the introitus. Mucocolpos should subside within 1 month as maternal estrogen exposure wanes; wait to perform hymenectomy until significant pubertal development unless symptoms of urinary obstruction

Without mucocolpos

- Wait until significant pubertal development to perform hymenectomy; procedure as with an adolescent

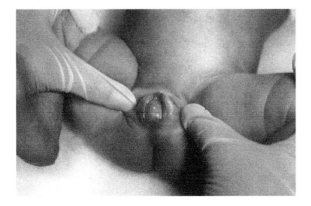

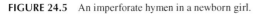

FIGURE 24.5 An imperforate hymen in a newborn girl.

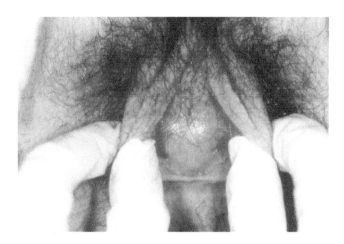

FIGURE 24.6   Imperforate hymen and hematocolpos in an adolescent girl.

Adolescent (Figure 24.6)

Presenting symptoms

- Asymptomatic: Found incidentally during well-child exam
- Symptomatic: Cyclic abdominal pain, urinary retention, back pain, and primary amenorrhea

Physical examination

- Asymptomatic: Labial traction, try probing with a lubricated swab or feeding tube. If unable to tolerate, follow with serial exams (and possibly a pelvic ultrasound) as Tanner staging progresses
- Symptomatic: Presents with hematocolpos (possibly hematometrocolpos), a bulging bluish mass at the introitus, typically the mass moves with Valsalva
  - If unclear diagnosis, try rectal exam
  - If still unclear, use pelvic ultrasound or MRI to distinguish from other outflow tract anomalies (i.e. transverse or longitudinal vaginal septum, distal vaginal agenesis, cervical atresia – also see Chapter 58, "Vaginal Tract Anomalies")

Treatment

- Hymenectomy
  - General anesthesia
  - Lithotomy position
  - Place indwelling urethral catheter to avoid injury secondary to distortion of urethra during the procedure
  - Use protective eye wear during procedure
  - Make cruciate or u-shaped incision using electrocautery (i.e. needlepoint bovie)
  - Suction the hematocolpos: Ideal to have irrigation fluid available as the old menstrual blood is quite thick and may require gentle irrigation to completely evacuate the vagina
  - After draining, excise remainder of excess hymen tissue (care taken to avoid the urethra and rectum)
  - Final introitus diameter should be adequate to accommodate two-finger breadths or a standard speculum
  - Vaginal mucosa can be sutured to hymenal ring using 3-0 or 4-0 absorbable interrupted sutures to reduce the risk of regression/stenosis

- Postoperative care
  - Comfort measures as needed
    - Cool compresses/ice packs to vulva/sitz baths
    - Use of oral nonsteroidal anti-inflammatory medications
    - Application of topical emollient or anesthetic daily
  - In prepubertal patients, estrogen cream applied to the area daily may aide in healing
  - Counsel patients
    - Regarding the extended course of vaginal bleeding after management of an imperforate hymen – This is normal as the uterus involutes from the hematometrocolpos
    - The patient should seek medical attention if they experience fevers/chills or malodorous vaginal discharge

Microperforate Hymen (Figure 24.7)

Definition

- Hymenal tissue completely covers the vaginal opening with a microperforate opening typically at the 12 o'clock position just below the periurethral tissue

Treatment

- Remove excess hymen tissue if requested to ease tampon use or permit penetrative vaginal intercourse. May also consider treatment if patient has incomplete egress of menses or vaginal discharge
- Hymenectomy performed similar to that outlined above for treatment of an imperforate hymen. Final introitus diameter accommodates two-finger breadths or a standard speculum. Postoperative care as with an imperforate hymen

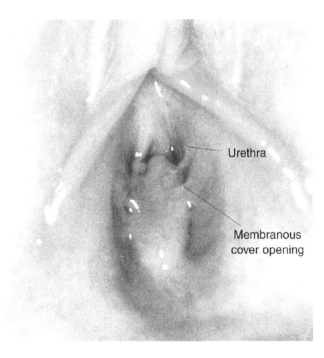

FIGURE 24.7 Eighteen month old with a microperforate hymenal orifice. Multiple periurethral and perihymenal bands. (From Kerns D, McCann D, Child Abuse Atlas, EvidentiaLearning.com, with permission.)

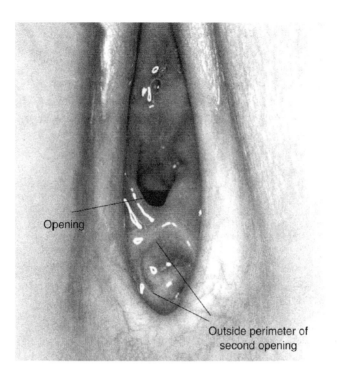

FIGURE 24.8 Three year old Anglo female with a midline hymenal defect; cribriform hymen, a congenital variation. (From Kerns D, McCann D, Child Abuse Atlas, EvidentiaLearning.com, with permission.)

Cribiform Hymen (Figure 24.8)

Definition

- Hymen stretches completely across the vaginal opening but has varied microperforate openings throughout

Treatment

- Remove excess hymen tissue if requested to permit tampon use or penetrative vaginal intercourse. May also consider treatment if patient has incomplete egress of menses or vaginal discharge
- Hymenectomy performed similar to that outlined above for treatment of an imperforate hymen. Final introitus diameter accommodates two-finger breadths or a standard speculum. Postoperative care as with an imperforate hymen

Septate Hymen (Figure 24.9)

Definition

- Bands of tissue that bisect the vaginal introitus, creating two or more openings
- Patient may present with difficulty inserting or removing a tampon. Often the patient is able to insert a tampon, but when the tampon expands with menstrual blood, the septum precludes easy removal. In this acute situation, deviation of the septum laterally will allow tampon removal

Treatment

- Remove if requested to ease tampon use or permit penetrative vaginal intercourse
- If patient is amenable and the septum is not too thick, in-office excision preferred
  - Topical anesthesia can be applied or can instill lidocaine at the anterior and posterior attachments
  - Suture ligate (using 4-0 absorbable suture) around the anterior and posterior aspect of the septum, then resect the intervening band of tissue. Alternatively, suture ligate around the middle of the band, and the septum should necrose at the suture line
    OR
  - Place curved hemostats around the anterior and posterior aspects of the septum and wait for 1 minute to allow for crush injury of tissue. Then remove hemostats and cut septum at site of crush injury using small Iris scissors. Silver nitrate may be used as needed for hemostasis. This allows for complete and immediate removal of septum in office and may be preferable to some
- If the patient is not cooperative, or the septum is too thick, perform removal under general anesthesia. Suture ligate around the superior and inferior aspect of the septum, then cut out the intervening band of tissue using electrocautery
- Postoperative care as with an imperforate hymen

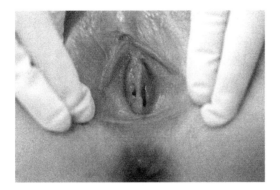

FIGURE 24.9 Septated hymen.

Hymen Tag (Figure 24.10)

Definition

- Pedunculated tissue extending from an area of the hymen. Variable in thickness and length

Treatment

- Remove if symptomatic
- If patient is amenable and the tag is thin, may remove in the office. Suture ligate around the base and allow to necrose off
- If the patient is not cooperative, or the band is too thick, perform removal under general anesthesia. Use electrocautery (i.e. needlepoint bovie) to resect the tag. Suture base using 4-0 absorbable suture
- Postoperative care as with an imperforate hymen

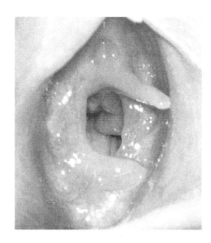

FIGURE 24.10   Ten-month-old Anglo female with a hymenal tag that appears to be an extension of a posterior vaginal column. (From Kerns D, McCann D, Child Abuse Atlas, EvidentiaLearning.com, with permission.)

Hymen Cyst (Figure 24.11)

Definition

- Cystic fluid collection within the hymen

Treatment

- Remove if symptomatic
- Perform removal under general anesthesia. Use electrocautery (i.e. needlepoint bovie). Suture base using 4-0 absorbable suture
- Postoperative care as with an imperforate hymen

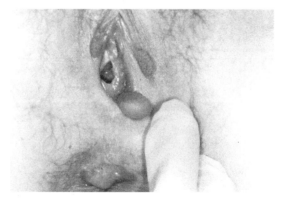

FIGURE 24.11   Hymenal cyst.

BIBLIOGRAPHY

Berenson AB, Grady JJ. A longitudinal study of hymenal development from 3-9 years of age. J Pediatr. 2002; 140:600–607.
Heger AH, Ticson L, Guerra, et al. Appearance of the genitalia in girls selected for nonabuse: review of hymenal morphology and nonspecific findings. J Pediatr Adolesc Gynecol. 2002; 15:27–35
Kerns D, McCann D, Child Abuse Atlas, EvidentiaLearning.com

25

Labial Disorders

Chelsea A. Kebodeaux and Jennifer E. Dietrich

ABSCESS

Key Points

- Labial abscesses (see Chapter 8, "Bartholin's Abscess" for discussion of glandular abscesses) originate in the skin and may result from some type of trauma (e.g. shaving, hair removal, piercing, damage to hair follicle) or exposure to MRSA
- Most labial abscesses are treated with incision and drainage +/– antibiotics
- Infection typically polymicrobial and often MRSA
- Noninfectious labial masses are mostly cystic or benign tumors
- Physical examination and laboratory and imaging studies will assist with evaluation of non-infectious labial masses to determine if observation is recommended or excision/biopsy is needed

Diagnosis

History

- Pubertal development
- Onset, duration, and change in size of mass over time
- Any associated pain, tenderness, erythema, drainage, or fever
- Review history for trauma or sexual abuse, previous labial/groin abscess, disorder of sexual or pubertal development, neurofibromatosis, inflammatory bowel disease, or dermatologic conditions
- Screen for Crohn's disease (review any gastrointestinal complaints, see Chapter 59, "Vulvar Disorders")

Physical Examination

- Evaluate vital signs for fever, hemodynamic stability, weight, and growth
- Perform thorough skin examination (noting any skin conditions, café-au-lait spots) and examine buccal mucosa for lesions
- Examine external genitalia and note location, size, color, tenderness, fluctuance, surrounding edema/induration, discharge, reducibility, and quality of mass

DOI: 10.1201/9781003039235-25

Management

Mainstay of treatment is incision and drainage (I&D) and should be performed in setting of

- Abscess >2 cm
- Failure of conservative treatment
- Systemic illness
- Risk factors for treatment failure (known or suspected MRSA carrier, immunosuppression, history of recurrent infection)

Conservative treatment (warm compresses or Sitz baths 3–4 times daily) can be used for abscess <2 cm with none of the above criteria

Can consider local anesthesia (EMLA® cream to skin (see Chapter 6, "Anesthetics in Pediatric Adolescent Populations") or local infiltration of lidocaine) in case of

- Older or more cooperative patient
- Abscess <5 cm
- Ability to achieve adequate exposure and debridement

General anesthesia should be used in case of

- Younger or uncooperative patient
- Abscess >5 cm
- Concern abscess may extend to another anatomic compartment

Incision and Drainage

- Perform incision in dorsal lithotomy position in the thinnest portion of the abscess (where it "points")
- Make incision large enough to place hemostat into abscess cavity
- Send drainage for Gram stain, aerobic and anaerobic culture, and susceptibility testing
- Drain and irrigate extensively, use hemostat to break up any loculations
- Make a separate stab incision with an 11 blade at the most superior margin of abscess and the most inferior margin then tie either a vessel loop or small caliber penrose drain through these openings to itself (see Figure 25.1)
  - Just as effective in maintaining the opening and allowing continued drainage as wet to dry dressing, but less painful to patient
- Have patient return to office within 5–7 days for removal of loop or drain

Antibiotics should be given if

- Treating conservatively (either initially or without improvement after 48 hours)
- After I&D if
  - Abscess >5 cm
  - Unable to drain completely
  - Abscess extends into another compartment
  - Extensive/rapidly progressing surrounding cellulitis
  - Suspicion for MRSA
  - Systemic infection

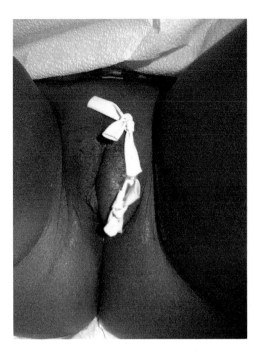

FIGURE 25.1 Drainage of labial abscess using penrose drain.

- Immunocompromised
- Recurrent abscess

Abscesses are typically polymicrobial (primarily *Staphylococcus aureus, streptococcus, Escherichia coli*, Gram-negative enteric microbes, or anaerobes).

Start with IV antibiotics if requires hospitalization or <5 years old

- Clindamycin 30–40 mg/kg per day IV in 3–4 doses
- Vancomycin 40–60 mg/kg per day IV in 4 doses (high dose only with severe illness)

After IV treatment or if requires only oral antibiotics, complete 7- to 10-day course with

- Trimethoprim-sulfamethoxazole 8–12 mg/kg per day in 3–4 doses
- Clindamycin 30–40 mg/kg per day in 3–4 doses
- Doxycycline 2–4 mg/kg per day in 1–2 doses

LABIAL ADHESIONS

Key Points

- Typically this is an asymptomatic condition but may present with genitourinary complaints
- Underlying cause may be related to vulvar inflammation in a hypoestrogenic environment, can also be caused by genital trauma
- Asymptomatic patients can be managed conservatively with observation until puberty
- Symptomatic patients may be treated with topical therapy (estrogen and/or steroid cream) or surgical separation

Definition

- Fusion of the labia minora in the midline, also known as labial agglutination
- Typically presents as a prepubertal condition with peak incidence 13–23 months of age

Diagnosis

History

- Often asymptomatic
- May have prior history with recurrence or persistence for several months
- If symptomatic may complain of
  - Abnormal voiding
  - Postvoid urinary dribbling
  - Vulvovaginitis
  - Urinary tract infections
  - Urinary retention
  - Dysuria

Physical Examination

- Perform gentle labial traction to evaluate
- Labial adhesions will appear as midline, linear tissue that is clear to gray and fibrotic (referred to as the raphe) extending from posterior fourchette anteriorly to the clitoral hood
- Partial adhesions typically occur posteriorly

Rule out other conditions such as

- Urogenital sinus
- Congenital absence of vagina
- Transverse vaginal septum
- Imperforate hymen

Management

Asymptomatic

- Observation, optimize vulvar hygiene with daily sitz baths, avoidance of harsh soaps and lotions, proper toileting hygiene
- Can apply topical emollient such as 40% zinc oxide, petroleum jelly, lanolin ointment, or coconut oil if desired (especially prior to urination if burning is present)

If symptomatic or persist into puberty

Topical steroids
- Recommended as first-line treatment
- Betamethasone dipropionate 0.05% cream

- Apply in scant amount to raphe with Q-tip or fingertip BID for 4–6 weeks, can apply gentle pressure for labial traction to promote separation
- Resolution in 68% of girls who had failed estrogen cream, may also have decreased recurrence risk compared to estrogen
- *Side effects*: Erythema, pruritis, folliculitis, and skin atrophy

Topical estrogens

- Conjugated estrogen vaginal cream or estradiol (0.01%) vaginal cream
- Apply in scant amount to raphe with Q-tip or fingertip BID for 2–6 weeks, use labial traction as above
- Resolution in 50–89% of patients
- *Side effects*: Erythema or hyperpigmentation of vulva, irritation, and breast budding

Manual separation

- Reserve for patients with urinary obstructive symptoms or urinary tract infections
- *Topical anesthetic*: Apply EMLA® cream (prilocaine 2.5%/lidocaine 2.5% combination cream) for 30 minutes or lidocaine jelly 2% for 5–10 minutes
- Medical sedation for patients unable to tolerate office procedure, especially children over 18 months
- Insert a lubricated or moistened Q-tip into the opening of the adhesions and apply gentle pressure along the raphe
- Postoperatively, apply estrogen cream daily or BID for 2–4 weeks between labia minora to promote healing

Recurrence

- Risk varies between 7 and 55%
- Parents should be informed of risk of recurrence
- Risk factors include:
  - Poor perineal hygiene
  - Vigorous cleansing techniques
  - Trauma
  - Recurrent genital infections
  - Persistent medical or dermatologic disorders
- Treat similarly to initial approach, conservative therapy first and can consider repeating topical therapy

LABIA MINORA ASYMMETRY/HYPERTROPHY

Key Points

- Extreme care should be taken prior to advising surgery for perceived abnormalities of the labia minora, as Federal Law 18 US Code § 116-Female Genital Mutilation (see Chapter 17, "Female Genital Mutilation") prohibits any removal of the labia minora for nonmedical indications, and labiaplasty in girls younger than 18 should only be considered under strict conditions
- Labia minora enlarge and darken during puberty and marked variation in size and enlargement or asymmetry is not generally pathologic
- Mostly asymptomatic but can present with irritation, pain with physical activity, difficulties with menstrual hygiene, or sexual intercourse

- Reassurance, education, behavior changes, and vulvar hygiene are the most important interventions
- Surgical correction (labiaplasty) is becoming more prevalent and is likely related to trends in pubic hair removal, idealized images of genital anatomy, and public awareness of cosmetic vaginal surgery

Definition

- Labia minora are two folds of hairless skin that border the vaginal vestibule, typical size of adult labia is 3–50 mm
- Labial asymmetry is common and may be seen as a normal variant
- No consensus in literature on definition of labial hypertrophy, some consider >4 cm from midline (see Figure 25.2)

Diagnosis

History

Often asymptomatic, but may have cosmetic concerns such as

- Visibility of labia through tight clothing
- Distress about appearance from adolescent
- Mother's concern that child has anatomical difference from her own anatomy due to lack of awareness of variation

If symptomatic, may complain of

- Local irritation
- Discomfort with tight clothing
- Pain with sitting or activity

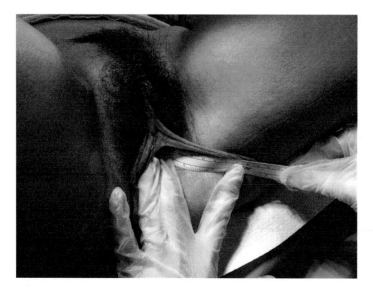

FIGURE 25.2   Labial hypertrophy.

- Menstrual or toileting hygiene issues
- Interference with sexual intercourse
- Review history for congenital malformations, vulvar trauma, infections, and inflammatory bowel disease
- Motivation for surgical intervention should be reviewed with parent and with adolescent alone
- Screen for body dysmorphic disorder and any other psychiatric conditions

Physical Examination

- Evaluate vital signs for weight and growth
- Perform routine external genital assessment, measure distance from base to the free edge of labia minora on each side
- Rule out other genital abnormalities such as labial mass, CALME (Childhood asymmetric labium majus enlargement), vulvar varicosities, skin conditions or infections, vulvar manifestations of inflammatory bowel disease

Management

Gold standard is conservative management

- Reassurance of normality for the individual
- Educate on concept of labial diversity (Petals by Nick Karras [shows vulvar photographs], The Labia Library at www.labialibrary.org.au, Great Wall of Vagina at www.greatwallofvagina.co.uk)
- Discuss federal law and that surgical removal of normal anatomy is prohibited
- Vulvar hygiene/comfort measures
  - Sensitive soap
  - Use of emollients
  - Loose cotton underwear or trialing several styles to find one that is comfortable
  - Avoid pubic hair removal
- Consider counseling/psychosocial support if significant distress is present

Surgical management

- Surgical correction (labiaplasty) should only be considered in girls younger than 18 with significant congenital or traumatic malformations and/or persistent symptoms directly related to labial anatomy
- Surgical alteration of the labia that is not necessary for the health of the adolescent is a violation of US federal criminal law
- Physicians should be aware of local, state, and federal laws that affect labiaplasty

Labiaplasty surgical techniques

- *Amputation*: The free edge of the labia is trimmed down and oversewn, resulting in scarring of the free edge of the revised labia minora
- *Removal of a section*: Either wedge resection or de-epitheliazation, resulting in scar within the labia with natural margins maintained

Surgical complications include wound dehiscence, hematoma, infection, bleeding, desire for additional revision, continued growth of labia after procedure, scarring/keloid formation, loss of sensation, and sexual dysfunction or pain.

LABIAL MASSES

Key Points

- Labial abscesses are the most common labial mass
- Noninfectious labial are uncommon and differential diagnosis is extensive
- Management depends on physical examination findings

Definition and Differential Diagnosis

Labial abscesses (tender, fluctuant/pus-filled, erythematous mass) result from infection of

- Skin/hair follicle
- Wound/hematoma
- Hidradenitis suppuritiva

Noninfectious labial masses have varied etiologies including

- Gonadal remnant
- Congenital or acquired hernia (failure of the processus vaginalis to close)
  - Can contain fluid, ovary or testicle (in case of DSD)
- Vulvar varicosity
- Embryonic remnants:
  - Mesonephric (Gartner duct) cyst
  - Canal of Nuck cyst
  - Bartholin's duct cyst
  - Paraurethral cyst
  - Hymenal cyst
- Mesenchymal tumors
  - Rhabdomyoma
  - Lipoma
  - Fibroma
  - Lymphangioma
  - Neural tissue
    - Granular cell tumor
    - Neurofibromatosis
  - Hemangioma
- Malignant tumors
  - Embryonal rhabdomyosarcoma (sarcoma botryoides)
  - Endodermal sinus tumor
  - Primitive neuroectodermal tumors (PNET)
  - Squamous cell carcinoma
  - Melanoma
- Rare causes
  - Hamartoma

- Precocious puberty
- Congenital adrenal hyperplasia (CAH)

Management

Treatment depends on diagnosis

- Infectious labial mass: See ABSCESS section at the beginning of this chapter
- Noninfectious labial mass
  - If physical examination is not diagnostic, begin with soft tissue ultrasound of the labia (and pelvis if indicated) to
    - Determine solid/cystic nature of mass (may visualize peripheral follicles if an ovary)
    - Document internal anatomy
    - Screen for concomitant pelvic tumors
  - Consider pelvic MRI to define a large mass
  - In cooperative and/or older patients, may be able to use topical EMLA® (see EMLA® use, Chapter 6) then infiltrate with lidocaine to perform in-office biopsy
- Precocious puberty or ambiguous genitalia: Obtain appropriate laboratory tests for these conditions (see Chapter 3, "Ambiguous Genitalia and Differences of Sexual Development" and Chapter 44, "Puberty")
- Hernia: Surgical repair should be performed, even if fluid filled, to prevent prolapse of ovary into hernia
- Neurofibromatosis (multiple café-au-lait spots): Mass may be the earliest clinical manifestation of neurofibromatosis, which is rarely malignant, observation appropriate
- Hemangioma (see Chapter 59, "Vulvar Disorders,"), lymphangioma, leiomyoma, and lipoma may be observed and do not require intervention unless symptomatic
- If mass is detected on ultrasound but etiology is still uncertain, biopsy and/or excision of mass is indicated
- Vaginoscopy/cystoscopy can be performed at the time of surgical excision if additional masses are suspected (neurofibromas can be found in the vagina or bladder)
- For nonmalignant tumors, excision is curative
- Malignant tumors of the labia are rare in children/adolescents they often have a poor prognosis

BIBLIOGRAPHY

Bacon JL, Romano ME, Quint EH. Clinical recommendation: labial adhesions. J Pediatr Adolesc Gynecol. 2015; 28:405–409.

Breast and labial surgery in adolescents. American College of Obstetricians and Gynecologists Committee Opinion No. 686. Obstet Gynecol. 2017:129:e17–9.

Lowry DLB, Guido RS. The vulvar mass in the prepubertal child. J Pediatr Adolesc Gynecol 2000; 13:75–78.

Runacres SA, Wood PL. Cosmetic labiaplasty in an adolescent population. J Pediatr Adolesc Gynecol. 2016; 29:218–222.

26

Menstrual Suppression in Special Populations

Y. Frances Fei and Elisabeth H. Quint

Key Points

- Menstrual suppression or management in adolescents is safe and may be indicated for a variety of reasons:
  - Hygiene issues for teens with disabilities
  - Myelosuppression due to cancer treatment
  - Bleeding disorders
  - Transgender care
- The goal of menstrual suppression can include complete amenorrhea, which may be hard to obtain, versus occasional, light scheduled bleeding.
- When choosing a method, contraceptive needs are important to consider.

Evaluation

History

- Needs and goals for suppression
- Physical safety, relationship status, and need for birth control
- Menstrual patterns, premenstrual and menstrual behaviors, and associated symptoms (dysmenorrhea, change in seizure frequency)
- Expected duration of myelosuppression (for patients with oncologic diseases)
- Mental health evaluation and counseling, planned timeline of transition, desire for pubertal or menstrual suppression (for transgender or gender nonbinary patients)
- Complete medical, surgical, social, and family history

Physical Examination

- Assess vitals, general appearance, thyroid, abdomen, extremities, heart, and lungs
- Breast and pelvic exams are generally not needed unless patient has specific complaints

Laboratory Tests and Imaging

- If normal periods: No labs
- If irregular bleeding, skipping cycles: Consider pregnancy test, thyroid-stimulating hormone, prolactin, bioavailable, and/or total testosterone (see Chapter 39, "PCOS")
- If heavy menses: Complete blood count, iron studies (see Chapter 1, "Abnormal Uterine Bleeding [AUB]")

DOI: 10.1201/9781003039235-26

- If concern for bleeding disorder, significant anemia: PT/PTT, von Willebrand disease panel (see Chapter 1, "AUB")
- If strong family history of venous thromboembolic (VTE) disease: thrombophilia workup (see Chapter 12, "Contraception")
- Pelvic ultrasound (usually transabdominal) generally only needed if patient has significant dysmenorrhea to rule out obstruction

Management

- See Table 26.1 for typical rates of amenorrhea per hormonal treatment option

For adolescents with cognitive and physical disabilities

- Menstrual suppression should not be initiated prior to onset of menses
- Establish goals: Complete amenorrhea, suppression of behavior changes or catamenial epilepsy, contraception
- Establish realistic expectations: It may take several methods and up to a year to achieve amenorrhea
- Hygiene concerns: For patients unable to tolerate pads, have difficulty maintaining hygiene, or play with body fluids, consider "period underwear." These look and feel like normal underwear but have an extra absorbent (often charcoal) layer to soak up menstrual blood instead of needing pads or tampons (e.g. Thinx®, Bambody®).
- If dysmenorrhea: Treat with nonsteroidal anti-inflammatory drugs (NSAIDs) (liquid form available for ibuprofen and naproxen)
- If periods affect quality of life (hygiene concerns, associated symptoms, etc.), consider hormonal management (see Chapter 12, "Contraception," for more detailed prescribing)
  - Continuous combined hormonal methods (CHC)
    - Oral contraceptive pills (OCP): Recommend monophasic 30–35 mcg estradiol, consider chewables
    - Extended cycling to decrease bleeding frequency (take pills in continuous fashion skipping placebo pills until breakthrough bleeding, then stop pills for 4 days and restart regardless of bleeding at that time)
    - Enzyme-inducing antiepileptic drugs may decrease serum levels of CHC, whereas lamotrigine levels are decreased by CHC
    - No data on VTE risk in patients with immobility concerns, assess other risk factors for VTE; however, less overall risk with progesterone-only options
  - Progestin methods
    - Oral progestins: Norethindrone (0.35 mg orally/day), medroxyprogesterone 10–20 mg orally/day, norethindrone acetate (2.5–15 mg orally/day), drospirenone (4 mg orally/day).
      Note, start at lowest doses and titrate up: contraception not established for all methods
    - Injectable depo medroxyprogesterone acetate (DMPA)
      - 150 mg/dose or subcutaneous 104 mg/dose, usually every 12–13 weeks
      - May need to alter frequency to less than 12 weeks if persistent breakthrough bleeding
      - Bone density concerns with long-term use
        - Calcium (1200–1500 mg/day) and vitamin D (600–1000 IU/day) supplementation
        - Consider bone density testing after years of suppression
        - No data on additional risks with immobility

- – Weight gain may be problematic for caregivers to perform activities of daily living (ADLs) and patients who transfer themselves
  - – Levonorgestrel IUD (52-mg dose provides most suppression and less bleeding)
    - – Often placed under anesthesia
    - – Does not suppress ovarian cyclicity and may not assist with catamenial symptoms or behavior changes (unless due to dysmenorrhea)
- • Surgical management
  - – Endometrial ablation and hysterectomy not recommended in young women, especially not as initial treatment.
  - – In many states, court approval is required for a minor or adult patient with cognitive delay to have procedures that affect fertility.

For adolescents with bleeding disorders

- • Establish goals: Complete suppression versus lighter, less frequent cycles; contraception
- • A combination of hormonal and nonhormonal options may be needed
- • Co-management with hematologist recommended
- • CHC: OCP, transdermal patch, vaginal ring
  - • Prevention of hemorrhagic cysts
  - • Extended cycling to decrease bleeding frequency
- • Progestin methods
  - • Oral progestins (see above):
    - – Starting dose is dependent on severity of bleeding and urgency of suppression
    - – Contraception not established for all methods
  - • Injectable DMPA
    - – Risk for intramuscular hematoma
    - – Emphasize weight-bearing exercise, calcium, and vitamin D supplementation
  - • Levonorgestrel IUD
    - – Consider prophylactic hemostatic agent (tranexamic acid, desmopressin, aminocaproic acid) prior to placement, consult with hematologist
    - – Does not suppress ovulation, may not prevent associated hemorrhagic cysts
- • Nonhormonal options
  - • Iron supplementation (60–120 mg every other day) and/or dietary increase in iron
  - • Consider using hemostatic agent (tranexamic acid, desmopressin, aminocaproic acid) for 3–5 days during cycle

For adolescents with oncologic disease

- • Establish goals: Menstrual suppression for thrombocytopenia due to cancer treatments, contraception
- • Caution with use of estrogen due to increased risk of thromboembolism
- • See Chapter 30, "Oncology Care and Gynecologic Concerns," for treatment options

For transgender or gender nonbinary patients

- • Establish goals: Suppression of menses, suppression of pubertal changes, contraception
- • See Chapter 51, "Transgender and Gender Diverse Care" for treatment options

TABLE 26.1

Amenorrhea Rates with Hormonal Treatment

	Type	Amenorrhea at 12 Months
Combined hormonal contraceptives	COC (30–35 mcg estradiol)	80%
	Vaginal ring	80%
	Transdermal patch	Not recommended[a]
Progestin only	Norethindrone 35 mcg	10%
	Norethindrone acetate 5 mg	76%
	IM Depot medroxyprogesterone 150 mg/mL	68%
	SubQ medroxyprogesterone 104mg/0.65mL	57%
	Etonogestrel implant	20%
	Levonorgestrel 52 mg	20%
	Levonorgestrel 19.5 mg	12%
	Levonorgestrel 13.5 mg	6%

Note: Amenorrhea rates based on product reporting.

[a] Not recommended for routine use continuously due to increased risk of thromboembolism.

BIBLIOGRAPHY

Hillard P. Menstrual suppression: current perspectives. Int J Womens Health. 2014; 6:631–637.

Hodax J, Wagner J, Sackett-Taylor A, Rafferty J, Forcier M. Medical options for care of diverse and transgender youth. J Pediatr Adolesc Gynecol. 2020; 33:3–9.

Options for prevention and management of menstrual bleeding in adolescent patients undergoing cancer treatment. ACOG committee opinion number 817. American College of Obstetricians and Gynecologists. Obstetrics Gynecol. 2021; 137:e7–e14.

Pradhan S, Gomez-Lobo V. Hormonal contraceptives, IUDs, GnRH analogues and testosterone: menstrual suppression in special adolescent populations. J Pediatr Adolesc Gynecol. 2019; 32:S23–S29.

Presky KO, Kadir RA. Women with inherited bleeding disorders – challenges and strategies for improved care. Thromb Res. 2020; 196:569–578. Doi: 10.1016/j.thromres.2019.07.004

27

Menstruation

Kimberly Huhmann

Key Points

- The average age of menarche is between 12 and 13 years
- Menarche typically occurs about 2 years after thelarche (breast budding) with range of 1–3 years
- Almost every girl has experience menarche by age 16

Normal Menstruation

In adolescents, the initial menstrual cycles (1–3 years after menarche) are more varied in interval than adult menstrual cycles because of the immature hypothalamic pituitary ovarian (HPO) axis.

The first 1–3 years of menstrual is a progesterone-deficient and estrogen-dominant state meaning cycles can be irregular but still considered normal.

By 3 years after menarche, 95% of periods are ovulatory (regular).

Even during this time of development

- The first day of a period occurs every 21–45 days
- Bleeding lasts 7 days or less
- Pad and tampon use
  - Six pads/regular tampons or less in a day
  - Four super tampons or less in a day
  - Heavier than expected bleeding may warrant an evaluation (see Chapter 1, "Abnormal Uterine Bleeding")
    - Using more products than listed above
    - Changing every 2–3 hours due to saturation
    - Flooding during the day or overnight
    - Passing blood clots larger than a quarter
- Cramping is common especially as cycles become ovulatory
  - NSAIDs and heat should provide adequate relief (see Chapter 14, "Dysmenorrhea")
    - Ibuprofen 600–800 mg every 6–8 hours starting the day before menses through the first 2–3 days of bleeding
  - Missing school because of cramping pain is considered out of the ordinary and should be evaluated

DOI: 10.1201/9781003039235-27

Tools to Track Menstruation

Providers should encourage adolescents and guardians to track menstrual cycles.

Identifying menstrual abnormalities during the adolescent years may help detect health conditions typically undiagnosed until adulthood.

There are numerous phone applications and paper charts that can be utilized to track period frequency, length, heaviness, and pain, can be found at Center for Young Women's Health: https://youngwomenshealth.org/wp-content/uploads/2014/08/Endometriosis-My-Symptom-Tracker.pdf.

BIBLIOGRAPHY

Graham RA, Davis JA, Corrales-Medina FF, The adolescent with menorrhagia: diagnostic approach to a suspected bleeding disorder, Pediatr Rev. 2018, 39 (12) 588–600. DOI: https://doi.org/10.1542/pir.2017-0105

Loveless M. Normal pubertal development and the menstrual cycle as a vital sign. In Sanfilippo JS, Lara-Torre, Gomez -Lobo (Eds) *Sanfilippo's Textbook of Pediatric and Adolescent Gynecology* (2nd ed.) (CRC Press, Boca Raton, FL, 2020), pp. 1–10.

Menstruation in girls and adolescents: using the menstrual cycle as a vital sign. ACOG Committee Opinion No. 651. American College of Obstetricians and Gynecologists. Obstet Gynecol. 2015;126(6):1328.

Pitts SAB, Gordon CM. The physiology of Puberty. In Emans SJ, Laufer MR, DiVasta AD (Eds) *Emans, Laufer and Goldstein's Pediatric and Adolescent Gynecology* (Wolters Kluwer, 2020), pp. 35–45.

28

Molluscum Contagiosum

Kaiane Habeshian and Kalyani Marathe

Definition

A common cutaneous viral infection caused by a poxvirus, which results in classic firm, waxy, dome-shaped, umbilicated lesions of the epidermis, that is spread by skin-to-skin contact with an infected person or material (e.g. clothing, towel).

Key Points

- Highly transmissible via autoinoculation or skin-to-skin contact, casual contact, fomite spread
- In adolescents often seen spread via shaving in vulvar area
- Usually a self-limited infection
- In immunocompromised patients, can be severely disfiguring and intractable

Differential Diagnosis

- Genital warts
- Atopic dermatitis
- Herpes simplex
- Herpes zoster

Diagnosis

History

- Single or multiple discrete painless papules
  - Lesions can be anywhere on the body, more likely to be on the extremities and can spread to vulva
  - Often pruritic
  - May spontaneously resolve
- May have bacterial superinfection
- Lack of systemic symptoms
- Patient/parent may recall contact with infected person – incubation period of about 2–6 weeks
- For lesions limited to the vulva without history of preexisting lesions elsewhere, ask about sexual abuse/consensual sexual contact

DOI: 10.1201/9781003039235-28

Physical Examination

- Well-defined pearly white or pink dome-shaped papules 2–6 mm in diameter with central umbilication that may occur anywhere on the body; predilection for existing eczema
- Beneath the umbilicated center is a white creamy core that appears cord-like if extracted
- Older lesions may become crusted and develop surrounding dermatitis as the body fights off the virus; may resolve with atrophic "chickenpox" like scars or hyperpigmentation
- Occasionally may become large, painful, inflamed; usually not true infection but rather the "beginning of the end" sign
- In immunocompromised patients, lesions are more widespread, larger, and may appear atypical
- In children, look for molluscum on other body parts as often autoinoculated to anogenital region
- In sexually active teens, check for other sexually transmitted diseases (chlamydia and gonorrhea)

Laboratory Tests

- Diagnosis usually clinical due to classic appearance
  - If diagnosis is uncertain, can examine contents with light microscopy:
    - Apply topical numbing medication for 10 minutes, clean with alcohol wipe, curette the molluscum, place contents on glass slide, apply KOH solution
    - Look for ovoid viral inclusion bodies termed Henderson-Paterson bodies
- Biopsy is not needed unless presentation is atypical (e.g. in immunocompromised patient)

Management

Disease is usually self-limited (often 1–2 years, may last 4 years)

- Observation/Conservative management is often treatment of choice, especially in younger children, but adolescents will not often be comfortable with waiting
  - Avoid picking/scratching, use moisturizer to repair skin barrier, sparse use of hydrocortisone ointment as needed for itching

Medical/Alternative therapies

- Quality evidence for most treatment modalities is lacking; risk of side effects is greater in the anogenital region
- There are no United States Food and Drug Administration (FDA)-approved treatments for molluscum
- Curettage or enucleate the central plug of lesion: for those who desire immediate removal or have only a few lesions
  - May apply EMLA® cream (see EMLA® use, Chapter 6, Anesthetics in the PAG populations) before curettage
- Imiquimod 5% cream: Immunomodulatory
  - Topical imiquimod is commonly used, but unpublished randomized controlled trials demonstrate lack of efficacy
  - Erythema at lesion is a positive response
  - Side effects include irritation, burning, flu-like symptoms, and leukopenia
  - Can cause significant erosion/irritation to vulvar epithelium

- Side effects may be more severe in prepubertal child
  - Apply test dose with a cotton-tipped swab to one lesion first week of therapy and then reevaluate before slowly extending area of treatment
- Decrease frequency of use if severe irritation occurs
- Treatment regiment
  - Adolescent: Apply tiny amount over molluscum at bedtime and rub in, wash off in the morning. Repeat 3×/week for 6–12 weeks
  - Pediatric/early adolescent: use once/week to twice/week
- Cantharidin: Stimulates breakdown of keratinocyte adhesion
  - Currently banned by the FDA in the United States; however, pure cantharidin and flexible collodion can be purchased in the premeasured amounts to be combined for use to treat (see Epstein 2001)
  - Adult (adolescent)/pediatric regiment
    - Apply sparingly with a wooden toothpick or the blunt wooden end of a cotton-tipped applicator to each lesion, avoiding contact with normal skin
    - Have patient sit still and wait 5 minutes to allow cantharidin to completely dry. Maximum treatment to 20 lesions per visit
    - Wash off in 4–6 hours or sooner if severe burning/irritation or vesiculation noted
    - Follow-up/repeat therapy every 2–4 weeks
  - Can cause significant local irritation with blister; initially try on one or two lesions to test patient's sensitivity and utilize extreme caution near mucosal surfaces

Alternative medical treatments

- Cimetidine: H2 blocker with immunomodulatory effects
  - Adult (adolescent > 45 kg) dose: 1600 mg divided BID-QID
  - Pediatric dose: 30–40 mg/kg/day po divided qid (max doses as above)

Immunocompromised patients

- Seek assistance from pediatric dermatology with use of antiviral drugs
  - Cidofovir: Selective inhibitor of viral DNA
    - Topical use of 1% or 3% preparation applied to lesion then occluded with tape once daily for 5 days/week for 8 weeks
    - IV use is associated with: Renal toxicity (must prehydrate with normal saline and monitor renal function), Granulocytopenia

BIBLIOGRAPHY

Chen X, Anstey AV, Bugert JJ. Molluscum contagiosum virus infection. Lancet Infect Dis. 2013;13(10):877–888.

Dohil M, Prendiville JS. Treatment of molluscum contagiosum with oral cimetidine: clinical experience in 13 patients. Pediatr Dermatol. 1996;13:310–312.

Epstein E. Cantharidin therapy for molluscum contagiosum in children. J Am Acad Dennatol. 2001;45:638

Katz KA, Williams HC, van der Wouden JC. Imiquimod cream for molluscum contagiosum: neither safe nor effective. Pediatr Dermatol. 2018;35(2):282–283. doi:10.1111/pde.13398.

Koning S. Interventions for cutaneous molluscum contagiosum. Cochrane Database Syst Rev. 2017;5(5):CD004767. Published 2017 May 17. doi:10.1002/14651858.CD004767.pub4

van der Wouden JC, van der Sande R, Kruithof EJ, Sollie A, van Suijlekom-Smit LW, Koning S. Interventions for cutaneous molluscum contagiosum. Cochrane Database Syst Rev. 2017;5(5):CD004767.

29

Obesity

Angie Hamouie and Maggie L. Dwiggins

Key Points

- Obesity affects almost 20% of U.S. children and adolescents ages 2–19 years
  - More common in the black (22%) and Hispanic (25.8%) population as compared to the white (14.1%) and Asian (11%) population
  - More prevalent in low-income groups and in children from families with low level of education (https://www.cdc.gov/obesity/data/childhood.html)
- Childhood obesity is a serious problem associated with long-term morbidities including
  - Gynecologic issues (e.g. anovulation, PCOS)
  - Nonalcoholic fatty liver disease (may have issues metabolizing hormonal contraceptives)
  - Depression
  - Hypertension
  - Type 2 diabetes
  - Coronary heart disease
  - Stroke
  - Gallbladder disease
  - Sleep apnea
  - Respiratory problems
  - Orthopedic conditions (e.g. slipped capital femoral epiphysis, tibia vara, genu valgum, musculoskeletal pain, increased susceptibility to fractures)
- Evaluation of obesity in childhood offers the best hope for preventing disease progression and associated morbidities; genetic and hormonal causes, while rare, warrant consideration
- Has a negative impact on the self-esteem of children and adolescents, with potential implications for long-term happiness and success in life
- Directed sessions that emphasize healthy eating and exercise habits for children and their families may have lasting effects on the lifestyle of these patients
- Pharmacologic and surgical options may be considered in patients with severe or refractory cases

Definition (Table 29.1)

Body mass index (BMI) is defined as weight in kilograms divided by height in meters squared.

- Inexpensive tool to identify adolescents at risk of weight-related diseases.
- The standard BMI weight-status categories used for adults are not dependent on age or sex and, therefore, cannot be used in the interpretation of BMI in adolescents.

DOI: 10.1201/9781003039235-29

TABLE 29.1

Weight Categories in Adults

Overweight	BMI greater than or equal to 85th percentile to less than 95th percentile
Class I	BMI greater than or equal to 95th percentile to less than 120% of the 95th percentile
Class II	BMI greater than or equal to 120% to less than 140% of the 95th percentile, or BMI greater than or equal to 35, whichever is lower
Class III	BMI greater than or equal to 140% of the 95th percentile, or BMI greater than or equal to 40, whichever is lower

- To account for normal sex-specific changes in weight, height, and adiposity up to the age of 19 years, BMI should be interpreted after it is plotted on growth charts to determine BMI-for-age and BMI-for sex percentile (https://nccd.cdc.gov/dnpabmi/calculator.aspx).
- Does not directly measure adiposity; therefore, it is not accurate in predicting health risk in athletic adolescents with increased muscle mass OR in sedentary adolescents with reduced muscle mass.

Overweight is defined as a BMI at or above the 85th percentile.

- Obesity is a BMI at or above the 95th percentile.
- Severe obesity is a BMI greater than or equal to the 99th percentile for age.
- Extreme obesity has been used to describe adolescents who are at or above 120% of the sex-specific 95th percentile for age.
- While the definitions of obesity and severe obesity are listed, when documenting in patient record, consider using obesity in terms of BMI percentile rather than morbid obesity terms.

Differential Diagnosis

Endogenous, Iatrogenic, and Environmental Factors Causing Obesity

Endogenous Causes

- Either hormonal or genetic defect
- Affects a very small percentage of children
- Can be inferred by a careful history and physical exam
- Characterized by growth failure; usually at or under the 5th percentile of height for age or significant drop off from the child's previous growth curve
- Hypothyroidism is the most frequent defect
  - Diagnosed with elevated thyroid-stimulating hormone (TSH) and/or low free thyroxine level
  - Associated with constipation, cold intolerance, and dry skin
- Hypercortisolism (Cushing's syndrome)
  - If highly suspected, should undergo at least two highly sensitive screening tests and should have at least two different, unequivocally abnormal results:
    - Late-night salivary cortisol
      - Cortisol levels should nadir in the evening, however do not in those with Cushing's syndrome
      - Lack of suppression of late-night salivary cortisol is considered a positive test but specific cutoff levels have not been determined
    - 24-hour urine free cortisol
      - Basal urinary cortisol excretion >3× the upper limit of normal (depending on the assay) is considered a positive test

    – Dexamethasone suppression test

      – Give 1 mg or 0.3 mg/m^2 of dexamethasone orally at 11:00 pm and draw a plasma cortisol at 8:00 am

      – A value of

          <1.8 mcg/dL rules out Cushing's syndrome

          1.8–7.2 mcg/dL makes Cushing's syndrome unlikely

          >7.2 mcg/dL makes Cushing's syndrome likely

- Other causes include growth hormone deficiency and pseudohypoparathyroidism type 1a (aka Albright hereditary osteodystrophy)

Iatrogenic Causes

- Antidepressants (e.g. MAOIs, TCAs, SSRIs, SNRIs)
- Antipsychotics (e.g. first generation and atypical antipsychotics)
- Diabetes medications (e.g. insulin, sulfonylureas, thiazolidinediones, meglitinides)
- Glucocorticoides (e.g. prednisone)
- Hormonal agents, especially progestins (e.g. medroxyprogesterone)
- Neurologic and mood-stabilizing agents (e.g. lithium, carbamazepine, gabapentin, valproate)
- Antihistamines (e.g. cyproheptadine)
- Alpha blockers (e.g. terazosin)
- Beta-blockers (e.g. propranolol)

Environmental Causes

- Consumption of sugar-sweetened beverages
- Increased screen time (e.g. video gaming, television watching)
- Irregular and shortened sleep schedule
- Decreased activity

Evaluation

Office Evaluation

- Initial visit and yearly, measure height and weight and graph on age-appropriate curve (see Figures 29.1–29.3)
- At each visit, check blood pressure with age appropriately sized blood pressure cuff; if abnormal, refer to primary care provider

At each yearly visit

- Evaluation for cardiac disease risk factors: Family history of early (less than age 55) cardiovascular disease, high cholesterol, hypertension, and type 1 or 2 diabetes; cigarette smoking or smoke exposure; level of physical activity
- Evaluation for orthopedic issues: Back or extremity problems
- Evaluation for dermatologic problems: Monilia, acanthosis nigricans in axillary and perineal intertriginous areas
- Evaluation for depression and other emotional issues (PHQ-9 form – see Chapter 13, "Depression")
- Evaluation for menstrual disorders
- If abnormal finding, refer to appropriate specialist for further evaluation and management

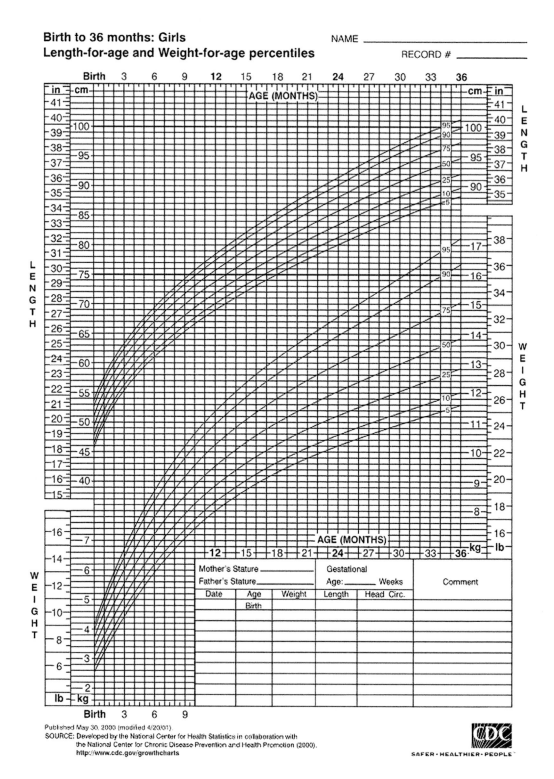

FIGURE 29.1   Girls' length-for-age and weight-for-age growth curves: birth to 36 months (5th–95th percentile). (From https://www.cdc.gov/growthcharts/data/set1clinical/cj41l018.pdf.)

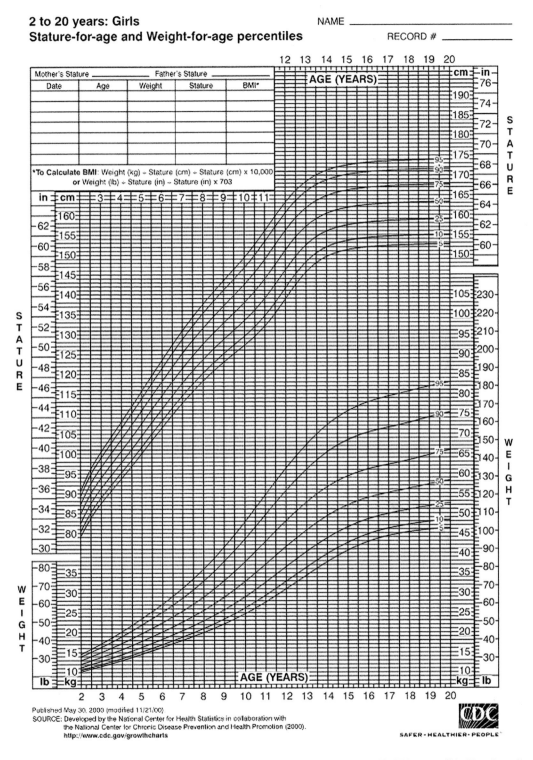

FIGURE 29.2 Girls' stature-for-age and weight-for-age growth curves: 2–20 years (5th–95th percentile). (From https://www.cdc.gov/growthcharts/data/set1clinical/cj41l022.pdf.)

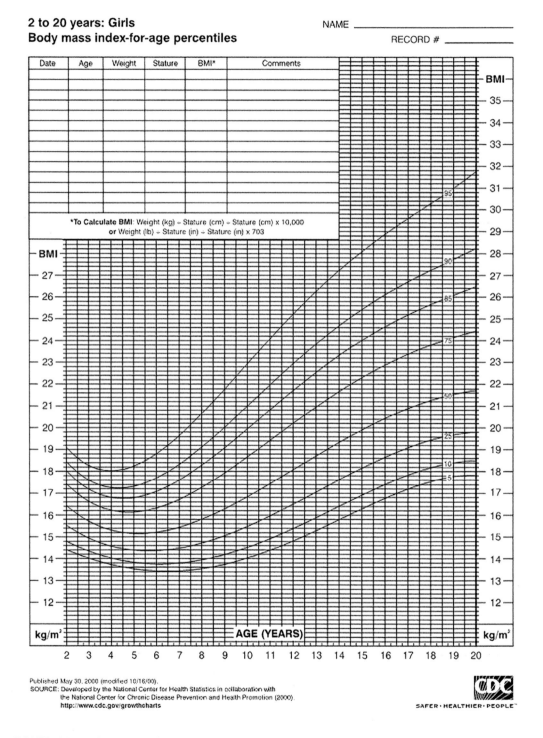

FIGURE 29.3 Body mass index for age. (From https://www.cdc.gov/growthcharts/data/set1clinical/cj41l024.pdf.)

Laboratory Tests

Lipid Screening

- No screening <2 years.
- Ages 2–8 years: No routine screening. Obese children or normal weight children with more than one risk factor for cardiovascular disease should have lipid screening performed every 1–3 years. This is done by measuring fasting lipid profile twice within a two week to three month span and average results.
- Ages 9–11 years: Universal lipid screening is recommended in *all* children within this age range, regardless of BMI or other risk factors for cardiovascular disease.
- Ages 12–16 years: Lipid screening is *not* recommended during this age range as the pubertal period causes changes in lipid levels that decrease the sensitivity and specificity of screening.
- Ages 17–21 years: All adolescents in this age range should undergo lipid screening once. For those with obesity or other risk factors for cardiovascular disease, guidelines are the same as for children ages 2–8 years, as outlined earlier.

Consider screening at initial visit for hyperinsulinemia and glucose intolerance and as indicated in future visits; if abnormal, refer to primary care provider or consult with pediatric endocrinology.

Intervention (Management)

- Early intervention is critical to prevent progression of disease and establish healthy habits
- Parents play a pivotal role in the success of these interventions (see Moran 1999 for tips for parents and components of a successful weight loss plan)

Role of Pharmacologic and Surgical Interventions in Treatment of Obesity

Medications

- Orlistat (tetrahydrolipstatin) 120 mg 3× per day
  - Lipase inhibitor that blocks fat absorption
  - The only weight loss medication FDA approved for adolescents ≥ age 12 years
  - Associated with a mean BMI reduction of $0.7–0.85 \text{ kg/m}^2$
  - Adverse effects include
    - Malabsorption of fat-soluble vitamins and therefore a multivitamin that includes vitamins A, D, E, and K should be prescribed concomitantly
    - Fecal urgency and soiling, which may limit its tolerability by adolescents
- Metformin
  - Biguanide insulin-sensitizing agent FDA approved for the treatment of type 2 diabetes mellitus in children of age ≥10
  - **Not** FDA approved for weight loss, however may play a role in BMI reduction in nondiabetic children
- Octreotide
  - Somatostatin analog that suppresses insulin secretion
  - Has been used in children with hypothalamic obesity
  - Has been associated with weight stabilization and BMI reduction
  - Not FDA approved and should be considered investigational

Surgery

- Weight loss surgery can be considered in adolescents with severe obesity and additional criteria
  - BMI >35 with severe comorbidities
  - Type 2 DM
  - Moderate-to-severe obstructive sleep apnea
  - Severe nonalcoholic fatty liver disease
  - Pseudotumor cerebri
  - BMI >40 with one mild comorbidity:
    Hypertension, dyslipidemia, mild obstructive sleep apnea, mild nonalcoholic fatty liver disease, prediabetes, panniculitis, urinary incontinence, venous stasis disease, weight-related arthropathies, impairment in activities of daily living, severe psychosocial distress
- Additional requirements
  - Tanner stages 4 and 5 pubic development and completion of 95% of anticipated growth
  - Improvement refractory to 6 months of organized, medically supervised attempts at weight loss
  - Underlying psychiatric conditions are stable
  - Evidence of maturity and understanding of risks/benefits of surgery
  - Able to provide informed consent
  - Demonstrated adherence to follow-up visits
  - Demonstrates understanding of short- and long-term lifestyle changes that will be required postoperatively
  - Supportive social environment
  - Willingness to avoid pregnancy for 1 year after surgery
- Types of weight loss surgery include
  - Roux-en-Y gastric bypass
    - Combined restrictive and malabsorptive procedure
    - Associated with the most robust and long-term reduction in BMI in the adolescent population (mean reduction 17.2 kg/m^2) at 12 months post surgery
    - Comorbidity resolution rates: 67–100%
  - Adjustable gastric band
    - Restrictive procedure with implantable device
    - Associated with 10.4 kg/m^2 reduction of BMI at 12 months
    - Long-term complications: Erosion of device in one-third of the patients, requiring surgical removal
  - Vertical sleeve gastrectomy
    - Restrictive but not malabsorptive procedure
    - Does not require implantable device
    - BMI reduction of 14.5 kg/m^2 at 12 months
    - Has more benefits/less risk than Roux-en-Y and gastric band with similar results; now used more frequently in adolescents

Gynecologic Issues of the Obese Adolescent

Abnormal uterine bleeding (amenorrhea, heavy menstrual bleeding; see Chapter 1, "AUB")

- Can result from increased free testosterone
- Increased risk of eventual endometrial cancer if this unopposed estrogen state untreated

Polycystic ovarian syndrome (see Chapter 39, "PCOS")

- Even if uncertain that patient has true diagnosis of PCOS, treatment is warranted
- Use of combination oral contraceptive pills to regulate menses and normalize androgens can be effective

Contraceptive concerns (see Chapter 12, "Contraception")

- Oral contraceptive pills, DMPA, contraceptive implant, intrauterine devices – Not contraindicated in the obese patient
- Contraceptive patch (150 mcg/day norelgestromin and 35 mcg/day ethinyl estradiol) contraindicated in BMI >30 or weight >90 kg due to increased risk venous thrombotic event in obese patients
- Emergency contraceptive – May be less effective with the exception of the copper intrauterine device, but no safety concerns exist

BIBLIOGRAPHY

Expert Panel on Integrated Guidelines for Cardiovascular Health and Risk Reduction in Children and Adolescents, National Heart, Lung, and Blood Institute. Expert panel on integrated guidelines for cardiovascular health and risk reduction in children and adolescents: summary report. Pediatrics. 2011; 128 Suppl 5: S213.

Moran R. Evaluation and treatment of childhood obesity. Am Fam Physician. 1999;59:861–868.

Obesity in adolescents. American College of Obstetricians and Gynecologists Committee Opinion No. 714. Obstet Gynecol. 2017; 130: e127–e140.

Skinner AC, Perrin EM, Moss LA, Skelton JA. Cardiometabolic risks and severity of obesity in children and young adults. N Engl J Med. 2015; 373: 1307–1317.

Wickham EP, DeBoer MD. Evaluation and treatment of severe obesity in childhood. Clin Pediatr (Ohila). 2015; 45(10): 929–940.

30

Oncology Care and Gynecologic Concerns

Maggie L. Dwiggins

Key Points

- Many cancer treatments, especially those involving alkylating agents, bone marrow transplant (BMT), or pelvic radiation, can damage reproductive function — Early referral for fertility preservation prior to treatment is necessary.
- Menstrual disorders such as heavy bleeding and amenorrhea are common during cancer treatment.
- Adolescents undergoing cancer treatment should not be assumed to be abstinent; sexual health counseling and contraception if needed should be provided.
- About 75% of pediatric cancer survivors will experience at least on late effect — Endocrine dysfunction, infertility, breast cancer, ovarian cancer, sexual dysfunction.
- Cancer treatment may have an immediate or delayed effect on reproductive function, and the gynecologist must be prepared to manage puberty induction, hormone replacement therapy, and fertility preservation along with sexual dysfunction and chronic vulvovaginal disease.
- A multidisciplinary approach to cancer treatment and survival is encouraged.

Specific Concerns

Fertility Preservation/Reproduction

Many treatments for childhood cancers result in gonadal damage (see Chapter 18, "Fertility Preservation")

- Initial referral prior to start of treatment is optimal
- Due to rapidly changing evidence and practices, referral to specialist in oncofertility is preferred
- For the adolescent female, oocyte/embryo and ovarian tissue cryopreservation are standard of care
- For the prepubertal girl, only ovarian tissue cryopreservation is an option
- Even if menses initially returns after treatment, some may experience primary ovarian insufficiency (POI) several years later
  - Patients should track menses, and if irregular, proceed with evaluation of ovarian function with FSH, estradiol, AMH, ± antral follicle count

Menstrual Irregularities

Acute uterine bleeding

- Consult with oncology team to determine safety of estrogen use
- Medical management
  - Estrogen therapy
    - Combined oral contraceptives tid×7 days
    - Premarin 25 mg IV q4 hours until bleeding stops

DOI: 10.1201/9781003039235-30

- Progestin therapy
  - Medroxyprogesterone acetate 60–80 mg twice daily until bleeding stops, then taper
  - Norethindrone acetate 10–20 mg q8 hours until bleeding stops, then taper
- If poorly controlled with one therapy, try switching to other
- Consider addition of antifibrinolytics
- The use of longer acting methods (e.g. depot medroxyprogesterone acetate, intrauterine device) may be required if other methodologies fail, but the onset of action is delayed and bleeding pattern more unpredictable; may be better used in combination with shorter acting hormonal therapy
- Consider placement intrauterine foley balloon tamponade if unresponsive to medical management
- AVOID surgical approaches such as uterine artery embolization and endometrial ablation
- Maintenance therapy to prevent future bleeding as detailed below

Heavy menstrual bleeding (see Chapter 1, "AUB")

- Heavy bleeding can place patients at risk for anemia or worsen anemia already present and impact treatment
- Common in patients with platelet dysfunction or thrombocytopenia and may be difficult to manage once present; therefore, prevention may be more successful
- Use of estrogen may increase risk of thromboembolic events and should be avoided unless benefits outweigh the risks as determined with collaboration from oncology provider
- Progestin-only oral therapies
  - Medroxyprogesterone acetate 10–20 mg daily
  - Norethindrone acetate 5–15 mg daily
  - Drospirenone 4 mg daily (also provides contraception)
  - Norethindrone 0.35 mg daily (also provides contraception)
- Injection
  - Depot medroxyprogesterone acetate 150 mg IM q3 months
  - Can cause difficult to manage breakthrough bleeding and weight gain
  - Concern for bone density with long-term use, therefore, add vitamin D and calcium supplement
- Long-acting reproductive contraception (LARC)
  - Can be safely used in women with immunosuppression due to cancer treatment per World Health Organization and Centers for Disease Control
  - Levonorgestrel 52 mcg intrauterine is FDA approved for treatment of menstrual bleeding
  - Etonogestrel subdermal implant commonly associated with side effect of continued bleeding
- Gonadotropin releasing hormone (GnRH) agonist
  - Most commonly used formulation leuprolide acetate 11.25/22.5 mg IM q3 months or 3.75 mg IM monthly
  - If low platelets, make sure to hold pressure on injection site for 30 minutes to avoid hematoma formation
  - Expect transient activation of ovaries and withdrawal bleeding 2–3 weeks after first injection
  - Use in conjunction with norethindrone acetate 5 mg for bone protection and consider 1200 mg calcium supplementation
  - Side effects include vasomotor symptoms, bone density loss
  - Only to be used for ≤2 years

Amenorrhea

- Chronic disease such as cancer and various treatments may lead to transient amenorrhea
- If amenorrhea persists >1 year after completion of therapy, may require evaluation for POI (see below)
- Avoid serum screening for POI during active treatment as results may be falsely low
- Counsel that pregnancy prevention is still needed even if no regular periods

Contraception

- Cancer patients may be told that treatment will lead to infertility, and many assume that means they are unable to become pregnant
- This is an incorrect assumption, and if pregnancy is not desired, reliable contraception is needed
- Consider LARC for all sexually active adolescents (see Chapter 12, "Contraception")
  - No contraindication for IUD despite previous concerns regarding foreign body
  - Concurrent use of levonorgestrel IUD with immunosuppressants is considered safe by the Centers for Disease Control and Prevention Medical Eligibility Criteria for Contraceptive Use (CDC MEC)
  - Consider bleeding profile and low rates of amenorrhea with the etonogestrel subdermal implant and if benefits outweigh potential bleeding risks prior to insertion
- Estrogen-containing contraceptives should be avoided due to increased risk of thromboembolic events
  - Refer to the CDC MEC for more information regarding patient eligibility (see Chapter 12, "Contraception") https://www.cdc.gov/reproductivehealth/contraception/mmwr/mec/summary.html
- Counsel regarding benefits of continuous abstinence while undergoing treatment
  - Only way to guarantee avoidance of pregnancy
  - May be more susceptible to infection
  - Theoretic risk of chemotherapy exposure in partner as these agents are excreted in oral and vaginal mucous
- GnRH agonists and norethindrone acetate are NOT considered contraceptives

Sexual Dysfunction

- Screening at every annual exam at a minimum
  - Cancer treatment may negatively affect sexual activity and response due to mucositis, vulvovaginal atrophy, graft versus host disease
- Consider use of validated screening tools such as the Female Sexual Function Index
  - Questions regarding desire, arousal, lubrication, orgasm, satisfaction, and pain
  - Can diagnose global sexual dysfunction as well as specific areas
  - Score of ≤26 is diagnostic of sexual dysfunction
- Consider management with referral to sexual health specialist, encourage use of lubrication and foreplay, and add medical management when necessary
  - Topical vaginal estrogen 1 g 3× per week
  - Ospemifene 60 mg oral daily
  - Caution in patients with hormone receptor positive breast cancer

Puberty

- Treatment may alter pubertal development — Can have precocious or delayed puberty, arrest of pubertal development, or POI
- Precocious puberty is more common in those who receive more than 24 Gy of cranial radiation or are <4 years at start of radiation therapy
  - Typically central/isosexual
  - Suspicion should be high if rapid pubertal development ensues
  - Treat in conjunction with endocrinology (see Chapter 44, "Puberty")
- Delayed puberty or arrest of pubertal development may warrant hormonal induction (see Chapter 40, "POI")
- If patient is 2–5 years after treatment and no signs of pubertal development or return of menses
  - Check FSH, estradiol, and AMH
  - If abnormal, repeat in 4–6 weeks
  - If remains abnormal, treat (see Chapter 40, "POI")
  - Note ovaries may have decreased function for 1 year after completion of therapy normally, avoid excessive serum monitoring and treatment prior to 1 year

Vaginal Graft versus Host Disease (GVHD)

- Complication especially following BMT
- More likely in patients experiencing chronic oral, eye, or gastrointestinal tract graft versus host disease (GVHD)
- Symptoms can be nonspecific and are often missed
  - Dyspareunia, vaginal dryness, vaginal discharge, and vulvar pain are common presenting symptoms
  - Noted to have vulvar erythema, localized tenderness (especially over Bartholin's or Skene's glands), white/reticulated patches or plaques on labia minora, perineum, clitoral prepuce, and vestibule, sparing labia majora
  - Should be suspected in any patient with oral GVHD
- Can lead to excoriations, chronic ulceration, thickened mucosa, narrowing of introitus, or complete obliteration of introitus due to scar tissue formation
- Management
  - Examination should be conducted yearly and tailored to age, comfort level of patient, and history of sexual activity
    - Prepubertal patients-external exam may be sufficient
    - Pubertal patients
      - Genital traction on labia majora to visualize labia majora, minora, clitoris, clitoral hood
      - Use cotton swab to gently touch vulva/vestibule for pain
      - Moisten cotton swab to place into vagina to assess for vaginal length and caliber
      - If tolerable, single-digit exam can assess vaginal caliber
      - Consider use of small speculum if exam tolerated to assess vaginal walls and cervix for mucositis
      - Consider rectal exam if bimanual not possible IF need to assess for hematocolpos
  - High-potency topical steroid (clobetasol 0.05%) twice daily for 4–6 weeks
    - Monitor for response every 4 weeks and continue as needed
    - Taper to maintenance regimen of 2–3× per week

- Topical tacrolimus 0.1% ointment may be used in unresponsive cases
- Consider moderate potency steroid such as hydrocortisone acetate rectal suppositories 25 mg plus clindamycin 2% both placed intravaginally
- Vaginal stenosis can be treated with vaginal dilator treatment, emollients, local estrogen or steroids or combination
- Thin adhesions can be managed with vaginal dilators or lysis of adhesions under anesthesia with postoperative vaginal dilator use
- Stenosis unresponsive to dilator therapy requires referral to clinical centers of expertise as these cases may require tissue grafting in addition to menstrual suppression

Breast and Cervical Cancer Screening

- Previous chest irradiation leads to 13–20% increased risk of breast cancer
  - Screening should begin by age 25 or 8 years after radiation, whichever occurs last
  - Continue annually until age when screening would be stopped in general population
  - Preferred screening modality breast MRI or mammography
- Cervical cancer screening same for general population unless chronically immunosuppressed
  - Consider screening as per CDC recommendations in those immunocompromised due to HIV
  - Encourage HPV vaccination

BIBLIOGRAPHY

Debiec KE, Todd N. Gynecologic care for pediatric and adolescent patients undergoing hematopoietic stem cell transplantation. J Pediatr Adolesc Gynecol. 2021; 34:112–116.

Gynecologic issues in children and adolescent cancer patients and survivors. American College of Obstetricians and Gynecologists Committee Opinion no 747. Obstet Gynecol. 2018; 132(2):e67–e77.

Kornik RI, Rustagi AS. Vulvovaginal graft-versus-host disease. Obstet Gynecol Clin North Am. 2017; 44(3):475–492.

Mulder RL, Kremer LCM, Hudson MM, et al. Recommendations for breast cancer surveillance for female childhood, adolescent and young adult cancer survivors treated with chest radiation: a report from the International Late Effects of Childhood Cancer Guideline Harmonization Group. Lancet Oncol. 2014; 14(13):621–629.

Options for prevention and management of menstrual bleeding in adolescent patients undergoing cancer treatment. American College of Obstetricians and Gynecologists Committee Opinion no 817. Obstet Gynecol. 2021; 137(1):e7–e15.

31

Operative Care

Katherine Hayes

Key Points

- Surgical principles are similar to adults, although some alterations are needed based on patient size
- Children should be included in the preoperative process as developmentally appropriate
- Weight-based dosing must be used for intraoperative and postoperative medications

Preoperative Care

- Prior to day of surgery
  - Review the indications, risks, benefits, and alternatives of the planned procedure(s) with the patient and the family
    - Include both medical and surgical alternatives, as well as the risk of not doing surgery if applicable
    - Discuss the possible need for blood transfusion
  - Consider using visual aids including videos, diagrams, and anatomically correct dolls
  - Allow the entire family to ask their questions
  - Obtain consent from the legal guardian and assent from the patient as age and circumstances allow
- On the day before surgery
  - Consider having patients bathe the evening before surgery to decrease the risk of surgical site infection postoperatively
  - Usually patients should stop solid food 8 hours prior to surgery
  - Newer protocols may allow for consumption of clear liquids up until 2 hours prior to surgery (see also ERAS in pediatric populations, Chapter 32, "ERAS")
  - Bowel preparations are not indicated for routine gynecologic surgery but may be considered if bowel surgery is planned
- On the day of surgery
  - Consider scheduling younger patients and special needs patients earlier in the day
  - Consider involving child life services if available, especially for younger patients
  - Lab testing
    - Pregnancy testing for perimenarchal and postmenarchal patients
    - Consider complete blood count (CBC) and type and screen (T&S) if significant blood loss is expected
    - Other testing needs determined by the patient's comorbidities

Intraoperative Care

- Prevention of venous thromboembolism
  - Sequential compression devices should be used for major surgeries including laparoscopy, laparotomy, and vaginal reconstructive procedures or procedures longer than 30 minutes in duration
  - Consider heparin prophylaxis if the patient is at high risk of thromboembolism
    - Children are at lower risk of thromboembolism, so consider preoperative hematology consultation for recommendations
  - Estrogen-containing contraceptives
    - It takes 4–6 weeks for changes in prothrombotic clotting factors to disappear after stopping estrogen-containing contraceptives
    - The risk of thromboembolism must be weighed against the risk of pregnancy
- Prevention of surgical site infection
  - Abdominal surgery-skin preparation should be with alcohol-based agents unless contraindicated
  - Vaginal surgery can be betadine or chlorohexidine (<4% alcohol preparation), based on physician preference
  - Weight-based antibiotics for procedures that are clean-contaminated, most frequently cefazolin 30 mg/kg (not to exceed 2 g for patients less than 120 kg or 3 g for patients more than 120 kg)
    - Hysterectomy
    - Reconstructive vaginal surgery
    - Consider for laparotomy without entry into bowel or vagina
- If hair removal is indicated, hair should be removed with electric clippers
- Intraoperative hypothermia should be avoided
  - Operating room temperature set based on patient's needs
  - Warming blankets to prevent heat loss through exposed skin
  - Heat lamps for neonates and young infants

Examination under anesthesia

- Positioning
  - Dorsal lithotomy with boot or candy cane stirrups
    - Be sure to use the appropriate size
    - Care should be taken to position without extreme flexion and extension to prevent nerve injury
    - Bony sites should be padded to prevent nerve injury
  - Frog-legged position with or without gel rolls can be used depending on the planned procedure and the patient size
- If a thorough exam was not obtained in clinic, consider examining skin, thyroid, breasts, and abdomen
- Perform a systemic evaluation of the external genitalia (see Chapter 20, "Gynecologic Examination")
- Consider collection of genital cultures, nucleic acid amplification testing for gonorrhea/chlamydia/trichomonas, cervical and/or vaginal cytology, and vulvar and/or vaginal biopsies as appropriate

Vaginoscopy

- Positioning is the same as examination under anesthesia, as these procedures are frequently performed together
- Cystoscope or hysteroscope can be used to perform vaginoscopy; size should be based on the size of the child with 3–5 mm scopes for smaller children and 6–10 mm scopes for older patients
- Sterile saline is most frequently used as the distension media
- Gentle pressure on the labia will occlude the vaginal opening and allow for vaginal distension and visualization of the vagina and cervix

Laparoscopy

- Positioning
  - If uterine manipulation will not be performed, supine position is appropriate
  - If vaginal access is required, dorsal lithotomy position with boot stirrups should be utilized
  - Consider an orogastric tube to decompress the stomach prior to entry
  - Consider a urinary catheter to decompress the bladder prior to entry (in-dwelling or in and out)
- Entry
  - Open
  - Veress needle
  - Direct and optical direct
  - Based on surgeon's personal preferred technique
  - Open entry should be used in neonates to decrease the risk of air embolism through patent umbilical vessels
- Insufflation
  - In children under 2, the pressure should be kept to less than 10 mmHg
  - In children 2–10, use pressures between 10–12 mmHg
  - Children over 10 usually can tolerate a pressure of 15 mmHg
  - Morbidly obese patients may require higher pressures for adequate visualization, this must be balanced with the ability of anesthesia to ventilate them appropriately
- Port placement
  - Utilize the smallest ports allowable for safe completion of surgery (available sizes include 2-, 3-, 5-, 10-, 11-, 12-, and 15-mm ports)
  - Consider portless 2-mm instruments if appropriate and available to decrease the number of accessory ports needed
  - Accessory ports often need to be placed higher on the abdomen in children to allow for appropriate triangulation and surgical ergonomics
- Specimen removal
  - Small biopsies can be removed directly through a port
  - Larger specimens can be removed with a specimen retrieval bag
  - Larger specimens may require in-bag mechanical morcellation and/or extension of the incision to remove
- Port closure
  - Fascial closure required at pediatric port placement even if port <5 mm size in order to prevent postsurgical port hernia formation

Laparotomy:

- Positioning
  - Supine position unless vaginal access is needed
  - If vaginal access is required, position in dorsal lithotomy with boot stirrups
- Incision
  - Based on size and location of pathology
  - If concern for malignancy or very large adnexal masses, vertical midline incision should be utilized
- Incision closure
  - Delayed absorbable suture should be utilized for vertical midline incisions
  - Consider delayed absorbable suture for Pfannenstiel incisions as children are more active postoperatively than adults
  - Close dead space to decrease risk of seroma formation and to decrease tension on the skin closure
  - Consider skin closure with absorbable subcuticular suture to improve cosmesis

Postoperative Care

- Pain management
  - Alternate acetaminophen and a nonsteroidal anti-inflammatory for laparoscopy and laparotomy
    - Acetaminophen dosing 10–15 mg/kg every 4–6 hours (not to exceed standard adult doses)
    - Ketorolac dosing 0.5 mg/kg (intravenously) every 6 hours (not to exceed 30 mg per dose)
    - Ibuprofen dosing 5–10 mg/kg every 6 hours (not to exceed standard adult doses)
  - Narcotic should be used sparingly, but if needed prefer immediate release oxycodone (0.05–0.15 mg/kg every 4–6 hours, maximum of 5 mg per dose)
  - Refer to ERAS in pediatric populations, Chapter 32 for additional pain management modalities postoperatively (i.e. epidurals, TAP blocks, gabapentin, etc.)
- Diet
  - Patients can resume diet immediately after surgery
  - Should advance as tolerated to minimize nausea and vomiting
  - Intravenous fluids should be stopped as soon as the patient is tolerating oral liquids well
- Incision care
  - Bandages can typically be removed on postoperative day #1
  - Patient can shower on postoperative day #1
  - Typically, incisions should not be submerged in water for 2 weeks postoperatively
- Postoperative restrictions
  - Patients with 5-mm incisions or less typically will have no restrictions past 48 hours
  - Patients with 10- to 12-mm incisions should avoid lifting more than 10–15 lb for 2 weeks postoperatively
  - Patients with laparotomy incisions should avoid lifting more than 10–15 lb for 4–6 weeks postoperatively
  - Patients who can drive should avoid driving until they feel they can slam on the brakes and steer the wheel hard to avoid an accident without hesitation

- Postoperative clinic visit
  - Ask the patient how she is recovering, including any residual pain and return to normal activities
  - Examine the incisions
  - Review the procedure in detail, include pictures taken if the patient/family is interested
  - Review the pathology results if applicable
  - Discuss the next steps in management as appropriate

BIBLIOGRAPHY

ACOG Practice Bulletin No. 195: prevention of infection after gynecologic procedures. Obs Gynecol [Internet]. 2018/05/26. 2018; 131(6):e172–e1789. Available from: https://www.ncbi.nlm.nih.gov/pubmed/29794678

American College of Obstetricians and Gynecologists' Committee on Gynecologic Practice. Perioperative pathways: enhanced recovery after surgery. Obstet Gynecol [Internet]. 2018; 132(3):120–30. Available from: https://www.acog.org/-/media/Committee-Opinions/Committee-on-Gynecologic-Practice/co750.pdf?dmc=1&ts=20180822T2127336408

Hewitt G. Pediatric and Adolescent Gynecologic Surgery. In Handa VL, Van Le L, eds. *TeLinde's Operative Gynecology* (12th ed., pp. 732–745). Wolters Kluwer, 2020.

Practice Bulletin No. 84: prevention of deep vein thrombosis and pulmonary embolism: correction. Obs Gynecol [Internet]. 2016/11/29. 2016; 127(1):166. Available from: https://www.ncbi.nlm.nih.gov/pubmed/27892904

32

Operative Care

Enhanced Recovery after Surgery (ERAS)

Krista J. Childress

Definition

Enhanced recovery after surgery (ERAS) is a tool to optimize perioperative care with the aim to maintain homeostasis as well as reduce surgical trauma, inflammation, and stress in order to facilitate faster return to baseline for patients after surgical procedures.

Key Points

- Has been shown to improve patient satisfaction, decrease postoperative pain, reduce length of hospitalization
- Encompasses protocols with preoperative, intraoperative, and postoperative components
- Focuses on maintaining homeostasis and reducing surgical trauma, inflammation, and stress

ERAS Protocol Instructions

The components of ERAS include

- Preoperative counseling
- Limited perioperative fasting
- Early postoperative oral intake and mobilization
- Scheduled pre- and postoperative opioid-sparing analgesia
- Use of regional anesthesia during procedure
- Use of minimally invasive surgery
- Use of goal-directed and judicious intravenous fluids
- Limited use of surgical drains and tubes

The ERAS Society has published guidelines for adult gynecologic surgery based on successful implementation in gynecologic surgery and other specialties including colorectal surgery (Table 32.1). ERAS protocols have also been successfully implemented in specialties of pediatric surgery including colorectal surgery, plastic surgery, otolaryngology, urology, and pediatric and adolescent gynecology.

DOI: 10.1201/9781003039235-32

TABLE 32.1

Components of ERAS to Be Considered for Perioperative Management

Surgical Phase	Intervention
Preoperative	
Fasting	Dedicated counseling on expectations of surgery
	NPO recommendations
	• Solids 6 hours before procedure
	• Liquids 2 hours before procedure
	Carbohydrate loading drink 2 hours before procedure
Analgesia	Day before procedure
	• Gabapentin 5 mg/kg TID
	Day of procedure
	• Gabapentin 15 mg/kg PO×1
	Acetaminophen 10 mg/kg PO×1
Intraoperative	
Analgesia	Regional anesthesia (nerve blocks i.e.: transversus abdominis block)
	Minimization of opioids
	Ketorolac
Fluids	Maintenance of zero fluid balance
	Decrease crystalloid administration
	Increase colloid administration
Antiemetics	Dexamethasone and/or ondansetron
Drains	Avoid bladder foley or remove at end of case
Thromboprophylaxis	Sequential compression devices where indicated
Antimicrobial therapy	• First generation cephalosporin or amoxicillin-clavulanic acid within 60 minutes of procedure where indicated
	• Re-dose antibiotics if blood loss > 1,500 mL
	• Skin cleanse: alcohol-based agent
	• Vaginal cleansing: 4% chlorhexidine gluconate or povidone-iodine
	• Hair clipping (no shaving)
Temperature	Maintenance of normothermia
Postoperative	
Activity/diet	Early mobilization and oral intake
Analgesia	Scheduled multimodal pain medications
	• Gabapentin 5 mg/kg TID PO×3–7 days
	• Acetaminophen 10 mg/kg PO every 6 hours
	• Ibuprofen 10 mg/kg PO every 6 hours
	• Lidocaine transdermal patches as needed
	• Opioids only for breakthrough pain (e.g. oxycodone)
Fluids	Limit fluid boluses

Abbreviations: TID: three time daily; PO: taken by mouth.

BIBLIOGRAPHY

Perioperative pathways: Enhanced Recovery after Surgery. ACOG Committee Opinion No. 750. American College of Obstetricians and Gynecologists. Obstet Gynecol. 2018;132(3):e120–e130.

Smith AE, Heiss K, Childress KJ. Enhanced recovery after surgery in pediatric and adolescent gynecology: a pilot study. J Pediatr Adolesc Gynecol. 2020;33(4):403–409. 10.1016/j.jpag.2020.02.001

33

Osteoporosis

Kelsey Shnaekel and Kathryn Stambough

Definition

- Low bone mineral density (BMD) in the pediatric and adolescent population is defined as Z score < −2. SD adjusted for age, gender, race, and ethnicity
- Note that normative BMD values for adults do not apply to the pediatric adolescent population because of dramatic and variable rates of bone mineral acquisition that take place throughout adolescence
- Slightly low BMD is defined as Z score between −1.0 and −1.9 SD
- The diagnosis of osteoporosis in patients younger than 20 requires both imaging consistent with low BMD and clinically significant fracture history

Key Points

- Adolescence is a critical time for peak bone accrual during which approximately 40% of adult bone mass is established.
- The major statistical predictors of lumbar spine BMD and femoral neck BMD in adolescents are race, chronologic age, and weight.
- Every 10% increase in bone mass acquired during adolescence translates to a potential 50% reduction in future fracture risk.
- Dual energy X-ray absorptiometry (DEXA) is the preferred method for assessing BMD and bone mineral content (BMC) in children and adolescents.
- Osteoporosis and low BMD are associated with poor nutrition, chronic disease states, genetic disorders, prolonged corticosteroid use, primary ovarian insufficiency (POI), cancer, renal disease, and certain other medication use.

Diagnosis

History

Menstrual history: Absence of menses for more than 6 months is concerning for decreased estradiol and potential bone loss

Medication use

- Antiseizure medications
- Chronic steroid use
- Long-term (>2 years) use of depot medroxyprogesterone

DOI: 10.1201/9781003039235-33

Past medical history

- Immobility (e.g. wheelchair dependent)
- Cancer
- Renal disease
- Severe asthma
- Primary ovarian insufficiency (POI)

Family history

- Osteoporosis
- Fractures

Physical Examination

- Measure height, weight, blood pressure, heart rate
  - Significant weight loss
  - Bradycardia often associated with caloric underfueling
- Look for signs of hypoestrogenism (e.g. breast or vaginal atrophy)

Laboratory Testing

If signs of amenorrhea, infrequent menses >90 days apart, hypoestrogenism

- Obtain FSH, TSH, prolactin, estradiol, 25 hydroxy vitamin D

Imaging

Dual-energy X-ray absorptiometry (DEXA)

- Preferred method for testing bone density for children and adolescents
- Typically measures lumbar spine and hip in adolescent (hip not useful in children)
- Z-score, which compares bone mass to similar age, gender, and ethnicity, is the appropriate reference for the pediatric and adolescent population
- T-score is not useful in pediatric and adolescent population as they have not reached peak bone density
- Pitfalls with DEXA
  - Provides only a two-dimensional measurement of bone in g/cm^2 with no information about bone depth
  - May help to recognize if pubertal delay is possible in patient of concern and check bone age first, then adjust DEXA to bone vs chronologic age

Quantitative computed tomography (QCT) and peripheral QCT (pQCT)

- Newer modalities to assess BMD
- Offer three-dimensional imaging that will circumvent influence of bone size on measures by quantifying true volumetric BMD in g/cm^3
- Used primarily in research and not widely available clinically

Diagnosis

In individuals less than 20 years of age, the diagnosis of osteoporosis requires both imaging criteria and clinically significant fracture history.

1. Imaging consistent with low BMD
2. Clinically significant fracture defined as one or more of the following
   a. Two or more long bone fractures by 10 years of age
   b. Three or more long bone fractures at any age up to 19 years
   c. One or more vertebral compression fractures.
3. Low bone density is defined as Z score < −2. SD adjusted for age, gender.
4. Slightly low bone density is defined as Z score between −1.0 and −1.9 SD.

Note: There is no fracture threshold established based on Z scores in children and adolescents.

Management

Pediatric endocrinology consultation

- Can also consider multispecialty approach with involvement of geneticist and other specialists as appropriate for management of comorbid conditions to improve bone health

Supplement calcium (1300 mg/day) and vitamin D (600 IU/day)

- Weight-bearing exercise
- Bisphosphonate therapy is reserved for severe cases refractory to supplementation (e.g. osteogenesis imperfecta) and management of comorbid medical conditions
- Not indicated for first-line use in otherwise healthy pediatric patients with low BMD
- Uncertainty regarding optimal bisphosphonate dose, frequency, and duration of treatment in pediatric population
- Reported side effects include hypocalcemia, musculoskeletal pain, gastrointestinal side effects, delayed healing after osteotomy, bisphosphonate-induced osteopetrosis, skeletal modeling defects, and teratogenicity
- Atypical fractures and osteonecrosis of the jaw have been reported in adults, but these side effects have not been reported in children or adolescents
- No long-term studies of effects on future pregnancies, fetus of females using bisphosphonates as children or adolescents

In adolescents with POI, hormone replacement therapy with estradiol is associated with improvement in BMD:

- Transdermal 17β estradiol 0.1 mg continuously with cyclic micronized progesterone preferred treatment as this method has been shown to significantly increase Z-score

Hormonal contraception and impact on bone health

- Use is not recommended to increase bone mass, NOT shown to increase BMD
- Long-acting reversible contraceptives do not affect peak bone mass acquisition and should be considered first-line contraceptive choice in individuals with low BMD and osteoporosis
- Combined oral contraceptive pill (OCP) use is not associated with increased fracture risk
  - Consideration of an OCP with at least 30-mcg ethinyl estradiol, as lower doses are insufficient to support peak bone mass acquisition

- Contraceptive patch and vaginal ring do not adversely affect bone health in adult women, but data is limited in adolescents
- Depot medroxyprogesterone (DMPA) decreases BMD
  - The deleterious bone effects are reversible if discontinued within 2 years of initiation
  - Complete bone recovery may not occur if discontinued after more than 2 years of use
  - Concerns about BMD should not preclude use in adolescents who prefers this method as the benefit of unintended pregnancy prevention far outweighs the risk
  - Routine DEXA assessment is not recommended for adolescents based solely on DMPA use
  - In individuals with osteoporosis or low BMD, consideration should be given regarding avoidance of DMPA if possible to avoid exacerbating underlying bone loss

Monitoring

- Initial DEXA should be considered a baseline for future comparison

Surveillance with serial DEXA

- Consider imaging at 12-month intervals to detect meaningful changes
- The minimal interval between scans should be not less than every 6 months

Prevention

- Identify risk factors such as chronic disease states, medication use, poor nutrition, family history of fractures, and POI
- Optimize modifiable and nonmodifiable risk factors

Counseling

Modifiable risk factors

- Optimize nutritional status including maintaining a healthy body weight and consuming the recommended dietary intake of calcium and vitamin D
- Participate in adequate weight-bearing exercise
- Avoid the use of tobacco and alcohol
- Limit carbonated beverages (soda)

BIBLIOGRAPHY

Cromer, BA, Binkovtiz L, Ziegler J, Harvey R, Debanne SM. Reference values for bone mineral density in 12-to-18-year-old girls categorized by weight, race and age. Pediatr Radiol. 2004 Oct; 34(10):787–792.

Golden, NH. Bones and birth control in adolescent girls. J Pediatr Adolesc Gynecol. 2020 Jun; 33(3):249–254.

Golden, NH and Abrams, SA. Optimizing bone health in children and adolescents. Pediatrics. 2014 Oct; 134(4):e1229–e1243.

Steffey, CL. Pediatric osteoporosis. Pediatr Rev. 2019; 40(5): 259–261.

34

Ovarian Cysts

Dana Elborno, Sari Kives and S. Paige Hertweck

Key Points

- Most commonly are functional cysts (i.e. the consequence of normal follicular growth and development)
- Ultrasonographically simple ovarian cysts have a very low incidence of complications including malignancy
- Ovarian cysts are common in premenarcheal and adolescent girls
- Less than 20 mm is considered physiologic and does not need follow-up
- The majority of functional cysts (simple and complex) resolve in 6 months without treatment
- Modern management of ovarian cysts in neonates, prepubescent, and adolescent girls is based on conservative treatment and close observation
- Surgical intervention is indicated for acute symptoms, solid or complex masses, and large (>5 cm) masses that do not undergo regression

Fetal Ovarian Cysts

- Prenatal ultrasound allows opportunity to diagnose in utero-ovarian cysts that would have otherwise gone undetected
- Up to 98% of female fetuses have small physiologic cysts detected by US around 28–32 weeks gestation
- In the fetus, follicular stimulation of the ovaries occurs as a result of stimulation from maternal estrogen, placental human chorionic gonadotropin, and fetal gonadotropins
- Complex cysts have echogenic appearance on ultrasound, may contain septa, debris-filled fluid levels, or clot, and often represent neonatal torsion or hemorrhage
- Malignancy is extremely rare in neonate/fetus

Differential Diagnosis of Cystic Masses in Female Fetus/Newborn

Gastrointestinal (GI) etiology

- Intestinal duplication
- Intestinal obstruction
- Cystic meconium peritonitis
- Omental cyst
- Mesenteric cyst
- Choledochal cyst

DOI: 10.1201/9781003039235-34

Gynecologic

- Hydrometrocolpos
- Ovarian cysts

Urologic

- Urachal cyst
- Hydronephrosis
- Renal cyst
- Bladder distention

Complications

- Most common complication is antenatal torsion +/− autoamputation (occurs 25–54% of the time)
    - Rapid increase in size and change in features from simple to complex is suggestive of torsion
    - More common if more than 5 cm
    - If decrease in size with change in location, suspect autoamputation
- Rarely mass effect may cause GI/GU compression +/− polyhydramnios

Management in Antenatal Period

- Observation
    - High-resolution rate in neonatal period
    - Low risk of antenatal complications
- Antenatal aspiration: Not indicated
- Defer treatment until neonatal period
- Allow spontaneous vaginal delivery
    - No support to indicate need for operative vaginal delivery or cesarean delivery

Neonatal Ovarian Cysts

- Usually unilateral
- Can be simple/complex
  Complex cyst characterized by: Fluid-debris level

  Retracting clot

  Septated with/without internal echoes
- Complex ovarian cysts: Usually represent in utero/neonatal torsion+/− autoamputation or hemorrhage
- Differential diagnosis same as for fetal cysts (see earlier)
- Both simple and complex cysts well documented to undergo regression within first 4 months of life
- Malignancy risk essentially nonexistent, so tumor markers are not routinely evaluated

Complications

- Ovarian torsion +/− autoamputation and necrosis
- GI/GU obstruction or respiratory distress from mass effect
- Incarceration in inguinal hernia

Management

- Serial ultrasounds every 4–6 weeks
- Educate caregivers on signs of acute torsion: Acute abdominal pain
      Nausea/vomiting
      Fever
- Percutaneous aspiration: Consider for large cysts (>5 cm)
- Surgical indications: Recurrent cysts after aspiration
      Complex adnexal masses without involution over 4–6 months (if autoamputated, may take 1 year to resolve)
      Acute abdominal symptoms
- Surgical technique: Laparoscopic ovarian cystectomy

Childhood Ovarian Cysts

- Ovarian cysts are least common in this age group due to low gonadotropin and sex hormone levels
- Microcysts (<9 mm) resolve over 6 months
- 10% of cysts >9 mm persist beyond 6 months
- Can be associated with precocious puberty
  - Autonomously functioning ovarian cyst (e.g., McCune-Albright syndrome or hypothyroidism) or gonadotropin induced (see Chapter 44, "Puberty")
- Most simple and complex masses in this age group resolve, even when >5 cm
- Most solid masses or simple/complex masses that do not regress are mature cystic teratomas
- Malignancy possible in approximately 10% cases with germ-cell tumors most common

Presentation

- Asymptomatic mass
- Increasing abdominal girth
- Acute abdominal pain with nausea, vomiting, fever (think torsion)
- Signs of precocious puberty
  - Breast development
  - Vaginal discharge or bleeding

Evaluation

Physical Examination

- Rule out precocious puberty
  - Increase in height curve
  - Breast development
  - Signs of estrogenization at hymen
  - Vaginal bleeding

Ultrasound

- For US features concerning for malignancy, see Figures 45.5 and 45.6 and Chapter 35 Ovarian Masses for further evaluation

Management

Based on size, symptoms, and composition seen on ultrasound

Small, simple cysts (<2 cm):	Normal findings
	Require no intervention
More than one small cyst:	If associated with precocity, see Chapter 44, "Puberty" for management
If cyst >2 cm:	Monitor q 4–8 weeks by ultrasound
	Regression likely
Surgical indications:	Acute symptoms or concern for torsion
	Solid or complex masses (see Chapter 35, "Ovarian Masses,")
	Cysts (>4 cm) that fail to undergo regression over several months
Surgical technique:	Laparoscopic ovarian cystectomy gold standard

Adolescent Ovarian Cysts

Presentation

- Asymptomatic
  - 12% of patients 10–19 years of age with US had incidentally found asymptomatic cysts
- Menstrual irregularities
- Abdominal/pelvic pain
- Urinary frequency
- Constipation
- Increasing abdominal girth

Differential Diagnosis for Ovarian Cysts

Functional Cysts
- Follicular cysts
- Corpus luteum cysts
- Hemorrhagic cysts
- Endometriomas
- Tubo-ovarian abscess (TOA)

Benign Ovarian Neoplasms
- Dermoid cysts
  Most common neoplasm in this age group
- Epithelial cystadenomas

Malignant (see Chapter 35, "Ovarian Masses")

Pathology mimicking ovarian cysts:

Disorders of the fallopian tube
- Hydrosalpinx
- Pyosalpinx
- Paratubal cyst
- Ectopic pregnancy
- Tubal torsion

Obstructive genital lesions
- Imperforate hymen
- Non-communicating uterine horn
- Müllerian remnants
- Peritoneal cysts
- Periappendiceal abscesses

Evaluation

History

- Menstrual history: Progressive dysmenorrhea may suggest congenital obstructive lesion
- Obesity and hyperandrogenism have been correlated with presence of paratubal cysts
    - Derived from stimulation of Wolffian remnants in females
    - May be hormonally sensitive
- Confidential sexual history: May suggest infectious process (i.e., tubo-ovarian abscess)

Physical Examination

- Abdominal examination — Abdominal tenderness
- Consider pelvic examination in sexually active patients

Laboratory Tests

- Human chorionic gonadotropin (hCG)
- If concern for TOA: CBC/STI testing
- If concern for malignancy, tumor markers (see Chapter 35, "Ovarian Masses")
- Recent studies have shown coexistence of mature dermoid with non-germinoma ovarian cell tumors
    - Obtain tumor markers for suspected mature dermoid as well

Imaging (See Chapter 45, "Radiologic Imaging" for Additional Information on US Imaging)

- Ultrasound
    - Modality of choice for evaluation of ovarian cyst/masses
- Ultrasonographic patterns
- Ovarian follicles (see Figure 45.1)
    - Normal follicles: Appear unilocular, anechoic
    - Corpus luteum: Thick-walled cyst ≤3 cm may have crenulated inner margins, internal echoes and intense peripheral color Doppler flow *or*
    - Hypoechoic area with peripheral flow

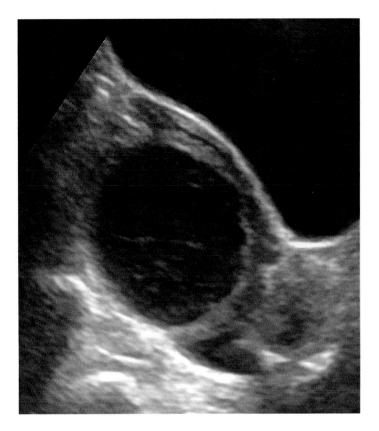

FIGURE 34.1 Hemorrhagic cyst.

- Hemorrhagic cyst (see Figure 45.3)
  - Reticular pattern of fine thin intersecting lines representing fibrin strands (see Figure 34.1)
  - Can have retracting clot: Avascular echogenic component with angular strait or concave margins
- Dermoid cysts (see Figures 34.1 and 45.3)
  - Typically are less than 10 cm
  - Have hyperechoic lines and "dots and dashes" appearance to fluid
  - Floating echogenic spherical structures can be seen
  - Often have hyperechoic components with acoustic shadowing
- Endometriomas (see Figure 45.3)
  - Commonly had homogenous low-level or ground-glass internal echoes with no internal flow
- Extraovarian cysts (see Figure 45.3)
  - Paratubal cysts
    - Typically unilocular with thin smooth wall +/- enhancement, no enhancing solid tissue
    - Can exert mass effect and moves separate from ovary when pressure is applied
    - Can cause torsion of tube and/or ovary
      - Tube may appear as solid non-enhancing tissue if torsed
    - Are almost certainly benign (O-RADS 2)

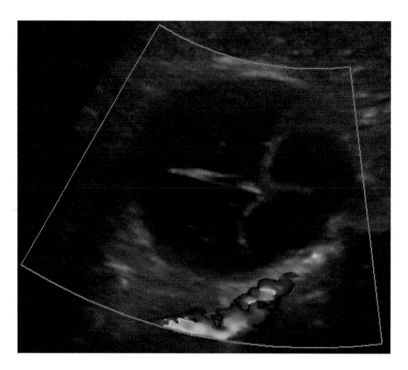

FIGURE 34.2   Dermoid cyst.

- Peritoneal inclusion cysts:
  - Follows contour of adjacent pelvic organs
  - Does not exert mass effect
  - Typically has septations
  - The ovary is at the margin or suspended within the lesion
- Hydrosalpinges
  - Incomplete septation noted
  - Tubular
  - Endosalpingeal folds: Short round projections around the inner wall of a fluid
    - Distended tubular structure in a "cog wheel" pattern
- Ultrasonographic tools
  - Morphology index (MI) (see Table 34.1)
    - A tool to relate US findings to tumor histology
    - A score of 7–10 is concerning for malignancy
  - Ovarian crescent sign (OCS) (see Figure 34.3)
    - Another new ultrasonographic tool used to evaluate ovarian neoplasms
      - May indicate normal ovarian tissue surrounding a cyst or
      - May assist in excluding an invasive ovarian malignancy
      - Can be present in cases of borderline malignancy and in ovarian metastases
      - Present in 96% of benign masses, 3% with microscopic malignancy
    - When used in conjunction with MI, OCS with emergent or nonemergent presentation in 19 year olds with ovarian tumors/torsion was noted to be a very accurate management tool: No malignancies were noted in asymptomatic patients with an ovarian mass that had an MI of 4 or less in a group of 1236 cases.

TABLE 34.1

Morphology Index (MI) Components

Structural Score	
0	Smooth wall, sonolucent
1	Smooth wall, diffuse echogenicity
2	Wall thickening (<3 mm), fine septa
3	Papillary projection (≥3 mm)
4	Complex, predominantly solid
5	Complex, solid and cystic areas with extratumoral fluid
Volume Score[a]	
0	$<10 \text{ cm}^3$
1	$10–50 \text{ cm}^3$
2	$>50–100 \text{ cm}^3$
3	$>100–200 \text{ cm}^3$
4	$>200–500 \text{ cm}^3$
5	$>500 \text{ cm}^3$

[a] Calculated using prolate ellipsoid formula ($L \times H \times W \times 0.523$).

Source: With permission from Stankovic ZB, et al. J Pediatr Adol Gynecol. 2017; 30:409.

Note: Structural score + volume score > 7 is worrisome in girls and adolescents.

CT Scanning: Can clarify images

Helpful to distinguish gastrointestinal disorders in case of surgical abdomen

MRI: Rarely indicated for benign pathology

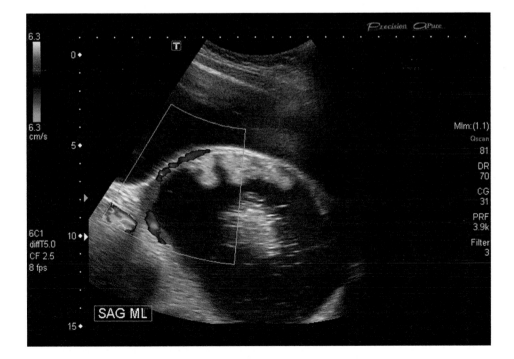

FIGURE 34.3 Ovarian crescent sign. (From Allen L, et al. 2E, OR Stankovic ZB, Sedlecky K, Savic D, et al.. J Pediatr Adolesc Gynecol. 2017; 30:405–412. With permission.)

Management

Functional Cysts (Follicular, Corpus Luteal, Hemorrhagic)

- Less than 5 cm less likely for torsion-observe, requires no future management
- Greater than 5 cm
  - May also spontaneously resolve
  - Can consider surgery at initial diagnosis vs repeat imaging in two cycles and proceed with surgery if persistent
  - Resolution occurs on average within 6 months of initial US
- Greater than 10 cm, would advocate surgical intervention
- Persistent simple cysts are more likely to be benign epithelial neoplasms like serous or mucinous cystadenomas
- Oral contraceptives do not hasten resolution of current cyst but may prevent new onset cysts

Dermoid Cysts (Benign or Mature Teratomas)

- Do not resolve spontaneously, need to be monitored even if small
- Benign, slow growth rate and, if asymptomatic, can be expectantly managed
- Resect if symptomatic or prophylactically if >5 cm or if growth rate >2 cm/year due to increased risk for torsion or rupture
- Rarely can contain functional thyroid tissue, i.e. struma ovarii
- Rarely may be associated with anti-NMDA receptor encephalitis
- Malignant transformation is extremely rare but coexisting benign teratoma with non-dysgerminoma ovarian germ-cell tumor foci has been reported
- Risk for recurrence within 1 year is about 10% after surgery — Monitor with US in 1 year

Paratubal Cysts

- Are not physiologic so do not spontaneously regress
- May be associated with hyperandrogenism
- Consider expectant management for cysts <5 cm and surgical intervention if >6 cm
  - Give torsion precautions
  - have high index of suspicion for less symptomatic isolated tubal torsion
  - Almost certainly benign

Surgical Principles

- Laparoscopic cystectomy is procedure of choice
- Laparotomy may be favored depending on size of lesion or patient comorbidities
  - Obtain peritoneal fluid for cytology
  - Inspect and document findings on omentum, peritoneal surfaces and opposite ovary
- Spillage at time of laparoscopy common, especially in large cysts
  - Dermoid cystectomy occurs 15–100% of the time and does not preclude laparoscopic approach
    - Risk for chemical peritonitis <1%
    - Complete removal of cyst contents and copious peritoneal lavage with normal saline recommended if spillage occurs

BIBLIOGRAPHY

Andreotti RF, Timmerman D, Strachowski LM, et al. O-RADS US risk stratification and management system: a consensus guideline from the ACR Ovarian-Adnexal Reporting and Data System Committee. Radiology. 2020; 294:168–185.

Anthony EY, Caserta MP, Singh J, et al. Adnexal masses in female pediatric patients. Am J Roentgenol. 2012; 198:W426–W431.

Aydin BK, et al. Evaluation and treatment results of ovarian cysts in childhood and adolescence: a multicenter, retrospective study of 100 patients. J Pediatr Adolesc Gynecol. 2017; 30(4):449–455. doi:10.1016/j.jpag.2017.01.011.

Ben-Ami I, et al. Long-term follow-up of children with ovarian cysts diagnosed prenatally. Prenat Diagn. 2010 Apr; 30(4):342–347. doi:10.1002/pd.2470.

Billmire D, Dicken B, Rescorla F, et al. Imaging appearance of nongerminoma pediatric ovarian germ cell tumors does not discriminate benign from malignant histology. J Pediatr Adolesc Gynecol. 2021; 34:383–386.

Multani J, Kives S. Dermoid cysts in adolescents. Curr Opin Obstet Gynecol. 2015 Oct; 27(5):315–319. doi:10.1097/GCO.0000000000000206.

Papic JC, et al. Management of neonatal ovarian cysts and its effect on ovarian preservation. J Pediatr Surg. 2014 Jun; 49(6):990–994. doi:10.1016/j.jpedsurg.2014.01.040.

Pienkowski C, et al. Ovariancysts in prepubertal girls. Pediatr Adolesc Gynecol Endocr Dev. 2012; 101–111. doi:10.1159/000326627.

Schallert EK, et al. Physiologic ovarian cysts versus other ovarian and adnexal pathologic changes in the preadolescent and adolescent population: US and surgical follow-up. Radiology. 2019; 292(1):172–178. doi:10.1148/radiol.2019182563.

Stankovic ZB, Djukic MK, Savic D, et al. Pre-operative differentiation of pediatric ovarian tumors: morphological scoring system and tumor markers. J Pediatr Endocrinol Metab. 2006; 19:1231–1238.

Stankovic ZB, Sedlecky K, Savic D, et al. Ovarian preservation from tumors and torsions in girls: prospective diagnostic study. J Pediatr Adolesc Gynecol. 2017; 30:405–412.

35

Ovarian Masses

Dana Elborno, Sari Kives and S. Paige Hertweck

Key Points

- **The majority of ovarian masses in PAG population are benign**
  - Only 10–20% are malignant
  - Advanced malignancies in children and teens are uncommon
  - In general, survival of ovarian malignancy is high
- Risk of malignancy increases with solid tumors.
  - 2/3 of solid masses are germ cell tumors
    - Encompass the majority of malignances in children and adolescents
      - Unlike adults for who epithelial origin are most common malignances
    - Dysgerminoma is the most common malignant germ cell tumor
  - The remaining 1/3 are sex cord tumors or epithelium tumors
- Children's Oncology Group staging (COG) is a modified FIGO staging system for this population that takes into account increased risk of recurrence in patients with positive washings
- Sex cord tumors are usually hormonally active and can present with precocious puberty, virilization, or dysfunctional bleeding

Differential Diagnosis

Classification of ovarian neoplasms

Germ cell tumors

- Benign
  - Gonadoblastoma
  - Embryonic origin
    - Mature teratoma (dermoid)
    - Polyembryoma
- Malignant
  - Embryonic differentiation
    - Embryonal carcinoma
  - Embryonic somatic origin
    - Immature teratoma
  - Extramembryonic origin
    - Endodermal sinus tumor(yolk sac tumor)
    - Choriocarcinoma

DOI: 10.1201/9781003039235-35

- • Pluripotent germinal state
  - – Dysgerminoma

Sex cord/stromal tumors

- • Benign
  - • Thecoma-fibroma
  - • Sclerosing stromal
  - • Gynandroblastoma
  - • Sex cord tumors with annular tubules
- • Malignant
  - • Granulosa cell (adult and juvenile type)
  - • Sertoli-Leydig cell
  - • Gynandroblastoma
  - • Sex cord tumor with annular tubules

TABLE 35.1

Ovarian Tumor Markers

	CA-125	HE4	AFP	hCG	INH	E2	TT	17-KS	Gn	MIS
Germ cell tumors										
Dysgerminoma	–/↑			–/↑	–/↑	↑/–				
Yolk sac tumor (endodermal sinus tumor)	–/↑		↑↑							
Choriocarcinoma	–/↑			↑↑		↑/–			↑	
Embryonal carcinoma	–/↑		↑/–	↑/–		↑/–				
Immature teratoma	–/↑		↑/–			↑/–				
Mixed germ cell tumor	–/↑		↑/–	↑/–		–/↑				
Epithelial-stromal tumors										
Serous carcinoma	↑↑	↑↑								
Mucinous carcinoma	↑	↑↑			↑↑					
Endometrioid carcinoma	↑↑	↑↑			↑					
Sex cord-stromal tumors										
Granulosa cell tumor	–/↑	↑			↑↑	↑			↓	↑↑
Juvenile granulosa cell tumor	–/↑	↑			↑↑	↑	–/↑^		↓	↑↑
Thecoma-fibroma	–/↑				↑	↑	–/↑^			
Sertoli-Leydig cell tumor	–/↑		–/↑^		↑	–/↑^	–/↑^	–/↑^	↓	↑
Sex cord tumor with annular tubules	–/↑				↑	↑				↑↑
Steroid cell tumor, NOS	–/↑						↑↑	↑↑	↓	
Other ovarian tumors										
Gonadoblastoma	–/↑					–/↑^	↑	↑	↓	

Note: Tumor markers may assist in diagnosis, as well as monitor response to therapy and detect relapse and/or progression. CA-125 levels may be slightly elevated in any of the ovarian tumors. HE4 is a newer tumor marker with improved sensitivity and specificity compared to CA-125. Lactate dehydrogenase (LDH) levels are useful for staging and risk assessment in germ cell tumors.

Abbreviations: AFP, Alpha-Fetoprotein; CA-125, Cancer Antigen 125; E2, Estradiol; Gn, Gonadotropin; hCG, Human Chorionic Gonadotropin; HE4, Human Epididymis Protein 4; INH, Inhibin; MIS, Müllerian Inhibiting Substance; TT, Testosterone; 17-KS, Urinary 17-Ketosteroid.

^ Indicates rare variant of the tumor.

Source: Courtesy of Dr. Robert Debski, Assistant Professor of Pediatrics and Pathology, University of Louisville, and Dr. Mary Fallat, Professor of Surgery, University of Louisville and Chief of Surgery for Norton Children's Hospital, Louisville, KY, USA.

Epithelial tumors: Serous, mucinous, endometroid, clear cell, transitional or mixed histology

- Benign
- Borderline
- Malignant

Other tumors

- Neuroblastoma
- Wilms' tumor
- Rhabdomyosarcoma
- Lymphoma/Leukemia

Diagnosis

Presentation

Most commonly asymptomatic, but may present with

- Abdominal pain
- Increasing abdominal girth
- Precocious puberty
- Virilization
- Dysfunctional uterine bleeding

NOTE: Symptomatology at presentation is not an accurate indicator of risk of preoperative malignancy

History

- Gastrointestinal/urologic symptoms
- Onset of pubertal development
  - Precocious (< age 8 years)
  - Contrasexual development
    - Hirsutism
    - Acne
    - Virilization
- Menstrual/sexual history

Family history

- Endometriosis
- Inflammatory bowel disease
- Ovarian tumors
  - Prior abdominal/pelvic surgery
  - Prior pelvic infections

Physical Examination

- Vital signs: General/pubertal development
- Abdominal exam: Assess for areas of tenderness/signs of peritonitis

                               Characterize mass (fixed, mobile, regular vs irregular and size)
- Pelvic exam: External genitalia (assess pubertal development: whether age appropriate)

Imaging (See Chapter 45, "Radiologic Imaging")

Ultrasound: Transabdominal without use of endovaginal probe is the initial imaging modality of choice to determine size of mass and characteristics (simple, complex, solid, bilateral, etc.)

In general, US features concerning for malignancy include

- Multilocular cysts
  - ≥10 cm smooth inner wall
  - Any size, smooth inner wall, color score=4
  - Any size, irregular inner wall and/or irregular septation, any color score
- Any solid component in a multilocular or unilocular cyst
- Ascites and/or peritoneal nodules
- Increased blood flow

MRI: Recommended if any of the above concerning features

- Further delineation of mass/liver/lymphatic involvement
- Helps with preoperative risk stratification and define full extent of disease if malignancy

Additional Testing

Tumor markers

Alpha-fetoprotein (AFP):	Endodermal sinus tumors (Yolk sac tumors)
	Mixed germ cell tumors
	Immature teratomas
	(**NOTE**: AFP can be increased until 8 months of age as a normal fetal antigen)
Lactate dehydrogenase (LDH):	Dysgerminomas
Human chorionic gonadotropin:	Dysgerminomas
	Choriocarcinomas
	Embryonal ovarian carcinoma
Carcinoembryonic antigen (CEA):	Epithelial ovarian carcinoma
Inhibin B:	Granulosa cell tumors
Müllerian inhibiting substance (MIS):	Granulosa cell tumors

CA-125:   Nonspecific marker for epithelial ovarian carcinoma, can be increased with many other intraperitoneal processes –e.g. endometriosis, PID, IBD, etc.

Karyotype: With concerns for dysgerminoma

NOTE: Estradiol/Testosterone/DHEA-S and androstenedione can be helpful in evaluating suspected sex cord stromal tumors.

Management

- Risk stratification for malignancy is a key component of evaluation
  - Use of tumor markers described above
  - Appearance on imaging (see Chapter 45, "Radiologic Imaging")
  - Helpful risk stratification tools include:
    - Morphology index (see Chapter 34, "Ovarian Cysts")
    - Ovarian crescent sign (see Chapter 34, "Ovarian Cysts")
    - O-RADS system
- Surgical staging for suspected germ cell tumor (GCT) malignancy
  - Less extensive than with epithelial malignancies
  - Includes
    - Collection of ascites or washings upon entering abdominal cavity
    - Evaluation of peritoneal surfaces with biopsy or excision of any nodules
    - Evaluation and palpation of any firm or enlarged nodes in retroperitoneum with
    - Sampling of any firm or enlarged nodes
    - Inspection and palpation of the omentum with removal of any adherent or abnormal areas noted
    - Inspection and palpation of the opposite ovary with biopsy of any abnormal areas
    - Complete resection of the tumor-containing ovary with sparing of fallopian tube if not involved.

Treatment Depends on Risk of Malignancy

- Low risk (imaging O-RADS 2, i.e. simple cyst, hemorrhagic, or dermoid)
  - Surgical intervention: laparoscopy/laparotomy for ovarian cystectomy
- Intermediate Risk (imaging O-RADS 3 or 4, i.e. equivocal imaging findings: cystic> solid components, complex > 8 cm; tumor markers negative/preoperative MRI without concern for extraovarian disease)
  - Consult pre-op with oncology and pediatric surgery
  - Surgical intervention laparoscopy vs open cystectomy
    - Discuss with patient and parents about option for and limitation of frozen section
    - Possible need for second surgery
- High risk (imaging O-RADS 5, i.e. irregular multiloculated solid tumors, papillary structures, solid components> cystic components, increased blood flow; elevated tumor markers, evidence of enlarged LN or extra-ovarian disease on MRI)
  - Consult preoperatively with pediatric surgery and/or oncology
    - Surgical staging

Staging

- Staged according to FIGO or COG classification
  - Note careful attention should be given to description of FIGO stage 1c or COG stage III patients

- Preoperative and intraoperative spill both fit the description of this stage, but details of spill and cytology results may have significant therapeutic implications

COG staging criteria: (Table 35.2)

TABLE 35.2

Ovarian Malignant Germ Cell Tumor Staging

Ovarian Malignant Germ Cell Tumors	
Stage	Extent of Disease
I	<ul><li>Ovarian tumor removed intact without violation of the tumor capsule.</li><li>No evidence of partial or complete capsular penetration.</li><li>Peritoneal cytology negative for malignant cells,</li><li>Peritoneal surfaces and omentum documented to be free of disease in operative note or biopsied with negative histology if abnormal in appearance.</li><li>Lymph nodes all < 1.0 cm by short axis on multiplanar imaging or biopsy proven negative (Note: Nodes 1 - 2 cm, require short interval follow-up in 4 - 6 weeks. If nodes are unchanged at 4-6 weeks (1 - 2 cm), consider biopsy or transfer to chemotherapy arm. If growing, transfer to chemotherapy arm.)</li></ul>
II	<ul><li>Ovarian tumor completely removed but with preoperative biopsy, violation of tumor capsule in situ, or presence of partial or complete capsule penetration at histology.</li><li>Tumor greater than 10 cm removed laparoscopically.</li><li>Tumor morcellated for removal so that capsule cannot be assessed for penetration.</li><li>Peritoneal cytology must be negative for malignant cells.</li><li>Lymph nodes, peritoneal surfaces and omentum documented to be free of disease in operative note or biopsied with negative histology if abnormal in appearance.</li></ul>
III	<ul><li>Lymph nodes ≥ 2 cm or lymph nodes > 1 -< 2 cm on short axis by multi-planar imaging CT that fail to resolve on reimaging at 4 - 6 weeks.</li><li>Ovarian tumor biopsied or removal with gross residual.</li><li>Positive peritoneal fluid cytology for malignant cells, including immature teratoma.</li><li>Lymph nodes positive for malignant cells, including immature teratoma.</li><li>Peritoneal implants positive for malignant cells, including immature teratoma.</li></ul>
III-X	Patients otherwise Stage I or II by COG criteria but with the following: <ul><li>Failure to collect peritoneal cytology.</li><li>Failure to biopsy lymph nodes > 1.0 cm by short axis on multiplanar imaging.</li><li>Failure to sample abnormal peritoneal surfaces or omentum.</li><li>Delayed completion of surgical staging at a second procedure for those patients who had only oophorectomy at first procedure.</li></ul>
IV	Metastatic disease to the parenchyma of the liver (surface implants are Stage III) or metastases outside the peritoneal cavity to any other viscera (bone, lung, brain) and pleural fluid with positive cytology
Bilateral ovarian tumors may be any stage as long as other stage criteria are met. Tumor staged according to ovary with most advanced features.	

Source: From National Cancer Institute, PDQ Cancer Information Studies, CDC, Bethesda 2002.

General Management Principles

- Treat all malignancies in conjunction with gynecologic/pediatric oncology/pediatric surgery
- Stage I GCT malignancies typically managed with surgical resection and active surveillance
  - Relapse rate up to 30%
    - All occurred within 1 year of initial surgery
    - 90% are successfully treated with salvage chemotherapy

- Adjuvant chemotherapy with platinum-based protocol usually indicated for advanced stage GCT malignancies
  - 3–4 cycles of PEb (cisplatin, etoposide, and bleomycin) is a common protocol
    - PEb has reduced frequency of bleomycin to limit pulmonary toxicity when compared to BEP for adults
  - Side effects/complications of chemotherapy include
    - Bleomycin: Pulmonary fibrosis
    - Etoposide: Acute myeloid leukemia
    - Cisplatin: Peripheral neuropathy and hearing loss
    - Note POI/infertility not a common side effect with this regimen
      - About 3% occurrence

General Prognosis

- Prognosis has improved vastly over the last 30 years

Cure rates

- Early stage: Approach 100%
- Advanced stage: 75%

Tumor Associations

Peutz-Jeghers syndrome:	Ovarian sex cord stromal tumors
	Granulosa cell tumors
STK11/LKB1 tumor suppressor gene mutation:	Sex cord stromal tumor-annualar tubules
DICER 1 mutations:	• Sertoli-Leydig cell tumors
	• Juvenile granulosa cell tumors
	• Gynandroblastomas
	• Rhabdomyosarcoma
	• Also seen with renal tumors, lung cysts, other sarcomas, and nodular thyroid disease
Gonadal dysgenesis:	Dysgerminoma

Specific Germ Cell Tumors

Dysgerminoma:	Most common subtype of malignant GCTs
	15% bilateral
Treatment:	Surgical resection and adjuvant chemotherapy (unless Stage 1A, removed intact, <10 cm and without evidence of metastatic spread)
	Very radiosensitive, though rarely needed
5-year overall survival:	Stage I – 96%
	Advanced stages treated with surgical resection and platinum-based therapy – 93.8%

Immature Teratoma (IT):	Graded from 1 to 3 based on degree of immature neural elements

- Most important risk factor for relapse is grade

In grade 3, stage impacts risk of relapse

- May occur with peritoneal gliomatosis
  - Mature glial tissue implants on the peritoneum
  - Does not upstage patient

Treatment: Complete surgical resection, staging with close surveillance

- Role of adjuvant chemotherapy current topic of controversy
- In children and adolescents, adjuvant chemotherapy does not seem to reduce risk of relapse

Second surgery and salvage chemotherapy for recurrence

4-year overall survival: If completely resected, 100% regardless of grade or presence of microscopic yolk sac tumor or elevated AFP

Endodermal sinus tumor: Also called yolk-sac tumor

- Most aggressive germ cell tumor
- Rapid spread via intraperitoneal seeding, hemotagenous and lymphatics and may more commonly present as advanced stage disease
- Propensity for liver/lung/central nervous system metastases

Treatment: Complete surgical resection and staging

- Adjuvant chemotherapy for stage II-IV
- If primary cytoreductive surgery not possible, may require neoadjuvant treatment

4-year overall survival: 96%

NOTE: Four-year **event-free** survival 52%

- Recurrences yield good outcomes with high successful salvage rate

Embryonal carcinoma: Very rare and highly malignant

- Typically occurs in the context of mixed malignant GCT

- b-hCG shared subunit with FSH/LH may result in precocious puberty, menstrual irregularity
- Intraperitoneal spread

Choriocarcinoma: Rare to present in a child

- Usually associated with a gestation
- Very aggressive and often occurs as a component of mixed malignant GCT
- hCG is good marker for response to treatment and recurrence
- Non-gestational form can involve other midline structures and has a poor prognosis

Non-Germ Cell Malignancies

Sex Cord Stromal Tumors (SCSTs)

History

- Obtain family history that might indicate DICER 1 syndrome
  - Colon polyps, pleuropulmonary dysplasia/lung cysts, sarcomas, thyroid disease, lung surgeries in early childhood, renal tumors like cystic nephromas

Physical exam

- Look for stigmata of Peutz-Jeghers syndrome
  - Melanocytic macules especially periorally
- Signs of enchondromatosis/Ollier disease – Can be associated with SCST
  - Hamartomatous proliferation of cartilage in metaphysis commonly in hands/feet
  - Causing distorted growth in length and pathologic fractures

Juvenile granulosa-thecal cell tumor: Most common sex cord stromal tumor

Malignancy related to amount of granulosa cells present 1/2 secrete estrogen and may present with precocious puberty/menorrhagia

Treatment: Stage I – treat with surgery alone; survival nearly 100%>

Stage I – multimodal therapy; survival 80%
Rarely recur and when they do, it is generally within 2–3 years after diagnosis

Sertoli-Leydig cell tumors: Rare

- Can secrete 17 OH Progesterone, testosterone, androstendione (rarely produce estrogen)
- May cause HTN
- Usually present with androgen excess (hirsutism, acne, amenorrhea, virilization)
- Vary in malignant potential

Treatment:	Surgical resection and staging
	Adjuvant chemotherapy recommended if beyond FIGO stage 1a or COG stage 1 or high-risk features (high mitotic activity/poorly differentiated)

Epithelial Tumors

Borderline Ovarian Tumors – BOT (Tumors of Low Malignant Potential):

- Usually unexpected finding on a pathology specimen
- Have cytologic features typical of malignant ovarian tumors (nuclear atypia, high mitotic index, epithelial hyperplasia) but lack stromal invasion by tumor cells
- More commonly seen in pubertal/menarchal girls, rare in premenarchal population
- Difficult to diagnose preoperatively
  - Suspect with increasing age, cyst size, presence of papillary or solid components, irregularity, presence of ascites, increased Doppler flow
- CA-125 can be elevated in about 50%

Treatment:

- If diagnosed incidentally on pathology, surveillance
  - Counsel recurrence rates are higher for patients who underwent cystectomy not USO
  - Does not affect overall survival
- If suspected pre-op
  - LSC or open unilateral salpingo-oophorectomy vs cystectomy
  - If bilateral, consider cystectomy
  - Accuracy of frozen section only 70%
- Mucinous BOT – appendectomy recommended
- Lymphadenectomy not recommended unless enlarged lymph nodes (LN) or frozen path consistent with micropapillary serous BOT
  - Repeat surgery for lympadenectomy on basis of final path has not been shown to improve outcome
- Typically diagnosed at early stage and curable using surgery alone
- Recurrence rate 30%
  Recurrence more likely in patients with:
  - Advanced stage at diagnosis
  - Invasive peritoneal implants
  - Micropapillary pattern of growth

- Follow-up
  - Sparse literature
  - Monitor every 3–6 months for 5 years then annually for 10–20 years
  - Follow physical exam, imaging, tumor markers if initially elevated

Epithelial invasive carcinoma:

- Very rare
- Patients with other than stage 1a tumors should be managed similarly to adult women

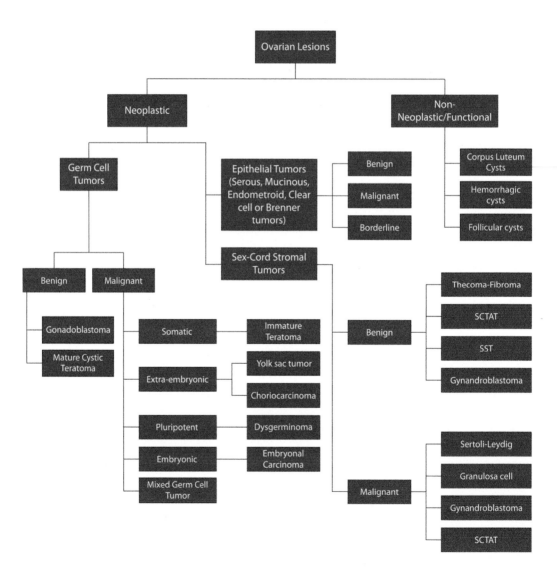

FIGURE 35.1 Classification of ovarian lesions (SCTATs, sex cord tumors with annular tubules).

BIBLIOGRAPHY

Childress KJ Patil NM, Muscal JA, et al. Borderline ovarian tumor in the pediatric and adolescent population: a case series and literature review. J Pediatr Adolesc Gynecol. 2018 Feb; 31(1):48–54. www.sciencedirect.com/science/article/pii/S1083318817304564

Goldberg HR, et al. Impact of introducing an evidence based multidisciplinary algorithm on the management of adnexal masses in the pediatric population. J Pediatr Adolesc Gynecol. 2017; 30(2):268–269. Doi:10.1016/j.jpag.2017.03.017.

Mahajan P, et al. (2020). Gynecologic Cancers in Children and Adolescents. In Emans SJ, Laufer ML, DiVasta (Eds). *Goldstein's Pediatric and Adolescent Gynecology* (7th ed., pp. 556–569), Wolters Kluwer.

Renaud EJ, Somme S, Islam S et al. Ovarian masses in the child and adolescent: An American Pediatric Surgical Association outcomes and evidence-based practice committee systemic review. J Ped Surg. 2019; 54:369–377.

Schultz KAP, Schneider DT, Pashankar F, et al. Management of ovarian and testicular sex cord-stromal tumors in children and adolescents. J Pediatr Hematol Oncol. 2012 May; 34(Suppl 2):S55–63. Doi:10.1097/mph.0b013e31824e3867

Shaikh F, et al. Paediatric extracranial germ-cell tumours. Lancet Oncol. 2016; 17(4),e149–e162. Doi:10.1016/s1470-2045(15)00545-8

Vaysse C, et al. Ovarian germ cell tumors in children. Management, survival and ovarian prognosis. A report of 75 cases. J Pediatr Surg. 2010; 45(7):1484–1490. Doi:10.1016/j.jpedsurg.2009.11.026

Von Allmen D and Fallat ME (2012). Ovarian Tumors. In Arnold C et al. (Ed.). *Pediatric Surgery* (7th ed., pp. 529–549), Elsevier Saunders.

36

Ovarian/Adnexal Torsion

Dana Elborno, Sari Kives and S. Paige Hertweck

Definition

Twisting of the adnexal pedicle due to laxity and/or presence of a mass resulting in obstruction of the arterial, venous, and lymphatic flow to ovary and eventual ovarian/tubal infarction if undiagnosed. Usually involves tube **and** ovary, but 5% of the time is isolated tubal torsion.

Key Points

- Ovarian/adnexal torsion is a surgical emergency due to the potential for
  - Infarction
  - Reproductive/hormonal compromise
  - Rare systemic infection/inflammation if left untreated
- Prompt diagnosis is important to provide intervention and salvage of involved structures
- The most common symptoms are sudden onset of abdominal pain that is intermittent, non-radiating, and associated with nausea and vomiting
- Transabdominal ultrasound is the imaging modality of choice – Decision to operate should **NOT** be based solely on sonographic findings and presence or absence of Doppler flow is not diagnostic
- Laparoscopy with untwisting +/– cystectomy is the preferred surgical approach
  - Ovarian function has been noted even in cases of blue-black appearing ovaries
  - Do not remove the ovary unless oophorectomy is unavoidable, such as when a severely necrotic ovary falls apart during the procedure
  - Risk of malignancy very low
- There is a predominance of right-sided torsion
- Most cases involve an underlying cystic or solid mass
  - Age <5, 25% of all cases are spontaneous without the presence of a mass

Common Presentation

- **Enlarged ovary** with or without mass with waves of **acute abdominal pain** often closely followed with onset of nausea and vomiting, eventual low-grade fever, and mildly elevated white blood cell count.

Differential Diagnosis

- Appendicitis
- Gastroenteritis – May see associated diarrhea or other family members with similar symptoms

DOI: 10.1201/9781003039235-36

- Ectopic pregnancy
- Pelvic inflammatory disease – Symptoms more gradual in onset vs torsion
- Hemorrhagic ovarian cyst
- Renal stone – More costovertebral angle tenderness; urine with large blood

Diagnosis

History

- Characterize pain: Location, quality, duration (can wax/wane), nausea/vomiting/anorexia (common)
- Past medical history: Previous torsion, abdominal surgery, inflammatory bowel disease, confidential sexual history

Physical Examination

- Vital signs: Look for fever/tachycardia
- Abdomen: Rebound tenderness/guarding, distention, aggravated by sitting up from supine position or with foot drop
  - Isolated tubal torsion may present with less-severe physical findings

Laboratory Testing

- **No** testing (i.e. leukocytosis, pyuria, C-reactive protein, ESR) is consistently useful in diagnosis

Ultrasound Findings

- Ovarian enlargement with or without mass
  - 70% of premenarchal patients have ovarian mass at the time of diagnosis
  - 80% of postmenarchal patients have ovarian mass at the time of diagnosis
  - Median volume of a torsed ovary without a mass is 12× that of the contralateral ovary in postmenarcheal females, as low as 3 times in premenarcheal girls
- Mass >5 cm (very unlikely in <5 cm or <125 mL in volume)
- Unilateral ovarian enlargement with ovarian edema characterized by peripherally displaced follicles giving a "String of pearls" sign-the appearance of multiple small follicles along ovarian periphery (see Figure 36.1)
- Complete absence of vascular flow is NOT necessary for diagnosis given dual vascular supply to the ovary from both ovarian and uterine vessels
- "Whirlpool sign" can sometimes be seen, is the appearance of twisted vascular pedicle
- Consider the use of prediction tool to score patients based on presentation and US findings
  - Includes menstrual status, presence of vomiting, adnexal volume, and adnexal size ratio (see Table 36.1)
  - Score of <3 there is <10% chance of torsion, expectant management may be appropriate

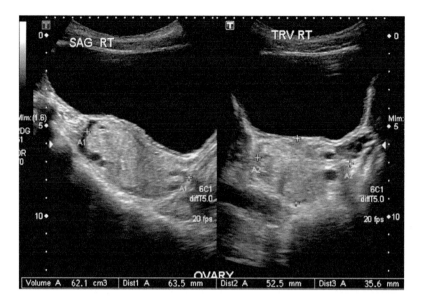

FIGURE 36.1   Unilateral ovarian enlargement with ovarian edema. (From Allen L, et al. Adnexal masses in the neonate, child, and adolescent, in Sanfilippo JS, et al., ed., *Sanfilippo's Textbook of Pediatric and Adolescent Gynecology*, CRC Press, 2019, with permission.)

Masses Associated with Torsion

- Typically benign cysts or neoplasm (commonly benign teratoma)
- Rates of malignancy are lower in ovarian masses that twist than in ovarian masses without torsion
- If torsion occurs in the presence of a mass with suspicious features for malignancy (see Chapter 35, "Ovarian Masses")
  - Recommended to complete urgent detorsion alone followed by routine evaluation with postoperative imaging and tumor marker analysis as indicated
  - It is NOT recommended to complete oophorectomy at the time of detorsion unless the malignancy workup has been completed preoperatively and is highly indicative of the presence of a malignancy

TABLE 36.1

Generation of Composite Scores

Independent Risk Factor	Value		Score
	Premenarchal	Menarchal	
Vomiting	No	No	0
	Yes	Yes	2
Adnexal volume (mL)	<6	>105	0
	6–17		1
	>17	105 or more	2
Adnexal ratio	<1–25	<2	0
	1.25–21	2–21	1
Composite score			Total (0–6)

Source: From Schwartz B, et al. Creation of a compositive score to predict adnexal torsion in children and adolescents. J Pediatr Adolesc Gynecol. 2018; 31(2):132–137, with permission.

- In cases of incomplete torsion, capillary hydrostatic pressure remains increased and obstructs lymphatic drainage, causing massive ovarian edema
- In cases of missed torsion, the ovary may autoamputate and resorb, calcify, or become a sessile complex mass within the abdominal cavity

Management

- If torsion is suspected, prompt surgical evaluation/management indicated
- Laparoscopy preferred surgical approach
  - Untwist and conserve tubo-ovarian tissue even if blue-black/necrotic in appearance
  - Decision to perform cystectomy can be at the discretion of the surgeon depending on edema/friability of the ovary, cystectomy will not affect future ovarian function
- Although ovarian bivalving after detorsion has been described as a possible technique to decrease ovarian intracapsular pressure, and allow for increased arterial perfusion, this is rarely performed clinically

Oophoropexy with permanent suture (e.g. 2-0 silk)

- No evidence that oophoropexy decreases incidence of recurrence or contralateral torsion/no literature to state that it causes harm
- Consider in cases of recurrent torsion of the normal ovary or absent contralateral ovary
- Theoretically could cause adhesions/distortion of ovary-tube relationship

Postoperative Course

- Patient likely to have slow recovery over 48–72 hours accompanied by fevers and increased white blood cell count that decreases over that time while the ovarian damage/tissue necrosis is corrected at the cellular level
- Should the patient worsen/not improve over 72 hours – repeat surgery with possible excision of affected adnexal structure would be indicated
- Recommend follow-up ultrasound at 4–6 weeks and 4–6 months

BIBLIOGRAPHY

Adnexal torsion in adolescents. American College of Obstetricians and Gynecologists Committee opinion no 783. Obstet Gynecol. 2019; 134(2):e56–e63. Doi:10.1097/aog.0000000000003373

Dasgupta R, et al. Ovarian torsion in pediatric and adolescent patients: a systematic review. J Pediatr Surg. 2018; 53(7):1387–1391. Doi:10.1016/j.jpedsurg.2017.10.053

Kives S. No. 341-diagnosis and management of adnexal torsion in children, adolescents, and adults. J Obstet Gynaecol Can. 2017; 39(2): 82–90.

Lawrence AE, Fallat ME, Hewitt G, et al. Factors associated with torsion in pediatric patients with ovarian masses. J Surg Res. 2021 Jul; 263:110–115.

Murphy DNC, et al. Post-operative ovarian morphology on ultrasound after ovarian torsion-Effect of immediate surgery: A retrospective cohort study. J Pediatr Adolesc Gynecol. 2021 Nov; 4:S1083-3188(21)00332-6. Doi: 10.1016/j.jpag.2021.10.013

Schwartz B, et al. Creation of a compositive score to predict adnexal torsion in children and adolescents. J Pediatr Adolesc Gynecol. 2018; 31(2):132–137. Doi:10.1016/j.jpag.2017.08.007

Tasset J, et al. Ovarian torsion in premenarchal girls. J Pediatr Adolesc Gynecol. 2019; 32(3):254–258. Doi:10.1016/j.jpag.2018.10.003

37

Pelvic Inflammatory Disease (PID)

Maggie L. Dwiggins

Key Points

- Spectrum of inflammatory disorders of the upper female genital tract
- Often caused by gonorrhea or chlamydia; however, only about half of women diagnosed with pelvic inflammatory disease (PID) will test positive for these two organisms
- Other causative organisms include *Mycoplasma genitalium, Gardnerella vaginalis, Haemophilus influenzae,* enteric Gram-negative rods, and other vaginal flora
- Screening for and treating gonorrhea and chlamydia reduces the risk of PID

Diagnosis

- Acute infection may be difficult to diagnose due to variation and subtlety of symptoms
- Clinical diagnosis has higher predictive value in the sexually active adolescent; however, no history, physical finding, or positive lab value is highly sensitive or specific for the diagnosis
- Must rule out other causes of pelvic pain (ectopic pregnancy, appendicitis, ovarian torsion, ovarian cyst, functional pain)

Minimum criteria (need at least 1)

- Cervical motion tenderness (CMT)
- Uterine tenderness
- Adnexal tenderness

Additional criteria that enhance specificity (at least 1)

- Oral temperature >38.3°C (>101°F)
- Mucopurulent cervical discharge or cervical friability
- Abundance of WBCs on saline microscopy of vaginal fluid
- Elevated erythrocyte sedimentation rate (ESR)
- Elevated C-reactive protein (CRP)
- Positive testing for gonorrhea or chlamydia

More specific diagnostic criteria include endometrial biopsy positive for endometritis, laparoscopic finding of salpingitis or positive intra-abdominal bacterial infection, however, are more invasive and not recommended in the setting of mild symptoms that are amenable to treatment.

MRI or transvaginal ultrasound may show thickened or fluid-filled fallopian tubes or tubo-ovarian abscess (TOA).

DOI: 10.1201/9781003039235-37

Treatment

- Should provide empiric, broad-spectrum coverage of causative organisms (if identified), anaerobes, plus gonorrhea and chlamydia

Hospitalization for

- Acute abdomen and the possible need for surgical intervention
- Tubo-ovarian abscess
- Pregnancy
- Severe illness, nausea, vomiting, or oral temperature >38.3°C (>101°F)
- Unable to follow or tolerate the outpatient oral regiment
- No response to outpatient therapy
- *NOTE*: There is no evidence that indicates adolescents have improved outcomes if hospitalized due to age alone

Parenteral treatment

- Ceftriaxone 1 g IV every 24 hours *plus* doxycycline 100 mg po/IV every 12 hours *plus* metronidazole 500 mg po/IV every 12 hours

  OR
- Cefotetan 2 gm IV every 12 hours *plus* doxycycline 100 mg po/IV every 12 hours

  OR
- Cefoxitin 2 g IV every 6 hours *plus* doxycycline 100 mg po/IV every 12 hours
- Alternate therapy: ampicillin-sulbactam 3 g IV every 6 hours *plus* doxycycline 100 mg po/IV every 12 hours OR clindamycin 900 mg IV every 8 hours *plus* gentamicin IV/IM 2 mg/kg loading dose followed by 1.5 mg/kg every 8 hours
- Continue for 24–48 hours after clinical improvement
- Transition to oral doxycycline 100 mg bid *plus* metronidazole 500 mg bid to complete 14 full days of treatment

IV/Oral treatment

- Ceftriaxone 500 mg (1g if weighing ≥150 kg) IM single dose *plus* doxycycline 100 mg po bid *and* metronidazole 500 mg po bid ×14 days

OR

- Cefoxitin 2 g IM single dose *and* probenecid 1 g po single dose *plus* doxycycline 100 mg po bid *and* metronidazole 500 mg po bid ×14 days
- Reevaluate within 72 hours to ensure clinical improvement; if no improvement, hospitalization and parenteral treatment is advised
  - *NOTE:* If IUD is used for contraception and is in proper location during acute PID infection, recommend treatment and continuing use of IUD, consider removal if no clinical improvement after 72 hours of parenteral treatment

For concomitant TOA

- Initial treatment is the same as for PID but also includes
  - Admit inpatient for at least 24 hours
  - If not responding within 72 hours, or clinically worsening in 24 hours, consider drainage

- Consider initial drainage if mass >7 cm
  – If locally available, drainage with interventional radiology (IR) is least invasive and recommended
  – Laparoscopic drainage otherwise preferred

Follow-Up

- Reevaluate within 72 hours for improvement in symptoms if treating outpatient
- Close follow-up after hospitalization is recommended
- Test for reinfection in 3 months
- Treat all sexual partners in last 60 days

Counseling

- 1 in 10 women with PID becomes infertile due to scarring of fallopian tubes; this number increases to nearly 50% after 3 infections
- Tubal scarring can lead to ectopic pregnancy
- Even one episode of PID can lead to chronic pelvic pain

BIBLIOGRAPHY

Centers for Disease Control and Prevention. Sexually transmitted diseases treatment guidelines 2021. MMWR Recomm Red. July 23; 2021;70(4).1–192.
Long-Acting reversible contraception: implants and intrauterine devices. American College of Obstetricians and Gynecologists Practice Bulletin No. 186. Obstet Gynecol. 2017 Nov;130(5):e251–e269.

38

Pelvic Pain

Amanda French

ACUTE PELVIC PAIN

Key Points

- The differential diagnosis for acute pelvic pain is long and varied (see "Differential Diagnosis" for examples, listed in no particular order, of common diagnoses. This list may not include all causes of pelvic pain)
- Common gynecologic causes include infection, ovarian cysts, endometriosis, ectopic pregnancy, or adnexal torsion
- Non-gynecologic sources include gastrointestinal, urinary, musculoskeletal, neurologic, and psychologic pathology
- Patients may have more than one diagnosis and one may potentiate pain from another

Differential Diagnosis

Gynecologic

- Pregnancy:
  - Ectopic pregnancy
  - Threatened abortion or miscarriage
- Ovary:
  - Cyst or mass
  - Torsion
- Fallopian tube:
  - Torsion
  - Hydrosalpinx or mass
- Cervix and vagina:
  - Obstruction
  - Foreign body
  - Mass
- Infection:
  - Endometritis
  - Cervicitis
  - Vaginitis and/or vulvitis
  - Pelvic inflammatory disease

- Cyclic:
  - Ovulatory pain (Mittleschmerz)
  - Dysmenorrhea
  - Endometriosis and/or adenomyosis
  - Obstructive Müllerian anomalies

Non-Gynecologic

- Gastrointestinal:
  - Appendicitis
  - Gastroenteritis
  - Inflammatory bowel disease
  - Meckel's Diverticulum
  - Intestinal Obstruction
  - Functional abdominal pain
  - Constipation
  - Hernia
  - Irritable bowel syndrome
  - Dietary (for example, lactose/gluten intolerance)

DOI: 10.1201/9781003039235-38

- Urologic:
  - Nephrolithiasis
  - Cystitis
  - Pyelonephritis
  - Painful bladder syndrome
- Musculoskeletal:
  - Acute muscle spasm (back, abdominal wall, pelvic floor, iliopsoas)
  - Trauma
  - Tumors
  - Bone or joint inflammation or infection
  - Trigger point/nerve entrapment
- Neurologic:
  - Nerve entrapment/neuralgia
- Pain amplification syndrome/nociplastic pain /other pain disorder
- Psychologic:
  - History of anxiety/depression
  - Physical or sexual abuse or trauma
  - Somatic pain
- Systemic illness:
  - Rheumatoid arthritis
  - Systemic lupus erythematosus
  - Fibromyalgia
  - Ehlers-Danlos
- Multiple concurrent diagnoses

Diagnosis

History

- When did the pain begin and when was the last menstrual period
- Onset of pain (gradual/sudden)
- Has this pain happened before
- Location of pain (right or left, periumbilical, upper or lower quadrants, vaginal, diffuse, etc.)
- Nature of pain (sharp, crampy, stabbing, constant, intermittent)
- Radiation (to back, down legs, to shoulder)
- Any medication or treatment (heat/cold, etc.) that helped or did not help
- Relieving/exacerbating symptoms
  - Walking/exercising/resting/eating/urinating/defecating
- Associated symptoms
  - Nausea, vomiting, fever, dysuria
  - When was the last bowel movement? Diarrhea? Constipation?

Gynecologic History

- Onset of menarche, when pain occurred in relation to menarche
- Menstrual history (last menstrual period, menorrhagia, dysmenorrhea)
- Sexual activity
- Contraceptive history
- Could patient be pregnant
- Vaginal discharge
- History of assault, abuse, or trauma
- History of sexually transmitted infection (STI)

Historical Clues

- Ovulatory pain: Typically dull pain at the time of ovulation lasting from minutes to hours (can be treated with nonsteroidal anti-inflammatory drugs or hormonal contraceptives)

- Dysmenorrhea: Cyclical pain with menses, could have associated nausea, vomiting, diarrhea, or constipation
- Torsion: Sudden onset of sharp pain, typically with nausea and/or vomiting.
- Musculoskeletal: Burning pain that is worse with movement, better with rest, history of injury preceding the pain. Can involve low back pain, could be worse with menses
- Gastrointestinal disease: Weight loss, diarrhea, constipation, symptoms that change with eating
- Appendicitis: Typically pain starts peri-umbilical and migrates to the right lower quadrant, associated with later onset of anorexia or nausea

Physical Examination

- A complete physical exam is ideal, if possible
- Vital signs including temperature
- Sexual Maturity Rating/Tanner staging
- Abdominal exam: Assess for masses, tenderness, hepatosplenomegaly, hernia, peritoneal signs, trigger points
- Back exam: Assess costovertebral angle (CVA) tenderness and muscle pain
- Pelvic exam (*Take into consideration age of patient, gender identity, any trauma history, and tailor the exam to the complaint and history – not all components of the exam are necessary for every patient, and patients may decline some or all of the exam. Obtain informed consent and explain the exam to the patient, keeping in mind confidentiality laws in your area with regard to adolescents and guidelines for chaperoning exams*)
  - External visual inspection of genitalia, including assessment of vulva, perineum, urethra, clitoris, hymen, and lower third of vagina, consider cotton swab to look for hymenal and vaginal anomalies and to ensure vaginal patency
  - If a bimanual exam is indicated
    - Assess the size, tenderness of uterus
    - Assess for vaginal mass or lesion, tenderness of urethra, bladder
    - Presence of cervical mass or cervical motion tenderness
    - Presence of adnexal mass or tenderness
    - Ensure patient not impacted with stool; heme test stool if indicated
  - If a speculum exam is indicated
    - Assess for bleeding, discharge, injury, other visible lesions, foreign body
    - Evaluate vaginal walls for bulging from an obstructive anomaly
  - If patient is prepubertal
    - An exam under anesthesia may be considered
    - A rectal exam may be considered and may be easier to tolerate than a vaginal exam
  - For cases where abuse is suspected, social services and local law enforcement must be involved, as well as providers with special training to evaluate victims of abuse

Laboratory Testing (Consider Based on Assessment)

- Complete blood count (CBC)
- Urinalysis
- Urine culture

- Nucleic acid amplification testing (NAAT) for gonorrhea and chlamydia (urine, vaginal, or cervical swab) or trichomonas
- Pregnancy test (urine or blood)
- Stool for occult blood
- Erythrocyte sedimentation rate (ESR)
- C-Reactive Protein (CRP)
- Vaginal culture

Imaging

- Pelvic ultrasound is preferred for evaluation of pelvic pathology and is first-line imaging for evaluation of possible appendicitis
  - Transabdominal imaging with a full bladder is the primary approach
  - Transvaginal approach may be considered for some older patients if appropriate
  - Transperineal approach can be useful when an obstructive anomaly is suspected
- Gastrointestinal films/skeletal films/other tests as indicated by history
  - Abdomen/pelvis radiograph to evaluate constipation, foreign body
  - Consult with pediatric surgery before recommending additional imaging such as CT for appendicitis
  - Occasionally MRI may be helpful, if available, and if previous imaging is confusing

Management

- Based on etiology of pain
- When diagnosis is not clear but exam is worrisome for acute abdomen
  - Diagnostic laparoscopy may help delineate cause by visualizing the pelvic and abdominal organs

CHRONIC PELVIC PAIN (CPP)

Key Points

- Endometriosis, musculoskeletal, and GI-related causes are the most common etiologies in the female adolescent
- The differential diagnosis is similar to that of acute pelvic pain, but the evaluation and treatment may proceed in a nonurgent fashion

Definition

- Lower abdominal menstrual or non-menstrual pain of at least 6 months duration

Common Causes

- Endometriosis
- Myofascial pain

- Pelvic inflammatory disease
- Irritable bowel syndrome
- Inflammatory bowel disease
- Constipation
- Pain disorders

Diagnosis

Assess for the major sources that might contribute to CPP (common examples are listed below; keep in mind that the differential diagnoses for acute pelvic pain also apply to chronic pelvic pain and that the patient may have more than one diagnosis).

Gynecologic

- Typically Cyclic
  - Dysmenorrhea
  - Ovulation pain
  - Endometriosis
  - Obstructive Müllerian anomalies
  - Ovarian cyst (physiologic/functional)
- Typically Noncyclic
  - Endometriosis
  - Ovarian Mass
  - Adhesions
  - Hydrosalpinx

Musculoskeletal and Neurological

- Myofascial pain
- Trigger points
- Anterior cutaneous nerve entrapment syndrome (ACNES)
- Fibromyalgia or other chronic pain syndromes

Gastrointestinal

- Irritable bowel syndrome
- Inflammatory bowel disease (Crohn's, ulcerative colitis)
- Constipation
- Lactose/gluten intolerance

Urologic

Psychologic

Systemic illness

History
- When was pain first noticed
- Localize pain: Groin, back, abdomen (right, left, upper, and/or lower quadrants, vaginal, umbilical, buttock, leg), abdominal wall
  - Radiation (does or does not?)

- Relation to menstrual cycles (cyclic or noncyclic?)
- Characterize pain: (Burning, sharp, stabbing, aching, squeezing, throbbing, steady, or intermittent)
  - Pain is worse at what time
  - Pain is worse with what position, activity
  - Pain is better with what position, activity
  - Does the pain awaken you from sleep? Can you sleep if you are in pain?
  - Does pain interfere with your normal activity? (school, sports)
- Any associated symptoms (nausea, vomiting, dysuria, diarrhea, constipation), what pain medicines or treatments have been used, and did they help?
- GI: How often do you have a bowel movement? Do you sit on the toilet for a long time? Diarrhea alternating with constipation? Blood in the stool? (Bristol Stool Scale – see Bibliography)
- Urologic: History of urinary tract infections, dysuria, frequency, incontinence, hematuria
- Substance use
- Psychologic: Depression or anxiety
- Sexual/physical/psychological abuse or trauma history
- Injury
- Family history (endometriosis, congenital anomaly, systemic illness)

Physical Examination

NOTE: A complete exam is ideal, if possible, and the sequence of the exam is important; if a bimanual is done, save for the final step as it incorporates multiple levels of tissue (e.g. uterus as well as abdominal musculature) and thus may have non-specific findings

- Observe self selected posture of the patient during an interview, walking to the exam room, moving onto an exam table
- Palpate lower back for pain or tenderness over bone (hip, spine)
- Abdomen
  - Have patient identify an area of tenderness and avoid that area at first
  - Try to locate any trigger points (often these are at muscle or fascia attachments or at lateral margins of rectus muscle – see Figure 38.1)
    - Cutaneous trigger point
      - With patient in supine position start at epigastric region and run fingers perpendicular to rectus muscle starting at the epigastric area and continuing vertical to the pubic bone
      - Ask patient to identify any area of tenderness along rectus – If trigger point is touched, though generally, the trigger point area is small (1–2 cm), the pain may radiate to other areas
      - If area of pain is located, hold pressure at the location of pain and have patient flex the neck to raise the head – If pain worsens, this is likely a rectus trigger point
    - Iliopsoas trigger point
      - At the level of umbilicus, palpate the lateral edge of rectus and press down medially into psoas muscle – If tender and pain worsens with ipsilateral straight leg lift – likely a psoas muscle trigger point
      - At the level of the anterior superior iliac spine, palpate inner border of ileum – If tender and pain worsens with ipsilateral straight leg lift – likely an iliacus muscle trigger point
      - Distal trigger point of iliopsoas can be appreciated by deep palpation at lesser trochanter along with the sartorius muscle

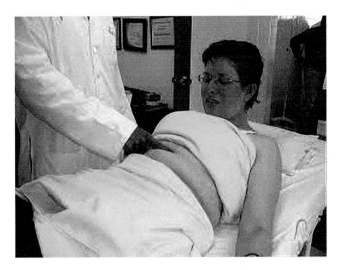

FIGURE 38.1 Locating trigger points along rectus muscle with head lift technique.

- Palpate each quadrant of abdomen for tenderness/fullness/masses
- Evaluate for hepatosplenomegaly/hernias
- Pelvic exam
  - Visual inspection of external genitalia including perineum, clitoris, and urethra
  - Perform cotton swab and/or a single digital exam of vagina (digital exam of vagina not possible in most prepubertal children, rectal exam may be considered instead)
  - Palpate anterior vagina, urethra, palpate lateral sidewalls of vagina to locate any levator muscle trigger point/tenderness
  - Palpate uterosacral ligaments
  - Check position/shape/mobility/tenderness of cervix and uterus
  - Speculum exam if appropriate based on age of patient, history and nature of complaint
  - Pap smear/NAAT STI testing if indicated
  - Bimanual exam if appropriate: Assess for location of tenderness, uterine enlargement, adnexal masses
  - Rectal exam (blood, fissures, stool impaction)

Laboratory Evaluation

- Complete blood count: Look for inflammation, anemia
- Urinalysis: Evaluate for renal/urinary tract disease
- NAAT testing: For gonorrhea and chlamydia (urine, vaginal or cervical specimen)
- Erythrocyte sedimentation rate (ESR): Check for inflammation, for example, inflammatory bowel disease
- Human chorionic gonadotropin (hCG): Rule out pregnancy

Imaging

- Pelvic ultrasound: Rule out pelvic mass/adnexal pathology, consider evaluation of kidneys and bladder
- Plain abdominal film: Rule out constipation
- Consider MRI if pelvic ultrasound is confusing

Management

- An empiric approach is generally preferred in children but management is tailored to the individual. While undergoing diagnostic testing, sequentially prescribe treatments for most likely causes and involve multidisciplinary evaluation (urology, gastrointestinal [GI], physical therapy)
    - If treatment relieves the pain, one can presume underlying cause and claim therapeutic success. If no relief, consider laparoscopy
- Diagnostic laparoscopy
    - Indications
        - Progressive dysmenorrhea without response to NSAIDs/hormonal treatment of menses with cycling or suppression
        - Suspected adnexal or uterine abnormalities
        - Unexplained painful, irregular bleeding
        - When diagnosis is unclear and pain persists
    - Look for evidence of endometriosis
        - Appearance may differ in adolescents as compared to adults (see "Endometriosis," Chapter 16)
- *NOTE*: A laparoscopy may be included as part of the initial workup for some patients
- *NOTE*: If laparoscopy is done and patient continues to have pain, the empiric approach may be continued; if organic pathology is not identified, consider referral to a pain management specialist

Treatment

- Primary dysmenorrhea: Painful menses in absence of specific pathologic cause
- Secondary dysmenorrhea: Painful menses due to specific gynecologic condition (e.g. endometriosis, obstructive Müllerian anomalies)
- See "Dysmenorrhea" (Chapter 14) for treatment
- Endometriosis: See "Endometriosis" (Chapter 16) for treatment
    - Base treatment on age of patient, severity of pain, any underlying medical condition, preservation of anatomy, and response to previous treatment
        - Medical suppression is mainstay of treatment in this age group (oral contraceptive pills/depot medroxyprogesterone acetate (DMPA)/long-acting reversible contraception such as subdermal implant or levonorgestrel releasing intrauterine device/GnRH agonist or antagonist)
        - Surgical (ablation/excision)
- GI symptoms: Gastroenterology referral
- Urinary tract symptoms: Urologic referral
- If pain worse with movement/better with rest, and/or identify muscle spasm/trigger point on exam and suspect musculoskeletal pain:
    - Refer for physical therapy (PT) and/or sports medicine/orthopedics
    - Even in cases of uncertain etiology or significant pathology, i.e. dysmenorrhea, endometriosis, a musculoskeletal component may be present, and pelvic floor physical therapy may be helpful

For intractable pain, consider a pain syndrome.

- Referral to a pain management specialist, use of alternative therapies such as acupuncture, yoga, Reiki, and massage, as well as psychological support (online resources, support groups, chat rooms) may be helpful

Always consider that patients may have more than one diagnosis, and thus one underlying process may potentiate the pain felt by a different organ system (e.g., a chronic back injury that is more painful during menses, constipation occurring concurrently with endometriosis, a co-existing trauma history).

BIBLIOGRAPHY

Chronic Pelvic Pain. ACOG Practice Bulletin number 218. American College of Obstetricians and Gynecologists Obstet Gynecol. 2020; 135(3):e98–e10. doi: 10.1097/AOG.0000000000003716

Dysmenorrhea and endometriosis in the adolescent. ACOG Committee Opinion Number 760. American College of Obstetricians and Gynecologists. Obstet Gynecol. 2018; 132:e249–e258.

Heaton KW, Lewis SJ. Stool form scale as a useful guide to intestinal transit time. Scand J Gastroenterol. 1997; 32(9):920–924.

International Pelvic Pain Society Research Committee Pelvic Pain Assessment. 2019. https://www.pelvicpain.org/IPPS/Content/Professional/Documents_and_Forms.aspx

Regino WO, Rodriguez EM, Mindiola AL. The cost of ignoring Carnett's sign: A case report and literature review. Rev Columb Gastroenterol. 2017; 32(1): 69–74.

39

Polycystic Ovary Syndrome (PCOS)

Lauren A. Kanner

Definition

A clinical syndrome of

- Ovulatory dysfunction — Either cycles <21 days or >35 days 2 years post-menarche *or* cycles <19 days or >90 days at any time post-menarche
- Clinical evidence of hyperandrogenism (hirsutism, acne, androgenic alopecia) and/or biochemical hyperandrogenemia via either elevated total or free testosterone
- Vaginal ultrasound evidence of polycystic ovarian morphology (**not** used in adolescents but can be used for diagnosis in adult women at least over 8 years post menarche or >age 21)
- Exclusion of other disorders (hyperprolactinemia, thyroid disorders, Cushing syndrome, non-classical congenital adrenal hyperplasia [CAH])

Key Points

- Also called chronic hyperandrogenic oligoanovulation (CHA), primary functional ovarian hyperandrogenism
- Many women have onset of symptoms during adolescence
- The most common cause of hyperandrogenism/hirsutism in adolescent girls
- The most common cause of infertility in young women
- Girls with idiopathic premature adrenarche are at increased risk of polycystic ovary syndrome (PCOS)
- Although PCOS is often associated with obesity, patients may be thin or normal in size

Pathophysiology

- Pathogenesis is multifactorial including genetic, neuroendocrine and environmental factors leading to altered ovarian steroidogenesis. Although there is familial clustering and genetic factors, less than 10% of PCOS heritability is accounted for by known genetic risk alleles.
- Basic defect is inappropriate gonadotropin (FSH, LH) stimulation of the ovary by the hypothalamic-pituitary unit leading to persistent anovulatory cycles.
  - Without proper signaling to the ovary, multiple small immature antral follicles (cysts) are present, hence, the term "polycystic ovary".
- The typical ultrasound ovarian appearance of "string of pearls" cysts is uncommonly seen in the adolescent, and therefore routine ultrasound for diagnosis is not recommended.
- PCOS patients are at risk for progression to metabolic syndrome, especially with concurrent insulin-resistant hyperinsulinism, dyslipidemia, nonalcoholic fatty liver disease, and psychiatric comorbidities of depression and anxiety.

DOI: 10.1201/9781003039235-39

Evaluation

History

- Menstrual pattern frequency, duration, age of menarche, primary/secondary amenorrhea (see Chapter 4, "Amenorrhea")
- Hirsutism-location, rapidity of onset, previous treatments, family history (differentiate hirsutism from hypertrichosis, which is not due to excess androgen)
- Premature adrenarche
- Acne specifically moderate-to-severe inflammatory acne which is persistent and poorly responsive to topical therapy
- Weight changes — Rapid gain, inability to lose weight despite diet/exercise
- Family history — Diabetes, gestational diabetes, PCOS, metabolic syndrome

Physical Examination

- Weight: Majority overweight but some may be thin, abdominal obesity common
- Blood pressure (BP): Rule out hypertension, elevations in BP may be due to CAH or obesity
- Skin: Hirsutism — Use Ferriman-Gallwey scoring (see "Hirsutism," Chapter 22), acanthosis nigricans (velvety, hyperpigmented, verrucous skin in the nape of neck, axilla, under breasts, in vulva and other body folds: associated with hyperinsulinemia), comedone and inflammatory acne unresponsive to topical medication
- Body habitus: Look for stigmata of Cushing's (violaceous striae, buffalo-hump, moon facies)
- Thyroid
- Abdomen: Look for male pattern midline hair growth, assess for abdominal masses
- External genitalia: Clitoromegaly, assess for signs of estrogenization (in severe hyperandrogenism, estrogen levels will be suppressed)

Laboratory Tests

- Rule out other causes of anovulation (see Chapter 1, "Abnormal Uterine Bleeding")

Baseline

- FSH, TSH, prolactin
- Total Testosterone: Many upper limits of normal 55 ng/dL, if >100 ng/dL rule out ovarian tumor with ultrasound
- Free testosterone (<9 pg/mL normal) plus sex hormone-binding globulin (SHBG)
  - If already on combined oral contraceptive pills, lab work may be falsely reassuring and should be rechecked off systemic medical treatment
- DHEAS
  - If > 700 ng/dL, rule out adrenal cause with CT of adrenals
- 17-hydroxyprogesterone acetate (17-OHP), best if drawn at 7 am and fasting
  - Normal <100 ng/dL
- If the level is 100–300 ng/dL, perform adrenocorticotropic hormone (ACTH) stimulation test to rule out CAHIf patient overweight, obese, or has acanthosis nigricans or if family history of diabetes or metabolic syndrome or if patient's mother had gestational diabetes
- Consider fasting hemoglobin A1c and/or oral glucose tolerance test, fasting lipid panel, AST, ALT

Management

Goals

- Whether diagnosed with PCOS or just considered "at risk", treatment should be started but individualized to optimize symptom relief
- Hormonal suppression to lower ovarian androgens, improve acne and hirsutism, prevent chronic estrogen exposure to the endometrium, and thereby prevent endometrial hyperplasia/carcinoma
- Address issue of hyperinsulinemia and obesity to decrease cardiovascular risk and risk of developing diabetes mellitus

Treatment Options

- First-line treatment: Cyclic combined oral contraceptives
    - Estrogens increase sex hormone-binding globulin, decrease free testosterone and decrease the production of adrenal androgens
- If irregular menstruation and unable to take estrogen-containing contraceptives use
    - Cyclic progestins: Provera 10 mg po cycle days 1–14 of the month
    - Continuous progestins for menstrual suppression
        - Includes continuous pills, LARC, subdermal implant, injection
        - Caution should be used with subdermal implant due to likelihood of irregular bleeding, as well as with injection due to possibility of weight gain
- If hirsute or severe acne
    - Add antiandrogen, such as spironolactone 100 mg po daily. Also, consider flutamide or finasteride but used less commonly
        - May not see decrease in hair for 3–6 months
        - Should be used with birth control due to antiandrogen effects on male fetuses impairing external genital development if used in pregnancy
    - Consider adjunctive hair treatments: Waxing, bleaching, electrolysis, laser removal
- If overweight/obese (see Chapter 29, "Obesity")
    - Strict caloric restriction with limited concentrated sugars intake, aerobic exercise of 150 minutes weekly according to the American Heart Association
    - Weight loss (even 5–10% loss) will decrease androgen production, improve insulin sensitivity, and reduce cardiovascular risk
- If evidence of insulin resistance or Hgb A1C >5.7%, consider the use of insulin potentiating medications
    - Referral to Endocrinology if lack of experience with these medications
    - Metformin (Glucophage®) XR
        - Start 500 mg po daily/bid and increase to 1000 mg bid as tolerable
        - Draw baseline electrolytes, BUN, creatinine, vitamin B12, ALT, AST
        - Common side effects: Heartburn, stomach pain, nausea, vomiting, bloating, gas, and diarrhea
        - Must temporarily discontinue use with dehydration/use of intravenous dyes as with radiographic studies until rehydrated and renal function recovers
        - Use contraindicated with renal insufficiency, congestive heart failure, hepatic dysfunction, metabolic acidosis, surgery, alcohol use

Long-Term Counseling

PCOS patients at risk of

Abnormal glucose metabolism, Type II diabetes mellitus, Non-alcoholic fatty liver disease, Dyslipidemia

- Emphasize weight reduction and exercise
- Assess for self-image issues and provide referral to psychotherapy as needed (see "Depression," Chapter 13)

Chronic anovulation leads to infertility or subfertility

- May need ovulation induction for pregnancy with use of aromatase inhibitor letrozole
- Consider referral to specialist after 6 months of inability to conceive as opposed to 1 year as per current definition of infertility
- If pregnancy is not desired, reliable contraception is recommended (menses occurs AFTER ovulation; therefore, there is a high risk of unintended pregnancy due to irregularity and unpredictability of ovulation)

Uterine health and risk of uterine cancer

- Unopposed estrogen increases the risk of uterine cancer, need progesterone support if fewer than 4 spontaneous periods per year

BIBLIOGRAPHY

Hoeger KM, Dokras A, Piltonen T. Update on PCOS: consequences, challenges, and guiding treatment. J Clin Endocrinol Metab. 2021:106(3);e1071–e1083.

Legro RS, Arslanian SA, Ehrmann DA, et al. Diagnosis and treatment of polycystic ovary syndrome: an Endocrine Society clinical practice guideline. J Clin Endocrinol Metab. 2013:98(12);4565–4592. Doi:10.1210/jc.2013-2350

Rosenfield RL. The diagnosis of polycystic ovary syndrome in adolescents. Pediatrics. 2015:136(6);1154–1165. Doi:10.1542/peds.2015-1430

Witchel SF, Burghard AC, Tao RH, Oberfield SE. The diagnosis and treatment of PCOS in adolescents: an update. Curr Opin Pediatr. 2019:31(4);562–569.

40

Premature/Primary Ovarian Insufficiency (POI)

Christina N. Davis-Kankanamge and Alla Vash-Margita

Definition

- Cessation of menstrual cycles prior to the age of 40
- Follicle-stimulating hormone (FSH) level and estradiol in the menopausal range two separate measurements 1 month apart
  - Numbers are dependent on the assay, typically
    - FSH > 30–40 mIU/mL
    - Estradiol <30 pg/mL
- Normal prolactin level and thyroid gland function

Key Points

- Can occur in the adolescent years.
- Can present with either primary or secondary amenorrhea, irregular menses ≥4 months apart, delayed or absent puberty.
- The incidence of primary ovarian insufficiency (POI) is not well established but has been estimated to be 0.9% among women under the age of 40 years.
- If POI presents as primary amenorrhea, up to 50% of those girls will have a chromosomal abnormality.
- Genetic causes account for approximately 20–25% of patients with POI
  - Use of next-generation sequencing (NGS) and whole-exome sequencing (WES) will lead to the discovery of the new candidate genes
  - A total of 10–15% of patients will have an affected first-degree relative

Differential Diagnosis

Genetic Causes

X chromosomal causes

- Turner syndrome (most common)
  - 45XO
    - Adolescents will present with absent or delayed puberty
    - Ovarian failure is due to accelerated atresia of the ovarian follicles
  - 45XO/46XX, mosaic pattern
    - Progressive loss of ovarian function
    - Ovarian tissue cryopreservation may be considered in selected cases in experimental setting

DOI: 10.1201/9781003039235-40

- POF1 in association with fragile X premutation
  - Trisomy X with or without mosaicism
- XY chromosomal causes
  - 46XY gonadal dysgenesis
  - 46XX gonadal dysgenesis
- Trisomy 21

Mutations in enzymes required in reproduction

- Carbohydrate-deficient glycoprotein deficiency
- Galactose-1-phosphate uridyl transferase (GALT) deficiency (galactosemia)
- 17 α-hydroxylase/17,20-desmolase deficiency
- Aromatase mutations

Mutations in hormone receptors/actions

- FSH/LH receptors

Iatrogenic

- *Effect of radiation*: Age- and dose-related (see Chapter 30, "Oncology Care and Gynecologic Concerns")
  - Prepubertal ovary is less sensitive to damage
- Bilateral oophorectomy
- Chemotherapeutic agents toxic to ovary especially alkylating agents (see Chapter 30, "Oncology Care and Gynecologic Concerns")

Autoimmune Disorders

- Associated with antibodies to other organs
  - Ovaries, adrenal, thyroid, parathyroid, pituitary glands, and smooth muscle
- Associated with other autoimmune states
  - Myasthenia gravis, diabetes mellitus, pernicious anemia, vitiligo, celiac disease, rheumatoid arthritis, systemic lupus erythematosus, congenital thymic aplasia, and IgA deficiency
  - Autoimmune oophoritis occurs in autoimmune polyendocrine syndromes (APS) I and II

Environmental Causes

Implicated Substances

- Phthalates
- Pesticides
- Bisphenol A (BPA)
- Cigarette (tobacco) smoking

Idiopathic Causes

- Diagnosis of exclusion, present in 85–90% of cases

Rare Causes

- Sarcoidosis
- Fanconi anemia
- Werner syndrome
- Bloom syndrome
- Ataxia telangiectasia
- Mumps
- Tuberculosis

NOTE: There is NO association between POI and receiving human papillomavirus (HPV) vaccine.

Diagnosis

Physical Exam

- Findings variable and dependent on whether the gonads have had some function
- Height and weight percentile with growth velocity
- *Breast exam*: Presence or absence, Tanner stage
- *Genital exam*: Assess Sexual Maturity Rating/Tanner stage pubic hair
  Assess for signs of estrogenization

Laboratory Tests

FSH level >30–40 mIU/mL

- Should be repeated if elevated with no explanation

Genetic testing: Should be done if elevated FSH with no explanation

Chromosome analysis

- If Y chromosome present, remove gonads to prevent malignant transformation
- Fragile X (FMR1) premutation carrier testing
- Chromosomal microarray analysis (CMA)
- Extended gene analysis (single-gene disorder)

If normal karyotype

- Check thyroid-stimulating hormone, thyroxine, complete blood count, calcium, phosphorus, 8 a.m. cortisol
- Consider antibody titers to thyroid, adrenal, ovary, islet, parietal cells to rule out further autoimmune disorders
- Screening for celiac disease: Transglutaminase antibodies and total IgA
- Check vitamin B12 level
- Screen for diabetes mellitus

Anti-Müllerian hormone (AMH) has been proposed as a quantitative marker of primordial follicles

- Can be a useful adjunct during ovarian tissue cryopreservation
- Not studied for use in adolescents

Not Recommended

- Anti-ovarian antibodies as not specific and not useful
- Inhibin B due to wide variation

Management

Consults with additional specialties may be helpful

- Pediatric endocrinology
- Genetics
- Psychology

Hormone Replacement Therapy (HRT)

Use estrogen and progestin medication to complete maturation of secondary sexual characteristics, individualized to particular patients' circumstances and pubertal progression (see Table 40.1).

- Induction of puberty
  - Estrogen only, start at a low dose and increase every 6 months
  - Use of transdermal preparations preferred to oral
- Establishment of menses and normal bone mineralization (12–18 months after induction)
  - Further increase estrogen
  - Add progesterone to protect endometrium (usually after first breakthrough bleeding, see in the succeeding sections)
- Long-term management
  - After breast development is finished
  - Maintenance dose of estrogen
  - Progestin cyclically: oral medroxyprogesterone 5–10 mg daily or micronized progesterone 200 mg daily for 12 days of the month
- Sexually active teens may switch to cyclic combined estrogen/progestin contraceptive formulations for long-term management
  - Pills, transdermal patch, or vaginal ring
  - Transdermal estrogen patch (long-term dose) and levonorgestrel intrauterine device (IUD), etonogestrel subdermal implant, or depot medroxyprogesterone is an alternative
- Although there are many options for HRT, there is no proven correct way

HRT Does NOT increase risk for VTE when used in physiologic doses.

TABLE 40.1

Sample Estrogen Dosing Schedules

Formulation/Route	Induction	Establishment of Menses	Long-Term Management
Micronized 17β-estradiol (oral)	0.5 mg daily	1 mg daily	2 mg daily
Micronized 17β-estradiol (transdermal)	0.00625–0.025 mg twice weekly	0.025–0.05 mg twice weekly	0.075–0.1 mg twice weekly

Additional Considerations

- Consider serial bone density evaluation (see Chapter 33, "Osteoporosis"):
  - Adolescents accrue peak bone mineral density in puberty; any interruption can have a negative impact, which should be documented, monitored, and addressed
- Administer 1,000–2,000 IU vitamin D3 (cholecalciferol) daily, along with 1200 mg of elemental calcium, either through dietary sources or supplements
- Monitor annual blood pressure, lipid levels every 5 years and nutritional counseling, vitamin D level assessment
- Thyroid gland function screening every 1–2 years
- Parathyroid gland function screening every 1–2 years (check calcium/phosphorus level)
- Patients with adrenal antibodies: Yearly screening to monitor for adrenal insufficiency
- Patients with Turner syndrome with or without cardiac pathology: Follow according to specific Turner syndrome guidelines (see Chapter 53, "Turner Syndrome")
- Counseling due to the stress and long-term fertility ramifications of POI for patient and family
- If sexually active, will need contraception (see in the preceding sections, Chapter 12, "Contraception")
  - Rare spontaneous ovulation has been reported (~5%)
- Family building: Spontaneous conception, child-free living, adoption, foster children, oocyte donation, and embryo donation
- Fertility preservation: Ovarian tissue cryopreservation may be a possibility in selected cases
- Continue HRT until the age of natural menopause (~50–51 yo)
- Increased risk for osteoporosis, cardiovascular events, and cognitive decline in untreated individuals as adults
- Can affect sexual functioning, mental health, and mood
- Increased risk for specific morbidity related to underlying etiology of POI

BIBLIOGRAPHY

Divasta, AD, Gordon, CM (2020). Primary Ovarian Insufficiency. In Emans SJ, Laufer MR, DiVasta AD, eds., *Pediatric and Adolescent Gynecology* (7th ed., pp. 409–417). Philadelphia, PA: Wolters-Kluwer.

Hormone therapy in primary ovarian insufficiency. Committee Opinion No. 698. American College of Obstetricians and Gynecologists. Obstet Gynecol. 2017; 129(5):e134–e141.

Primary ovarian insufficiency in adolescents and young women. Committee opinion no. 605: American College of Obstetricians and Gynecologists. Obstet Gynecol. 2014; 124(1):193–197.

Qin Y, Jiao X, Simpson JL, Chen ZJ. Genetics of primary ovarian insufficiency: new developments and opportunities. Hum Reprod Update. 2015; 21(6):787–808.

41

Premenstrual Dysphoric Disorder (PMDD)

Rachael L. Fisher

Definition

Distinct changes that occur during the last week of the luteal phase, including markedly depressed mood, anxiety, affective lability, and anhedonia, with these symptoms being minimal or absent in the week after menses. The timing rather than the nature of the symptoms is important.

Key Points

- PMDD is the most severe form of premenstrual syndrome (PMS) with the cyclical reoccurrence of severe and sometimes debilitating changes in affect, particularly mood lability and irritability.
- Symptoms occur in the luteal phase of the menstrual cycle and subside shortly after the onset of menses.
- Present in 2–5% of women overall.

Diagnosis

Confirmation requires at least two prospectively charted cycles (using diaries) that correlate periodicity with symptoms *and* presence of 5 of the 11 specific symptoms (see in the succeeding sections) *and* clear documentation of impairment. Diagnosis can be made provisionally prior to confirmation.

DSM-V criteria for PMDD:

In most menstrual cycles during the past year, five or more of the following symptoms are present during the week before menses, begin to improve within a few days after the onset of menses, and are minimal or absent in the week post menses.

At least one of the five symptoms must be one of the first four on the list

1. **Marked lability (e.g. sudden sadness or tearfulness, increased sensitivity to rejection, mood swings)**
2. **Persistent irritability, anger, or increased interpersonal conflicts**
3. **Feelings of marked sadness, hopelessness, or self-deprecating thoughts**
4. **Pronounced tension, anxiety, and/or feelings of being 'on edge'**
5. Decreased interest in usual activities (e.g. school, friends, work, hobbies)
6. Difficulty concentrating
7. Feeling fatigued, lethargic, or lacking in energy
8. Marked changes in appetite, which may be associated with binge eating or craving certain foods
9. Hypersomnia or insomnia
10. A subjective feeling of being overwhelmed or out of control
11. Other physical symptoms, such as breast tenderness or swelling, joint or muscle pain, weight gain, or a sensation of bloating

DOI: 10.1201/9781003039235-41

Evaluation

Before concluding PMDD is the sole diagnosis

- Need to investigate disturbance is not an exacerbation of symptoms of another disorder (e.g. major depression, bipolar, panic disorder, personality disorder) as PMDD can co-occur with any of these disorders
- Need to evaluate symptoms not attributed to physiologic affects from a substance (e.g. medication, drug abuse, other treatment) or another medical condition (hyperthyroidism)

History

- Ensure regularity of menstrual cycles
- If cycles irregular (<21 days or >45 days)
  - Perform appropriate endocrine evaluation (see "Abnormal Uterine Bleeding," Chapter 1)
- Obtain 2 months of prospective symptom rating
  - The Daily Record of Severity of Problems (DRSP) is a prospective validated rating tool
  - Premenstrual Symptoms Screening Tool (PSST) is a retrospective tool to make a preliminary diagnosis
  - Symptom recordings can be achieved online via an iPad, computer, or mobile phone or be paper based (consider the use of Me v PMDD app for smartphone, but need to help patient with use, consider downloading it during visit and review use as language is not adolescent-friendly)
  - Can print DRSP from the internet (RCOG 2007, Green-top Guideline no. 48 appendix 3)
- Obtain a confidential sexual history

Physical Examination

- Assess for medical conditions
- Evaluate for signs/symptoms of thyroid disease
  - *Hypothyroidism*: Dry skin, goiter, delayed deep tender reflex, constipation, hair loss
  - *Hyperthyroidism*: Tachycardia, tremors, exophthalmos, diarrhea, vomiting

Laboratory Tests

- Complete blood count, chemistry profile, thyroid-stimulating hormone to rule out other causes

Management

If no medical condition is identified

- Have patient record symptoms prospectively for 2 months with a prospective symptom rating scale. Example: DRSP

If *no* documented symptom-free interval in follicular phase

- Have patient evaluated for mood or anxiety disorder

If documented symptom-free follicular phase or significant reduction of symptoms in follicular phase

- Patient then qualifies for the treatment options listed next
  - If the patient is sexually active prescribe contraceptives in addition to treatment

- Continue to validate diagnosis through continued prospective charting, offer reassurance and education regarding the hormonal basis for symptoms
- Provide education regarding effects of ovarian hormones and menstrual cycle on mood and behavior in addition to the charting of symptoms to increase awareness and predictability.
- Recognition allows for better behavioral self-management and can be helpful for an adolescent and her family

Treatment

Pharmacologic treatment

Antidepressants: Selective serotonin reuptake inhibitors (SSRIs)

- First-line treatment in females 18 years of age and older

  Fluoxetine (Sarafem® or Prozac®)

  - A total of 20 mg dose daily (FDA-approved dose for PMS)
  - 15% of patients will experience side effects
  - Most common
    – Headache
    – Nausea
    – Insomnia
    – Anxiety/jitteriness
    – Sexual dysfunction
  - There is no evidence that increasing dose will improve response
  - Dosing options include
    – Intermittent dosing (begin at the time of presumed ovulation approximately 14 days before the next menstrual cycle and continue until 1–2 days after the onset of menses) *or*
    – Continuous daily dosing
  - Daily dosing best for patients with comorbid anxiety or mood disorders, difficulty remembering an atypical medication regimen, side effects from initiation or withdrawal of SSRIs

  Sertraline (Zoloft®)

  - May be effective
  - A dose of 50–150 mg/day throughout the menstrual cycle

NOTE: It is important to recognize the complexity of prescribing antidepressants in an adolescent population. A health-care provider with experience and training treating adolescents with mental health disorders should manage these patients.

Hormonal Options

Combined Oral Contraceptives

Use of cyclic 3-mg drospirenone/20-μg ethinyl estradiol (Yaz®)

May help PMDD

- Side effects include
  - Nausea
  - Intermenstrual bleeding
  - Breast pain

Use of a continuous oral contraceptive regimen (e.g. levonorgestrel (90 µg) and at least 20-µg ethinyl estradiol equivalent)

- Take pills daily skipping placebo pills

Gonadotropin-releasing hormone (GnRH) agonists

- Lupron Depot 3.75 mg IM monthly
- Counsel patient/parent about potential bone loss
- Give norethindrone acetate (Aygestin®) 5 mg PO daily
- Assess patient's vitamin D level to maintain normal intake
- Instruct patient to have 1000–1300-mg calcium intake daily (diet plus appropriate supplement) with 400-IU Vitamin D
- Encourage weight-bearing exercise

Non-Pharmacologic Treatment

- Cognitive behavioral therapy (CBT) as adjunctive therapy to medical management

BIBLIOGRAPHY

American Psychiatric Association (2013). *Diagnostic and Statistical Manual of Mental Disorders, 5th Edition (DSM-5).* Arlington, VA: American Psychiatric Association.

Endicott J, Nee J, Harrison W. Daily record of severity of problems (DRSP): reliability and validity. Arch Women's Ment Health. 2006; 9(1):41–49.

Lopez LM, Kaptein AA, Helmerhorst FM. Oral contraceptives containing drospirenone for premenstrual syndrome. Cochrane Database of Systematic Reviews. 2012; (2). Art. No.: CD006586. DOI: 10.1002/14651858.CD006586.pub4

Marjoribanks J, Brown J, O'Brien PMS, Wyatt K. Selective serotonin reuptake inhibitors for premenstrual syndrome. Cochrane Database of Syst Rev 2013; (6). Art. No.: CD001396. DOI: 10.1002/14651858.CD001396.pub3

Nevatte T, O'Brien PMS, Bäckström T, et al. ISPMD consensus on the management of premenstrual disorders. Arch Womens Mental Health. 2013; 16:279–291.

Rapkin AJ, Mikacich JA. Premenstrual dysphoric disorder and severe premenstrual syndrome in adolescents diagnosis and pharmacologic treatment. Pediatr Drugs. 2013; 15:191–202.

42

Premenstrual Syndrome (PMS)

Rachael L. Fisher

Definition

Premenstrual syndrome (PMS) is a cyclic reoccurrence of severe physical or behavioral changes, which can result in interference with interpersonal relationships and normal activities. PMS occurs during the luteal phase of the menstrual cycle and resolves shortly after the onset of menstruation.

Key Points

- Three in four women will say PMS symptoms occur at some point in their lifetime with most having minimal symptoms
- Differs from premenstrual dysphoric disorder (PMDD) in that a minimum of five symptoms is not required (see Chapter 41, "PMDD") and does not have the required affective symptoms
- Diagnosis depends on exclusion of other medical and psychiatric disorders

Diagnosis

- Establish cyclic occurrence with the prospective recording of symptoms on a calendar for 2–3 cycles.
- Have the patient list three to five symptoms that are the most concerning and track them daily. Review the symptom diary in 2–3 months. Cyclical symptoms are severe enough to impair the adolescent's life.
- Example for recording symptoms can use Daily Record of Severity of Problems (DRSP) (see Chapter 41, "PMDD") and patients can also download a paper symptom tracker from the International Association for Premenstrual Disorders (IAPDMD) website at https://iapdmd. org/toolkit.

Symptoms

- PMS can be identified based on the presence of at least one behavioral symptom and one physical symptom during the 5 days prior to menses and relieved after the onset of menses (Table 42.1).
- Occur in the absence of hormone ingestion, pharmacologic therapy, or drug/alcohol usage.

History

- Menstrual history (menarche, cycle interval, length of flow)
- Associated menstrual symptoms
  - Dysmenorrhea
  - Nausea/vomiting/diarrhea

DOI: 10.1201/9781003039235-42

TABLE 42.1

PMS Symptoms

Behavioral	Physical
Anxiety	Abdominal bloating
Irritability	Breast tenderness or swelling
Depression	Headache
Expressed anger	Swollen extremities
Confusion	Weight gain
Social withdrawal	Joint or muscle pain

- Onset of time with PMS symptoms to menstruation
- Previous attempts at treatment
- Impact of PMS symptoms on activities (such as missing school or other life events)
- Past medical history:
  - Any past/chronic illnesses
  - Psychiatric disorders
  - Increased life stressors: change in school/divorce/death
  - Athletic endeavors

Physical Examination

While typically the exam is normal, look for any organic cause of symptoms

- Thyroid disorder
- Chronic diseases
- Pelvic pain due to ovarian cyst or endometriosis

Laboratory Tests

Laboratory testing is rarely needed but may consider on an individual basis

- Complete blood count (CBC), erythrocyte sedimentation rate (ESR) to evaluate for anemia, chronic disease
- Thyroid function tests (TFTs) – Evaluate thyroid status
- Other tests as indicated by exam (e.g. prolactin for galactorrhea)

Management

Treatments are used in a stepwise approach with increasing order of complexity. Suggest supportive measures first prior to medical management.

Non-pharmacologic treatments

- Educate about PMS disorder
- Encourage healthy diet (complex carbohydrates vs simple)
- Recommend regular aerobic exercise
- Identify stressors/refer for help with stress reduction
  - Relaxation measures: breathing exercises, yoga, meditation
- Obtain adequate sleep

- Consider initiation of cognitive behavioral therapy
- Nutritional supplementation with calcium 1200 mg total (divided in daily doses) can help reduce physical and mood symptoms

Pharmacologic treatments

- If non-pharmacologic treatment is unsuccessful then start with the medications with the lowest side effect profiles
- Start with oral contraceptive pills (OCPs) or spironolactone. If no success in three cycles, then try selective serotonin reuptake inhibitors (SSRIs)
- In severe cases, consider short-term use of gonadotropin-releasing hormone (GnRH) with add-back hormonal therapy, understanding the unknown full negative potential effect on adolescent and long-term bone density

Suggest obtaining a second opinion from an appropriate specialist regarding the patient's specific symptoms (i.e. gastroenterology for nausea, neurology for headaches, etc.).

NSAIDs

- Can be helpful for premenstrual headaches, breast pain, abdominal cramping

Spironolactone

- May alleviate breast tenderness/bloating/perceived weight gain
- 100 mg by mouth daily from cycle day 12 until onset of menses

Oral Contraceptives

- May improve physical symptoms
- Offer cyclical or continuous use
- May help especially teens with premenstrual seizures

SSRIs

Fluoxetine 20 mg/day continuously and/or luteal phase administration (14 days before next period expected and continued until 1–2 days after onset of menses)
- May increase does up to 60 mg/day if needed but may have increased side effects
- Side effects: Insomnia, sweating, gastrointestinal irritability, sexual dysfunction, mental disturbance
- Usually administered in the morning to reduce difficulty falling asleep
- A health-care provider with experience and training treating adolescents with mental health disorders should manage these patients

GnRH Agonists

Depot leuprolide acetate 3.75 mg monthly
- Counsel patient/parent regarding the risk of osteoporosis with use as well as side effect profile
- Give Aygestin (ESI Lederle, Inc., Philadelphia, PA) 5 mg by mouth daily
- Ensure calcium supplement plus diet is 1500 mg/day
- Give 400 IU vitamin D by mouth daily

- Encourage weight-bearing exercise
- Treatment for more than 6 months carries a significant risk of osteoporosis and limits long-term usefulness (see "Osteoporosis," Chapter 33)

BIBLIOGRAPHY

Premenstrual Syndrome. In American College of Obstetricians and Gynecologists' *Guidelines for Women's Health Care A Resource Manuel* (4th ed., pp. 607–610). Washington, DC: Amer College of Obstetricians & Gynecologists.

Rapkin AJ, Mikacich JA. Premenstrual dysphoric disorder and severe premenstrual syndrome in adolescents diagnosis and pharmacologic treatment. Pediatr Drugs. 2013;15:191–202.

U.S. Department of Health and Human Services, Office on Women's Health. Premenstrual syndrome (PMS). Available at: https://www.womenshealth.gov/menstrual-cycle/premenstrual-syndrome. Retrieved May 27, 2020.

Yonkers KA, O'Brien PM, Eriksson E. Premenstrual syndrome. Lancet 2008;371: 1200–1210.

43

Prolactin Disorders

Ann Marie Mercier and Kathryn Stambough

Definitions

- Hyperprolactinemia: Prolactin level greater than the upper limit of laboratory assay (typically >20–25 ng/ml)
- Hypoprolactinemia: Prolactin level less than the lower limit of laboratory assay (typically <2 ng/ml)

Key Points

- Prolactin is secreted from the anterior pituitary
- Primarily stimulates proliferation and differentiation of mammary cells; also contributes to metabolic homeostasis
- Production is predominantly regulated by a negative feedback loop involving dopamine
- Recommended to check AM/fasting prolactin level, as prolactin is typically lowest after fasting and in the morning. Can naturally increase after eating, stress, exercise, nipple stimulation, and coitus
- Hyperprolactinemia is more common; hypoprolactinemia is clinically very rare

Hyperprolactinemia

Evaluation

History

- Symptoms of menstrual abnormalities, galactorrhea, possible visual field defects, headaches, or pubertal delay or arrest

Physical Exam

- Visual field examination and possible ophthalmology consultation
- Skin exam; evaluate for evidence of hyperandrogenism and chest wall trauma
- Thyroid exam
- Breast exam
- Exam of the external genitalia for evidence of hypoestrogenemia

Diagnostic Testing

- Random prolactin level
  - If elevated repeat as AM fasting prolactin level
  - If elevation persists, or if levels >100 ng/mL, imaging may be warranted

DOI: 10.1201/9781003039235-43

- MRI of the hypothalamus and pituitary with gadolinium contrast is the preferred imaging modality
- Obtain TSH, pregnancy test, hepatic function panel with an assessment of renal and liver function

Most Common Causes

1. Physiologic (pregnancy, postpartum/postabortal/lactating, repetitive nipple stimulation)
2. Pathologic
   a. Cranial tumors (pituitary adenoma, prolactinoma, congenital colloid cyst)
   b. Systemic disease (PCOS, chronic renal failure, hypothyroidism, Cushing's, Addison's, hypothalamic diseases)
   c. Other (genetic causes, such as multiple endocrine neoplasias, and McCune-Albright, inflammatory diseases, such as sarcoidosis, pituitary infundibular injury, chest wall trauma such as herpes zoster or chest wall surgery)
3. Pharmacologic
   a. Dopamine antagonists, antihypertensives, H2-receptor antagonists, gastric motility medications, antipsychotics, antidepressants, opiates
4. Idiopathic

Management

- Treatment is based on the etiology of hyperprolactinemia
  - Asymptomatic children/adolescents due to idiopathic causes or pituitary adenoma can be offered expectant management
  - Symptomatic children need treatment. Consultation with a pediatric endocrinologist prior to management is imperative
- Goals: Resolve symptoms, normalize pubertal development, restore gonadal function, decrease tumor size, and maintain bone mass
- Medical treatment with Dopamine agonists (bromocriptine or cabergoline)
  - Dose monitored and adjusted based on prolactin level
  - Often requires long-term use
  - Bromocriptine: 2.5–15 mg/day
  - Cabergoline: Initial dose of 0.25–0.5 mg weekly and gradually increased every 4 weeks to 0.5–3.5 mg 1–2× per week
    - More expensive than bromocriptine but generally better tolerated with less-frequent dosing
- Treatment of hyperprolactinemia due to prolactinoma
  - Dopamine agonist
  - Surgical intervention if the absence of response to medical management, concern for visual impairment, or macroadenoma >10 mm
- If due to medication or other medical conditions, treat underlying cause
- If menstrual irregularities persist after treatment, consider menstrual regulation with exogenous hormonal therapy

Hypoprolactinemia

- Rarely diagnosed in children and adolescents. Most often diagnosed after deficiency of other pituitary hormones.

Most common causes

1. Empty sella syndrome
2. Medications (dopamine agonists)
3. Destruction of pituitary tissue (Sheehan syndrome, inflammation or autoimmune, tumor, post-operative, postradiation, infection)
4. Pseudohypoparathyroidism
5. Idiopathic

Management

- If accompanied by panhypopituitarism, replacement of deficient hormones (e.g. ACTH deficiency – hydrocortisone, TSH deficiency – levothyroxine, gonadotropin deficiency – estrogen/progestin)
- Treatment for macroadenoma destroying lactotroph cells: Neurosurgical consultation for likely surgical intervention
- Otherwise, there is no available treatment to replace prolactin

BIBLIOGRAPHY

Bernard V, Young J, Binart N. Prolactin—a pleiotropic factor in health and disease. Nat Rev Endocrinol. 2019; 15:356–365. https://doi.org/10.1038/s41574-019-0194-6

Hoffmann A, Adelmann S, Lohle K, et al. Pediatric prolactinoma: initial presentation, treatment, and long-term prognosis. Eur J Pediatr. 2018; 177:125–132. https://doi.org/10.1007/s00431-017-3042-5

Matalliotakis M, Koliarakis I, Matalliotaki C, Trivli A, Hatzidaki E. Clinical manifestations, evaluation and management of hyperprolactinemia in adolescent and young girls: a brief review. Acta Biomed. 2019; 90(1):149–157. https://doi.org/10.23750/abm.v90i1.8142

44

Puberty

Katherine L. O'Flynn O'Brien

Definition

Normal: Onset between ages 8 and 13 years

Delayed: Absence of breast development or secondary sex characteristics by age 13 *or*
Delay in menarche 4 years from thelarche *or*
Lack of menses by age 15 *or*
Lack of menses by age 14 and hyperandrogenic features (hirsutism, acne)

Precocious: Age cutoffs for evaluation are debated for precocious puberty (PP)

- Historically, considered the development of secondary sexual characteristics before age 8
- Newer definitions suggest evaluation for White girls ≤ 7 years old and Black girls ≤ 6 years old
- Proposed considerations for evaluation
Isolated thelarche **or** adrenarche younger than age 6 *or*
Thelarche **and** adrenarche younger than age 8

Isolated PP: Includes premature thelarche, premature pubarche, and premature menarche

- Characterized by a lack of linear growth or associated skeletal development or other pubertal characteristics
- All are diagnoses of exclusion, tailor workup to each clinical scenario

Key Points

- Average age of puberty has decreased over the past decades
- Constitutional delay of puberty is a diagnosis of exclusion
- PP may result in short stature due to early closure of epiphyseal plates if untreated
- Incomplete forms of PP, such as premature thelarche, may be benign variants or may progress to true PP
- Older age limits for evaluation of PP may miss a population of girls who have true pathologic PP; therefore, development of pubertal changes between ages 6 and 8 warrant a thorough history and physical to inform decision for close observation vs a limited initial workup
- In isolated PP, 1/3 of patients will progress to central PP, 2/3 remain as an isolated benign variant

     DOI: 10.1201/9781003039235-44

TABLE 44.1

Mean Age (in Years) of Pubertal Milestones by Racial/Ethnic Group

	Black	Mexican American	Non-Hispanic White
Thelarche	9.5	9.8	10.3
Pubarche	9.5	10.3	10.5
Menarche	12.1	12.2	12.7

Source: Data from NHANES III 1988–1994, https://wwwn.cdc.gov/nchs/nhanes/nhanes3/default.aspx

Normal Pubertal Development

Onset between ages 8 and 13 years

- Timing influenced by genetics, health status, and social and environmental factors (Table 44.1)
- Normal pubertal sequence: Thelarche, adrenarche, maximal growth velocity, menarche
- Total length of development is ~4.5 years (range: 1–6 years)

Delayed Puberty

Differential Diagnosis of Delayed Puberty

Subtype can be stratified by gonadotropin [follicle-stimulating hormone (FSH) and luteinizing hormone (LH)] and estradiol levels (E2); see Table 44.2.

TABLE 44.2

Stratification of Delayed Puberty

	Hypogonadotropic Hypogonadism	Hypergonadotropic Hypogonadism	Eugonadism
Lab results	Low-to-normal LH and FSH, low E2	High LH and FSH, low E2	Normal levels of LH, FSH, and E2
Conditions	*CNS causes*	*Gonadal causes*	*Anatomic causes*
	• Constitutional delay (most common, diagnosis of exclusion) • Chronic disease • Energy deficit (e.g. excessive weight loss/disordered eating/relative energy deficiency in sport (RED-S)) • Depression/stress • Genetic syndromes (e.g. Prader-Willi syndrome) • Defects in GnRH signaling (e.g. Kallman syndrome, GnRH receptor defects) • CNS tumors (e.g. craniopharyngioma) • Pituitary causes (e.g. infiltrative disease, prolactinomas, panhypopituitarism) • Medications (e.g. antipsychotic drugs) *Thyroid causes* • Hypothyroidism *Adrenal causes* • Congenital adrenal hyperplasia (CAH) • Cushing syndrome	• Primary ovarian insufficiency (idiopathic or autoimmune) • Turner syndrome • Fragile X carrier • Gonadal dysgenesis • Gonadotoxic chemotherapy or abdominal/pelvic radiation • Galactosemia • Oophorectomy *Peripheral signaling defects* • 17α-hydroxylase deficiency • Aromatase deficiency • LH and FSH receptor defects	• Imperforate hymen • Transverse vaginal septum • Lower vaginal atresia • Cervicovaginal agenesis • Müllerian aplasia syndromes (e.g. Mayer-Rokitansky-Kuster-Hauser syndrome or MRKH) • Androgen insensitivity syndrome

History

- *Age of initiation of any pubertal development and rate of development:* Distinguish between lack of development and halted development
- *Birth history:* Congenital anomalies, history of intrauterine growth restriction, neonatal hypoglycemia
- *Past medical history:* Chronic disease (e.g. inflammatory bowel disease, sickle cell disease), exposure to chemotherapy, thyroid disease, history of traumatic head injury
- *Past surgical history:* Anorectal anomalies, pelvic surgery
- *Family history:* Parental heights, age of menarche of close female relatives, family history of delayed menarche/puberty, androgen insensitivity, CAH, autoimmune conditions, fragile X premutation carriers, ovarian tumors
- *Medications:* e.g., antipsychotic medications

Review of Systems

- *Constitutional:* Weight changes, excessive exercise
- *HEENT:* Blurred vision, lack of smell
- *Gastrointestinal:* Chronic or cyclic abdominal pain, diarrhea
- *Genitourinary:* Sexual activity
- *Integumentary:* Hirsutism, acne
- *Neurological:* Headaches, lack of smell
- *Psychiatric:* Disordered eating habits, substance abuse
- *Endocrine:* Hot or cold flashes, galactorrhea

Physical Exam

- Review previous height and weight, compared with standard growth curves (see Chapter 29, "Obesity")
- *Blood pressure*
- *General:* Midline facial defects, short stature, webbed neck
- *Thyroid:* Assess for thyromegaly, goiter
- *Breast:* Sexual Maturity Rating/Tanner stage, galactorrhea, shield chest
- *Abdomen:* Pelvic masses
- *Genitourinary:* Tanner stage, evidence of estrogen effect, assess for patent hymen, clitoromegaly, urogenital sinus or ambiguous genitalia, determine the presence of a uterus, consider rectal exam to assess for pelvic mass and presence of uterus in nonsexually-active patients

Diagnostic Evaluation

Laboratory Assessment

FSH, LH, E2 levels
- See Table 44.2
- Elevated FSH results should be repeated for confirmation
   - Persistently elevated FSH signals gonadal level defect

TSH

Prolactin

Additional considerations

- Obtain karyotype for persistently elevated FSH

- *Virilization:* Check dehydroepiandrosterone sulfate (DHEA-S), 17-hydroxyprogesterone (17-OHP), testosterone panel
- Consider screening for chronic disease based on H&P (e.g. CBC, ESR, electrolytes, celiac testing, liver function testing)

Imaging

Bone age

- Menarche correlated more to bone age than chronological age
- Usually delayed in constitutional delay

Pelvic US

- To confirm uterine agenesis, Müllerian anomalies, or adnexal masses
  or
- To assess adolescents in whom a rectoabdominal or bimanual exam is not possible

NOTE*: Uterus/ovaries may not be well-visualized on ultrasound in a patient without pubertal estrogen levels and may be incorrectly assumed to be absent*

Additional considerations

- Consider brain MRI to evaluate neurologic symptoms or lab results concerning for CNS process
- Consider pelvic MRI if pelvic US unequivocal or structures require further delineation

Treatment

- Constitutional delay: Reassurance and support

Other causes

- Must address the underlying condition
  - Treatment of chronic disease
  - Turner syndrome patients require multispecialty follow-up in addition to hormone therapy for induction or continuation of pubertal development
  - Gonadal dysgenesis patients may require gonadectomy to reduce the risk of development of malignancy
  - Surgical management of obstructive anomaly
- Nonreversible causes will require estrogen therapy (+progesterone, if indicated) to achieve secondary sex characteristics and provide physiologic levels of hormones (see Chapter 40, "Primary Ovarian Insufficiency")

Precocious Puberty

Differential Diagnosis (Table 44.3)

History

- *Age of initiation of any pubertal development and rate of development:* Rapid development more associated with a hormone-secreting tumor than true PP

- *Birth history:* Neurological trauma at birth, prematurity
- *Past medical history:* Thyroid disease, history of traumatic head injury, seizures, encephalitis, meningitis, abdominal pain
- *Past surgical history:* History of pelvic/abdominal mass
- *Family history:* Parental heights, pubertal timing of family members, family history of CAH or neurofibromatosis, use of androgen- or estrogen-containing medications by household members
- *Medications:* Possible ingestion of exogenous hormones

Review of Systems

- *Gastrointestinal:* Chronic or cyclic abdominal pain
- *Genitourinary:* Clitoromegaly, pubic hair development, vaginal bleeding or discharge
- *Musculoskeletal:* Rapid growth
- *Integumentary:* Hirsutism, acne
- *Neurological:* Headaches, seizures, visual changes
- *Endocrine:* Hot or cold flashes, galactorrhea

Physical Exam

- *Review previous height and weight:* Examine growth curve for the acceleration of height velocity (see Chapter 29, "Obesity")
- *Blood pressure*
- *HEENT:* Visual field evaluation, evaluate for papilledema (sign of CNS tumor)
- *Thyroid:* Assess for thyromegaly, goiter
- *Breast:* Tanner stage, galactorrhea
- *Abdomen:* Abdominal and pelvic masses
- *Genitourinary:* Tanner stage, evidence of estrogen effect, vaginal discharge, clitoromegaly
- Consider rectal exam to assess for pelvic mass and presence of uterus in nonsexually-active patients
- *Skin:* Acne, apocrine odor, café au lait spots, axillary hair

Diagnostic Evaluation

Consider consultation with a pediatric endocrinologist.

Laboratory Assessment

- Basal FSH, LH, and E2
  - See Table 44.3
  - Order ultrasensitive E2 assay with pediatric reference values
- TSH
- HCG (elevated levels can trigger the secretion of ovarian hormones)
- Prolactin
- Additional considerations
  - Virilization: Obtain DHEA-S, testosterone panel, 7 am 17-OHP level (to evaluate for 21-hydroxylase deficiency)
  - Consider adrenocorticotropic hormone (ACTH) stimulation testing to confirm CAH

- Elevated basal gonadotropin levels: GnRH stimulation test to distinguish between central and peripheral causes of PP
- High stimulated LH level suggestive of central PP

Imaging

- *Bone age:* Accelerated skeletal maturation is evidence of sex hormone exposure
  - A total of >2 standard deviations above chronologic age is unlikely to be a normal variant
  - Can repeat every 6 months to monitor skeletal maturation
- *Pelvic US:* Evaluate for uterine size and shape, ovarian masses, ovarian follicles
- *Adrenal imaging:* US, CT, or MRI to evaluate for adrenal masses (if elevated adrenal androgens present)
- *CNS imaging:* CT or MRI to assess for intracranial lesion
  - Perform in patients < 8 years old with progressive central PP or any patient with neurological symptoms

Treatment

Overall goals

- Stop or delay pubertal progression until a normal age of puberty
- Maximize the likelihood of achieving genetic height potential
- Reduce psychosocial distress related to the early development of sexual characteristics

General considerations for initiation of treatment

- Bone age > 2 years older than chronologic age or predicted adult height is below genetic height potential
  - Predicted adult height based on the Bayley-Pinneau table using chronologic age vs bone age once patient > age 6
- Pubertal development in a patient less than 6 years old
- Menarche less than 8 years old

If not initiating medical treatment, continue serial evaluations with a physical exam, monitoring of height velocity, and bone age every 6 months.

Central PP

- If secondary to CNS pathology, manage in conjunction with the appropriate subspecialty (e.g. CNS tumor, prolactinoma)
- Treatment with GnRH agonist: Reversible suppression of LH and FSH secretion
  - E.g. Leuprolide acetate IM injection or histrelin subcutaneous implant
  - Monitor treatment effect with LH and FSH levels after GnRH agonist administration and serial physical exams
  - Continue until the patient reaches mean age for the stage of pubertal development
- After GnRH agonist discontinued
  - Pubertal changes proceed with the normal pace
  - Menarche occurs within 1–2 years

Peripheral PP: Treatment aimed at underlying pathology

- *Ovarian/adrenal functional tumors:* Surgical removal ± chemotherapy/radiation based on underlying tumor type
- *Ovarian cysts:* Monitor, may regress with the treatment of underlying condition or suppression of gonadotropins
- *Adrenal gland enzyme deficiency:* Replacement of mineralocorticoids and glucocorticoids
- *Severe hypothyroidism/Van Wyk-Grumbach syndrome:* Levothyroxine treatment
- *McCune-Albright*
  - Consult with an endocrinologist
  - Treatment with aromatase inhibitors or selective estrogen receptor modulators to inhibit peripheral effects of hormones and sex steroid synthesis
  - May require treatment with a GnRH agonist if progresses to central PP

TABLE 44.3

Subtypes of Precocious Puberty

	Central (Gonadotropin Dependent)	**Peripheral (Gonadotropin Independent)**
Lab results	High basal and/or stimulated LH and FSH levels, high E2	Low LH and FSH, normal-to-high E2 (plus additional findings below)
Characteristics	• Follows typical pattern and time course of pubertal development but at an early age • Isosexual development	• May follow an abnormal pattern (e.g. vaginal bleeding precedes thelarche, rapid onset/progression) • May be isosexual or contrasexual (e.g. virilization) development

Conditions	• Idiopathic (most common, diagnosis of exclusion)
	• Cerebral disorders
	  • Congenital defects (e.g. hydrocephalus)
	  • Brain tumors
	  • Cerebral infection/inflammation
	  • Head trauma
	• Neurofibromatosis
	• Tuberous sclerosis
	• Secondary central precocious puberty (e.g. progression from peripheral to central cause due to incompletely treated CAH or postexposure to androgen-secreting tumors)
		• Exposure to exogenous androgens or estrogens
		• Sex steroid-secreting tumors of adrenals or ovaries (e.g. granulosa cell tumor)
		• Gonadotropin-secreting tumors
		• McCune-Albright syndrome
		• Van Wyk-Grumbach syndrome
		• Severe hypothyroidism
		• Adrenal gland enzyme deficiencies (e.g. CAH)

Isolated Precocious Puberty

Premature Thelarche

Definition

Isolated breast development before 8 years old in the absence of other pubertal signs, growth spurt, or acceleration of skeletal maturation

- Two forms
  - *Classical:* Occurs during first 2–3 years of life secondary to activity of HPO axis
  - *Nonclassical:* Affects older girls, more associated with progression to PP
- Can be unilateral or bilateral

- Proposed mechanisms: intermittent HPO axis activation and secretion of FSH, transient E2 secretion from ovarian cysts, exogenous estrogen exposure, or increased sensitivity of breast tissue to E2

Differential Diagnosis

- Idiopathic/self-limited
- McCune-Albright syndrome
- True PP

Evaluation

Bone age
- If normal, can defer imaging and labs
- If advanced or is progressive, complete more extensive PP workup (see the previous section)

Laboratory evaluation
- *Gonadotropins:* Prepubertal LH, normal-to-elevated FSH
- *GnRH stimulation test:* Only FSH will be elevated

Pelvic US
- Evaluate for an ovarian cyst or pelvic mass
- Prepubertal appearance of uterus and ovaries

Management and Follow-Up

- Reevaluate every 6–12 months to assess for progression to PP

Premature Adrenarche

Definition

Development of pubic and/or axillary hair before 8 years old in the absence of other pubertal signs

- In African Americans, may normally occur before or concurrent with thelarche
- Can be associated with later development of PCOS
- *Proposed mechanisms:* Early increase in secretion of adrenal androgens (androstenedione, DHEA, and DHEA-S) or increased sensitivity of hair follicles to circulating androgens

Differential Diagnosis

- Pubic hair of infancy
- True PP
- Virilizing tumor
- Non-classic CAH

Evaluation

Bone age
- If normal, can perform limited lab evaluation: Testosterone, DHEA-S, and 17-OHP
- If advanced or progressive: Pursue complete PP workup (see the preceding section)

Laboratory evaluation
- If androgens and 7 a.m. 17-OHP levels are elevated or associated with advanced bone age, consider ACTH stimulation test

Management and Follow-Up

- Reevaluate every 3–6 months to assess for progression

Premature Menarche

Definition

Uterine bleeding in the absence of pubertal maturation

- Rare occurrence after 6–9 months of age
- Proposed mechanism: Activation of HPO axis and increased FSH levels and increased endometrial sensitivity to estradiol

Differential Diagnosis

- Rule out more common non-endocrine causes: Exogenous estrogen exposure, malignancy, vulvovaginitis, foreign body, trauma, or abuse
- McCune-Albright
- True PP

Evaluation

- History
  - Pattern of bleeding, associated vaginal discharge
- Physical exam
  - Assess for trauma, vaginal lesions, abdominal mass, estrogenization of vaginal tissues, vaginal discharge, foreign body
- Consider exam under anesthesia and/or vaginal irrigation
- Consider vaginal culture
- Bone age
  - If advanced or progressive, pursue complete PP workup (see above)
- Laboratory evaluation
  - Prepubertal E2 and gonadotropin levels
    - No change in response to GnRH stimulation test
- Pelvic US
  - Evaluate for ovarian cysts, pelvic mass
  - Prepubertal appearance of uterus and ovaries

Management and Follow-Up

- Reevaluate every 6 months for progression to PP
- Treat underlying etiologies (e.g. resection of tumor, treatment of vaginal infection)

BIBLIOGRAPHY

Chan, Y.M., Biro, F.M., & Emans, S.J. Delayed puberty. In Emans, S.J., Lauger, M.R., DiVasta, A.D. (Eds) (2020). *Emans, Laufer, Goldstein's Pediatric and Adolescent Gynecology* (7th ed., pp. 363–377) Philadelphia, PA: Wolters-Kluwer.

Dietrich, J.E. (Ed.). (2014). *Female puberty: A comprehensive guide for clinicians.* New York, NY: Springer Science & Business Media.

Fritz, M.A., & Speroff, L. (Eds.). (2011). *Clinical gynecologic endocrinology and infertility* (8th ed.) Philadelphia, PA: Lippincott Williams & Wilkins.

Pitts S.A., & Gordon C. The physiology of puberty. In Emans, S.J. Laufer, M.R., DiVasta, A.D. (Eds.) (2020). *Emans, Laufer, Goldsteins's pediatric and adolescent gynecology* (7th ed., p. 35) Philadelphia, PA: Wolters –Kluwer.

Stafford, D.E., & Mansfield, M.J. Precocious puberty. In Emans, S.J., Lauger, M.R., DiVasta, A.D. (Eds) (2020). *Emans, Laufer, Goldstein's Pediatric and Adolescent Gynecology* (7th ed., pp 351–362) Philadelphia, PA: Wolters-Kluwer.

Wu, T., Mendola, P., & Buck, G. (2002). Ethnic differences in the presence of secondary sex characteristics and menarche among US girls: The Third National Health and Nutrition Examination Survey, 1988–1994. Pediatrics. 110(4), 752–757.

45

Radiologic Imaging for Gynecologic Conditions

Charis Chambers and S. Paige Hertweck

ULTRASONOGRAPHY (US)

Key Points

- First line for diagnosis of benign abnormalities of the uterus, ovary, fallopian tube, cervix, and kidney

Types

- *Transabdominal*: Perform with a full bladder to improve image quality; most useful and widely used in evaluating female pelvic organs and kidneys
- *Transvaginal*: Perform only in the sexually active or tampon-using, cooperative, older adolescent; helpful in diagnosing tubo-ovarian abscess (TOA), and early pregnancy
- *Color Doppler*: Cannot be used to exclude or diagnose ovarian torsion but can help in diagnosis of ovarian torsion when additional morphological signs are present (i.e. ovarian stromal edema, an eccentric ovarian mass) and with high clinical suspicion
- *Three-dimensional rendering*: Useful in demonstrating malposition of an intrauterine device (IUD) and delineating anorectal malformations
- *Transperineal (translabial)*: Useful in defining abnormalities of urethra, periurethral soft tissues, anterior rectum, distal gynecologic tract

Advantages

- No radiation risk

Disadvantages

- Abdominal ultrasounds may be limited or require backfilling of the bladder for patients incontinent of urine

Interpretation of Ovarian and Adnexal Masses Seen on Ultrasound

Ovarian-Adnexal Reporting and Data System (O-RADS)
- Is a pattern recognition tool that is based on transvaginal ultrasound imaging in adults, may serve as a tool for pediatric and adolescent gynecologic (PAG) ultrasound imaging even though most PAG US imaging is abdominal

DOI: 10.1201/9781003039235-45

- Uses both internal ovarian content description and color score based on vascularity, from No Flow (score 1), and Minimal Flow (2), through Moderate Flow (3), to Very Strong Flow (4)
- It is designed to
  - Provide consistent interpretation
  - Decrease ambiguity in the US reports by using similar descriptions or lexicon
  - Provide higher probability of accuracy in assigning risk of malignancy to ovarian adnexal/masses
  - Aid in the management recommendation based on each risk category added:
    O-RADS 0 = Incomplete evaluation (due to technical factors, like bowel gas, inability to obtain transvaginal imaging)
    - *Management*: Repeat study
    O-RADS 1 = Physiologic category (normal premenopausal ovary)
    - *Management*: No follow-up is needed
    - Includes follicle (defined as cyst or corpus luteum ≤3 cm), see Figure 45.1
    O-RADS 2 = Almost certainly benign category (<1% risk of malignancy), see Figure 45.2
    - Includes unilocular cysts <10 cm
    - *Management*
    Simple cysts
    - <5 cm: No follow-up
    - >5 cm but <10 cm: Follow-up in 8–12 weeks if not surgically managed
    Non-simple unilocular cysts with smooth walls
    - ≤3 cm: No follow-up
    - >3 cm but <10 cm: Follow-up 8–12 weeks if not surgically managed

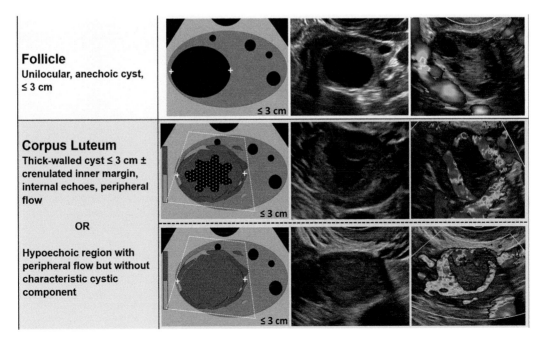

FIGURE 45.1 O-RADS 1: Normal ovary. (From Andriotti RF, et al. Radiology 2020; 294, with permission.)

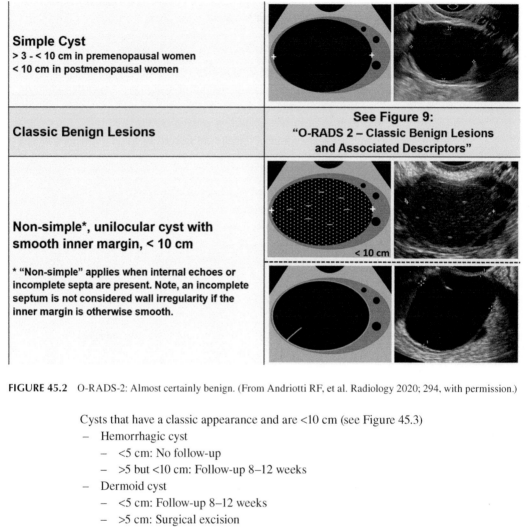

FIGURE 45.2   O-RADS-2: Almost certainly benign. (From Andriotti RF, et al. Radiology 2020; 294, with permission.)

Cysts that have a classic appearance and are <10 cm (see Figure 45.3)

- Hemorrhagic cyst
  - <5 cm: No follow-up
  - >5 but <10 cm: Follow-up 8–12 weeks
- Dermoid cyst
  - <5 cm: Follow-up 8–12 weeks
  - >5 cm: Surgical excision
- Endometrioma
  - <5 cm: Follow-up 8–12 weeks
  - >5 cm: Surgical excision
- Paraovarian cyst
  - <5 cm: Follow-up 8–12 weeks
  - >5 cm: Surgical excision
- Peritoneal inclusion cyst
  - Based on clinical presentation/scenario
- Hydrosalpinx
  - Based on clinical presentation/scenario

O-RADS 3 = Lesions with low risk of malignancy (1–10%) (see Figure 45.4)

Surgical management includes

- Unilocular cysts >10 cm
- Typical dermoid cysts, endometriomas, hemorrhagic cysts >10 m
- Unilocular cysts any size with inner wall <3 mm height
- Multilocular cysts <10 cm, with the smooth inner wall
- Solid smooth lesions of any size with a color score of 1

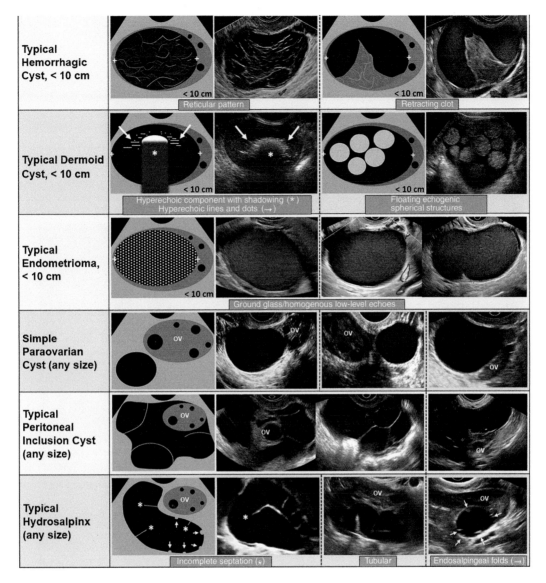

FIGURE 45.3 O-RADS-2: classic benign lesions and associated descriptors. (From Andriotti RF, et al. Radiology 2020; 294, with permission.)

O-RADS 4 = Lesions with intermediate risk of malignancy (10–50%) (see Figure 45.5)

Multidisciplinary care with pediatric surgery/pediatric oncology

Includes:

– Multilocular cysts with no solid component
  – ≥10 cm, smooth inner wall, color score = 1–3
  – Any size, smooth inner wall, color score = 4
  – Any size, irregular inner wall and/or irregular septation, any color score
– Unilocular cysts with solid component
  – Any size, 0–3 papillary projections, any color score

– Multilocular cysts with solid component
– Any size, color score = 1–2
– Solid lesions
– Smooth, any size, color score 2–3

O-RADS 5 = Lesions with a high risk of malignancy (>50%) (see Figure 45.6)

Multidisciplinary care with pediatric surgery/pediatric oncology

Includes:
– Unilocular cyst, any size, ≥4 papillary projections, color score = any
– Multilocular cyst with a solid component, any size, color score = 3–4
– Smooth solid, any size, color score = 4
– Ascites and/or peritoneal nodules

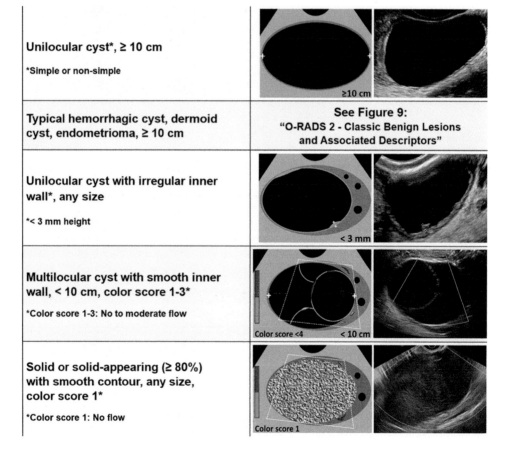

FIGURE 45.4   O-RADS-3: low risk of malignancy. (From Andriotti RF, et al. Radiology 2020; 294, with permission.)

MAGNETIC RESONANCE IMAGING (MRI)

Key Points

- Useful in defining congenital reproductive tract anomalies, especially Müllerian duct and vaginal defects (when ultrasound fails to do so), and vulvar masses

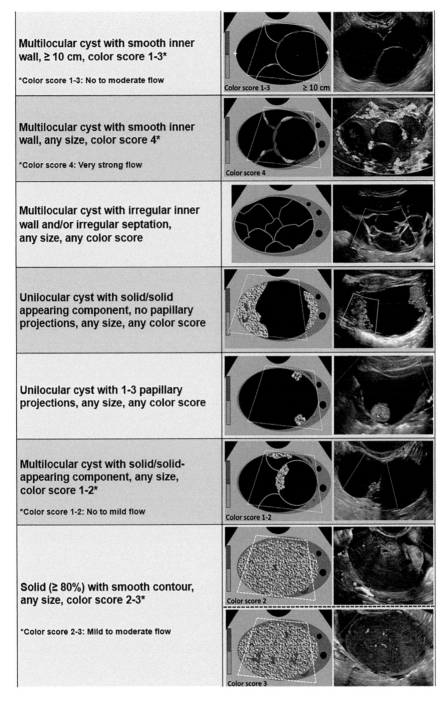

FIGURE 45.5 O-RADS-4: Intermediate risk of malignancy. (From Andriotti RF, et al. Radiology 2020; 294, with permission.)

- Abnormalities in external uterine fundal contour allowing differentiation between uterine didelphys and bicornuate uterus vs septate uterus; allows clear depiction of rudimentary uterine horns and whether they have functional endometrium
- Provides the ability to detect the renal anomalies that may accompany Müllerian anomalies

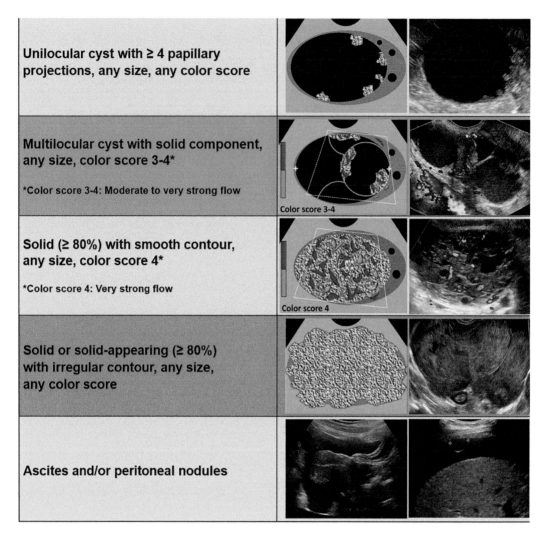

Unilocular cyst with ≥ 4 papillary projections, any size, any color score	
Multilocular cyst with solid component, any size, color score 3-4* *Color score 3-4: Moderate to very strong flow	
Solid (≥ 80%) with smooth contour, any size, color score 4* *Color score 4: Very strong flow	
Solid or solid-appearing (≥ 80%) with irregular contour, any size, any color score	
Ascites and/or peritoneal nodules	

FIGURE 45.6   O-RADS-5: High risk of malignancy. (From Andriotti RF, et al. Radiology 2020; 294, with permission.)

Specific Views Image Specific Organs

- *T1-weighted views*: Excellent for soft tissue evaluation and helpful in delineating hematometrocolpos
  - *Coronal*: Kidneys and ovaries
  - *Sagittal*: Uterus, vagina, and spine
- *T2-weighted views*: Superior for delineating uterine anomalies
  - *Sagittal*: Uterus and vagina
  - *Axial*: Ovaries, lower uterine segment, cervix, and vagina

Advantages

- Use of a perineal marker (typically a special gelatin capsule or gel inserted in the vagina) can help determine the extent of a vaginal obstruction

Disadvantages

- May require sedation for younger children (under the age of 7 years) to keep still for length of procedure

COMPUTED TOMOGRAPHY (CT)

Key Points

- Valuable in diagnosing major abdominal or pelvic trauma; pelvic or renal malignancies; post-operative complications (i.e. vascular/organ injuries, abscesses)

Advantages

- Spiral views are very helpful in ruling out appendicitis

Disadvantages

- Not helpful in routine screening of pelvic structures
- Radiation dose is significant to the gonads
- Although not as long as an MRI, may require sedation to allow young children to keep still
- Contrast is often required with an associated small risk of anaphylaxis and nephrotoxicity

GENITOGRAM

Key Points

- Valuable in defining anatomy in ambiguous genitalia and a single perineal opening

Advantages

- Useful in the very young child

Disadvantages

- Requires a procedure
- Uses radiation
- Opening has to be large enough to place catheter

Procedure Details

- Place 5 or 8 Fr feeding tube in orifice
- Inject Hypaque-cysto dye
- Use fluoroscopy to image passage of dye and map anatomy
- Use in conjunction with cystogram and/or rectal contrast in selected cases

BIBLIOGRAPHY

Andriotti RF, Timmerman D, Strachowski LM, et al. O-RADS risk stratification and management system: a consensus guideline from the ACR Ovarian-Adnexal Reporting and Data System Committee. Radiology. 2020; 294:168–185.

Behr S, Courtier J, Qayyum A. Imaging of Müllerian duct anomalies. Radiographics. 2012; 32:233–250.

Patel M, Young S, Dahiya N. Ultrasound of pelvic pain in the nonpregnant woman. Radiol Clin N Am. 2019; 57:601–616.

Yoo R, Cho J, Kim S, et al. A systematic approach to the MR imaging-based differential diagnosis of congenital Müllerian anomalies and their mimics. Abdom Imaging. 2015; 40:192–206.

46

Sexual Abuse, Sex Trafficking, and Rape

Jacqueline Sugarman and S. Paige Hertweck

SEXUAL ABUSE

Definitions

- *Sexual abuse* occurs when a child is engaged in sexual activities they cannot comprehend, for which they are developmentally unprepared, cannot give informed consent, and which violate social and legal taboos.
- *Sexual abuse* involves a wide spectrum of activities and encompasses fondling, oral and/or anogenital contact, as well as noncontact abuses (exhibitionism, voyeurism) and child exploitation (pornography, prostitution).
- *Incest* occurs when a perpetrator has sexual intercourse with a victim who is related by blood or marriage. Laws can vary by state.
- *Rape:* "penetration, no matter how slight, of the vagina or anus with any body part or object, or oral penetration by a sex organ of another person, without the consent of the victim." (FBI Uniform Crime Reports).
- *Acquaintance rape*: Perpetrator is known to the victim, common.
- *Statutory rape:* Laws define the age below which an individual is legally incapable of consenting to sexual activity. These laws can vary by state.

Key Points

- Approximately 1 in 13 boys and 1 in 4 girls are sexually abused before the age of 18 (Centers for Disease Control data).
- The majority of children who are sexually abused will have normal examinations.
- The diagnosis most commonly is made by history.
- Children present as a result of (1) disclosure (most common—although often delayed with abuse occurring long before), (2) sexually transmitted infection (STI), (3) injury, or (4) concerning signs and symptoms.
- The relationship to the perpetrator, age at first incident of abuse, use of physical force, the severity of abuse, demographic variables, and how the disclosure is received by caretakers all impact a child's willingness to disclose.
- One in 5 women have experienced completed or attempted rape.
- One in 3 female rape victims experienced it for the first time between the ages of 11 and 17 years old and one in 8 reported that it occurred before age 10.

DOI: 10.1201/9781003039235-46

Clinical Indicators

- Behavioral signs and symptoms
  - Nightmares, trouble sleeping, changes in behavior, aggression, sexualized behaviors, regression, eating disturbances, depression, isolating from others, self-harming behaviors
- Physical signs and symptoms
  - *Recurrent somatic complaints:* headaches, abdominal pain, enuresis, encopresis, dysuria, anogenital pain, anogenital bleeding, anogenital discharge, anogenital bumps, or sores
  - *Accidental genital trauma:* Injury should match history (e.g., straddle injuries typically do not result in penetrative injury).
  - *STI:* Implications of STI and sexual abuse vary by disease (Table 46.1)
    - HIV, gonorrhea, syphilis, and chlamydia infections (if not acquired perinatally, rare nonsexual vertical transmission, or by transfusion for HIV) are considered diagnostic of sexual abuse in a prepubertal child. This infection should be reported to the child protection hotline.
    - Trichomonas vaginalis (if perinatal transmission and rare nonsexual vertical transmission is excluded) is considered diagnostic for sexual abuse. This infection should be reported to the child protection hotline.
    - Genital herpes can be transmitted via autoinoculation, however, if no clear history exists, it is considered suspicious for sexual abuse and should be reported to the child protection hotline.
    - Anogenital warts may be transmitted sexually as well as perinatally and horizontally. If there is no clear mode of transmission or the warts are believed to be the result of abuse, report to the child protection hotline.
- Prior history of STI, previous sexual intercourse, previous or current pregnancy should prompt the healthcare provider to discuss the age and use of coercion by previous sexual partners.

Mimics of Sexual Abuse

Conditions that may present with bleeding:

- Group A strep vulvovaginitis
- Shigella vulvovaginitis
- Urethral prolapse
- Vaginal foreign body
- Straddle injury or other accidental trauma
- Bleeding associated with precocious puberty

Conditions that resemble genital injury or trauma:

- Lichen sclerosus (subepithelial hemorrhages)
- Failure of midline fusion
- Labial adhesions (confused with scarring and/or may bleed)
- Linea vestibularis

Conditions that can mimic STI:

- Genital aphthous ulcers

Vaginal discharge from other infectious causes:

H. flu

TABLE 46.1

Sexually Transmitted Infections in Prepubertal Children: Interpreting Their Significance and Taking Appropriate Action after Their Recognition

Infection Diagnosed by Appropriate Testing (Exclude False Positive Tests and Perform Confirmatory Testing If Indicated)	Significance	Recommended Action
Gonorrhea, Chlamydia trachomatis, syphilis, Trichomonas vaginalis	These infections are considered **diagnostic for sexual abuse** if perinatal transmission and rare vertical transmission are excluded as likely modes of acquisition.	Report to local or state child protection agency
HIV	This infection is considered **diagnostic for sexual abuse** if it is not perinatally acquired or acquired from transfusion.	Report to local or state child protection agency
Anogenital herpes	This infection is considered **suspicious for sexual abuse** if there is no clear history of autoinoculation.	Report to local or state child protection agency if no clear history of autoinoculation exists, therefore warranting further investigation
Anogenital warts (Condyloma acuminata)	This infection is considered **suspicious for sexual abuse**. Perinatal transmission, horizontal transmission or autoinoculation should be excluded as modes of acquisition.	Report to local or state child protection agency if no clear mode of transmission exists or evidence (history, physical examination, or additional sexually transmitted infections) exists to suspect abuse. Lesions appearing for the first time in a child aged >5 years are more likely to have been caused by sexual transmission
Molluscum contagiosum	This infection is considered **inconclusive for sexual abuse**. Can be transmitted via autoinoculation.	Medical follow-up. No report indicated in the absence of any additional evidence of abuse (concerning history or physical findings)
Bacterial vaginosis	This infection is considered **inconclusive for sexual abuse**.	Medical follow-up. No report indicated in the absence of any additional evidence of abuse (concerning history or physical findings)

Source: Adapted from Kellogg N; American Academy of Pediatrics Committee on Child Abuse and Neglect. The evaluation of child abuse in children. Pediatrics. 2005;16:506–12; Adams JA, Farst KJ, Kellogg ND. Interpretation of medical findings in suspected child abuse: an update for 2018. J Pediatr Adolesc Gynecol. 2018;31:225–31; Workowski KA, Bachmann LH, Chan PA, et al. Sexually transmitted infections treatment guidelines, 2021. MMWR Recomm Rep. 2021;70(No. RR-4):1–187. Doi: http://dx.doi.org/10.15585/mmwr.rr7004a1; and American Academy of Pediatrics. Red Book: 2021–2024 Report of the Committee on Infectious Diseases. 32nd ed. American Academy of Pediatrics; 2021.

History (See Table 46.2)

- History should be obtained for the purpose of medical decision-making and to ensure the child's safety.
- Ideally history should be obtained from the child or adolescent by a trained forensic interviewer (usually at a Children's Advocacy Center).
- When in the ER or clinic setting, try to obtain most of the history of abuse from the parent or caregiver **(without the child present)**. Then, if possible, from the child separately not in the presence of the caregiver.
- Should focus on
  - Medical issues: Oral or anogenital concerns (vaginal discharge, new anogenital bumps or sores, presence of pain, dysuria, and/or bleeding)
  - Mechanism of injury/type of contact (to guide testing and explain medical findings)

- Whether the child is safe in her current environment
- Questions to address
  - Is the child safe in her current environment?
  - Who was involved?
  - When did it happen?
  - When was the last contact with the perpetrator?
  - What happened?
  - Is the child having any symptoms and could these symptoms be related to the history of abuse?
  - Has the abuse been reported?

- To assist in history, ask and document what terminology the child uses to identify private parts and use that terminology when asking child questions related to a private area.
- Acknowledge that you are asking difficult questions.
- Remain unbiased and objective.
- Use open-ended statements and nonleading questions to obtain the history, such as "Tell me about coming here today. Tell me why you are here today."
- See Table 46.2 for more sample questions to aid in history taking.

"Clarify what the child has told you by repeating, but not suggesting. Be concrete. Make sure you understand what the terminology the child uses means (for example, if a child says she has been raped, you might tell her that rape means many things to different people. What does it mean to her?)

Document any statements made by the child verbatim and place in quotations in the medical record; record questions asked to elicit those statements.

In preteens and teens, assess for human trafficking, substance abuse, and self harm (see Sex Trafficking section below and Chapter 21, "High-Risk Behaviors").

Physical Examination

Timing

- **Nature of abuse, timing, and chronicity are important in determining where and when the examination should be performed, whether forensic evidence collection is necessary, and what tests should be sent.**
- Each state has specific time frames recommended for when evidence is collected. Evidence is collected if the possibility for recovery of biological or trace evidence exists. In general, this possibility is most likely if the most recent abuse occurred within the last 72–96 hours.

Indications for an acute exam are to

- Recover evidence
- Assess for injury
- Assess for etiology of any pain or bleeding
- Screen for STI
- Detect any suicidal ideation, pregnancy, or transmission of HIV

Indications for immediate examination for injury and *evidence* collection

- An event that occurred within an acute time frame and included vaginal and/or anal penetration with a penis.
- Situations in which there is potential to recover biological or trace evidence: There was contact with the reported perpetrator's genitalia, blood, semen, saliva, or skin cells.

TABLE 46.2

Interviewing Children about Sexual Abuse

I	Initial procedure
	1. Obtain information from the parent, social worker, or caretaker without the child present
	2. Ask child's terminology for genitalia
II	Interview child alone in the non-threatening environment (if possible, not in examination room)
III	1. Establish rapport with child (play, color, ask child's name and age)
	2. Ask about the household
	a. Where does the child live?
	b. Who else lives there?
	c. Where does the child sleep?
	d. Does the child go to school? Where?
	3. Identify body parts
	a. Identify all body parts – eyes, nose, hair, hands, belly button, as well as genitalia
IV	Begin to focus on the possibility of abuse
	1. 'Do you know why you came to see me?'
	2. 'Do you know what kind of doctor I am? I am a doctor who checks children's hearts, listens to their lungs, and also checks their private parts. Do you need your private parts checked?'
	3. 'Some children who come to see me tell me that something has happened to their bodies that made them feel uncomfortable/didn't like. Has anything like that happened to you?'
V	What happened?
	1. Where were you?
	2. Who was there?
	3. Where was Mommy? Daddy?
	4. Who did it?
	5. What did he/she do?
	6. Where were your clothes? Panties? His/her clothes?
	7. Does anyone else know what happened? How do they know?
VI	Concluding the interview
	1. Thank the patient for speaking with you
	2. Reassure the child that they did a good job speaking with you and it was not his/her fault that something happened
	3. Tell the child that you believe what he/she said
	4. Tell the child, "you were very brave to tell me what happened. Talking about this is not an easy thing to do."
VII	Explain the examination
	a. 'Now we need to check you out – listen to your heart, lungs; feel your tummy; and look at your private parts'
	b. Describe how the anogenital exam will be performed
VII	Don't
	1. Ask children leading questions (e.g. Johnny touched you here, didn't he?)
IX	Document
	1. Document questions asked and answers given
	2. Try to document exact words and phrases
X	Modifications for adolescent
	1. Obtain more specific information: date and time of the assault, history of assault (oral, rectal or vaginal penetration, oral contact by the offender, ejaculation if known, digital penetration or penetration with foreign object)
	2. Obtain a history of any self-cleaning activities (teeth brushing, urination, douching, changing clothes)
	3. Obtain menstrual history and whether the patient uses contraception. Were any lubricants or a condom used?

Source: From Sugarman JM, Evaluation of child sexual abuse, in: Giardino AP, Damer EM, Asher JB, eds, *Sexual assault: Victimization across the life span, A clinical guide,* GW Publishing Inc., St Louis, 1997; 58.

- Situations in which there is unclear history AND there is reason to believe that there was contact with the reported perpetrator's genitalia, blood, semen, and saliva or skin cells.
- History indicates there was a struggle that may have left some of the reported perpetrator's blood or semen on the victim's clothes or body.
- History indicates that saliva could be recovered from the neck or breast or other areas of the body.
- Oral penetration occurred within 24 hours.

Indications for immediate examination for injury and *likely evidence* collection

- An event occurred within acute time frame and included digital vaginal and/or digital anal penetration or vaginal or anal penetration with an object (strongly consider because digit or object could be contaminated with saliva, blood, or semen.)

Performing the examination

- Obtain consent/assent from the patient after offering an explanation of the exam
    - A patient can consent to some portions of the exam and decline others.
    - A patient who declines part or all of the exam may still return and receive additional components of the exam at a later time.

If possible, use clinical photography to document any injuries noted on the exam.
Try to coordinate physical examination/anogenital exam/STI testing, evidence collection (if necessary), and clinical photographs all at the same time to avoid multiple exams.
The exam can be performed with a caretaker or support person present if the patient desires one. Examiner **must have** a nurse or tech present to both assist and chaperone.
A complete physical exam includes a head-to-toe exam.

- Identify and document
    - Areas of tenderness
    - Abnormal findings
        - Bruising, bite marks, abrasions, petechiae, etc.
- Assess the oropharynx
    - Check for injuries to frenula, palatal petechiae, or abrasions to the buccal mucosa
- Assess the neck and breast, high yield areas for contusions and saliva
- Assess areas that might be hidden by the hair but are injured, i.e. ears and behind the ears
- Assess for signs of strangulation
    - Neck injuries, subconjunctival hemorrhage, facial petechiae, and hoarseness, difficulty or pain with swallowing
- Examine the abdomen for tenderness or masses
- Assess for other signs of nonaccidental trauma
    - Pattern injuries
    - Injuries to areas of the body that are not commonly accidental
        - Ears, neck, cheek, torso, genitalia, hands, and feet

Anogenital examination

- Prepubertal girl (vagina and anus)
    - Use the supine frog leg or supine lithotomy position
    - Can use the prone knee–chest position to better visualize the posterior hymen and vagina, if needed, as well as the anus.

- A difficult to visualize hymen can also be assessed by "floating the hymen" or squirting water or saline on the hymen.

NOTE: The hymen in prepubertal girls is very sensitive and touching of the hymen should be avoided.

- **Speculum and anoscopic exams are NOT indicated in prepubertal girls unless**
  - There is a concern for a laceration of the vagina
  - The source of vaginal or rectal bleeding is unknown
  - The presence of a foreign body is suspected
  - If a speculum exam is needed, sedation is required
- Postpubertal females
  - Use the supine lithotomy position
  - Can use prone knee–chest position to better visualize the posterior hymen and vagina, as well as the anus
  - The contour of the hymen can be further assessed by tracing the rim with a moistened cotton swab or placing a foley catheter behind the hymen (see Chapter 20, "Gynecologic Exam")
  - Use of speculum could cause pain and further trauma: Use only if absolutely needed
  - Indications for speculum use
    - To recover evidence of sperm in the cervical os
    - To identify vaginal lacerations or other sources of bleeding
    - To determine presence or absence of the foreign body in the vagina

Use photodocumentation of any findings, if possible, and when not, use chart illustration in medical record.

Diagnosis

Sexual abuse diagnosis is based on the history, examination, and laboratory findings.

The majority of children and adolescents who report sexual abuse and rape have normal examinations, for many reasons:

- The nature of the abuse may not leave injury.
- Injuries heal rapidly.
- Disclosures of sexual abuse are often delayed.
- There may be discordance between what a child perceives has happened and the actual event (remember that the law defines rape as penetration no matter how slight, of the vagina or anus with any body part or object, or oral penetration by a sex organ of another person, without the consent of the victim).
- Peer reviewed medical literature supports that healing is rapid, that exams are normal even in cases where perpetrators have confessed to sexual assault or in pregnancy.

Findings highly suggestive of abuse, (unless a clear and convincing history of accidental trauma, straddle injury, impalement injury, or crush injury is provided), include

- Acute injuries to the anogenital structures
- Injuries to the hymen, vagina, posterior fossa, perianal laceration with exposure to the tissues below the dermis, healed transections of the hymen)
- Presence of STI in prepubertal or nonsexually active females (see Table 46.1)

Laboratory Testing

- Perform STI testing in prepubertal children especially under the following circumstances (see Table 46.3)
  - Patient has experienced penetration of the vagina, anorectum, or oropharynx.
  - Patient exhibits signs and/or symptoms of an STI.
  - A sibling or adult in the house has a known STI.
  - The perpetrator has a known STI or is at high risk.
  - The perpetrator is a stranger.
  - The family is requesting testing.
  - Evidence of recent or old healed injury of genitals, anus, or oropharynx is present.
  - Unclear history and there is reason to believe the patient is at risk for acquiring an STI.
  - Follow-up is difficult or unlikely.
- Perform STI testing in **all** children who are pubertal.
- Obtain gonorrhea and chlamydia diagnostic evaluation from any sites of penetration or attempted penetration. Other STI testing may also be indicated (see chart - Table 46.3).
- Evaluation of sites other than those disclosed should be strongly considered since often the initial disclosure may be limited and does not represent the full extent of the abuse.
- Order pregnancy testing in pubertal females.

Consider obtaining a urine drug screen up to 120 hours after the event if there is a history of the patient being given drugs or alcohol or there is reason to suspect that this occurred. A positive screen could support the patient's history and the patient's inability to consent as a result of impairment due to drugs or alcohol.

TABLE 46.3

STI Testing and Other Testing

	Source	Test
Hepatitis B	Serum	Hepatitis B surface antibody, Hepatitis B surface antigen, Hepatitis B core antibody
Hepatitis C	Serum	Hepatitis C antibody
HIV	Serum	HIV Antibody
Herpes	Genital lesion (unroofed vesicle or base of ulceration)	PCR, culture
Syphilis	Serum	Syphilis IgG and IgM antibodies or RPR
Trichomonas	Cervical/vaginal/ urine	Prepubertal: NAAT and/or culture and wet mount. Testing for *T. vaginalis* should not be limited to girls with vaginal discharge if other indications for vaginal testing exist. Postpubertal: NAAT from vagina or urine.
N gonorrhea[a] C Trachomatis[a]	Pharyngeal Rectal Cervical/Vaginal Urine (prepubertal girls)	Culture, NAAT
Genital warts	Genital lesion	Visual confirmation
Urine		Urinalysis and culture
Drug screen (if indicated)	Urine, Serum	
Pregnancy	Urine Serum	PCOT urine Serum hCG confirmatory

[a] Although cultures have historically been considered the gold standard for the diagnosis of sexually transmitted infections in children, in some locations initial testing may be through NAAT testing if culture media is unavailable or there is difficulty in assuring that the sample is sent to the lab under appropriate environmental conditions.

Forensic Evidence

- Collect Evidence Kit (if **ACUTE event** – ideally within 72 hours but could be longer. Collection window may vary by state.)
  - The kit can be provided by local law enforcement.
  - Many emergency departments have unused kits stored to use when needed.
  - A description of the specimens to be taken and instructions on how to obtain the specimens are available in the kit.
- The kit should not be left unattended by medical personnel once it is opened. All persons handling the materials in the kit should be identified in the documentation that is placed in the kit to maintain a "chain of evidence." Once the specimens are collected and the documentation is completed, then the kit should be sealed and given to law enforcement.
- Specimens collected and placed in the kit include
  - Buccal swab (to identify the patient's DNA)
  - Underwear that the patient was wearing at the time of the assault
  - Swabs of any dried or moist secretions observed on the patient's body
  - Swabs of the oral cavity, vagina, and anorectum
- Kits vary by state and it is imperative that healthcare providers read and follow the directions carefully.
- Collect *ALL* evidence that the patient will consent to having collected. (Sometimes all the details and kinds of abuse are not disclosed immediately).
- Remember that bed clothes and underwear have a high yield for forensic evidence.
  - Collect underwear the patient is wearing even if the patient has changed them since the assault.
  - Have family keep unlaundered bedding and underwear/clothes that remains at home and save for law enforcement.
  - Provide paper bags to the family for items of clothing to be collected at home.

Management

Repair of injuries

- Fortunately, most victims do not sustain a serious physical injury as a result of sexual abuse or assault
- For genital trauma, see specific recommendations, Chapter 19, "Genital Trauma"

Treatment of STIs [see Table in Chapter 48, "Sexually Transmitted Infections" Chapter 23, "Human Immunodeficiency Virus (HIV)"]

- Prepubertal asymptomatic children
  - Defer STI treatment until testing is complete and positive test results are confirmed – except for HIV nPEP
  - Do not delay initiation of post-HIV-exposure prophylaxis (nPEP)
- Pubertal child
  - Provide STI prophylaxis, if the event was recent or the patient is symptomatic or follow up is unlikely
  - Provide emergency contraception
  - When emergency contraception and STI treatment are provided, also provide antiemetic
  - Offer HIV nPEP when indicated

HIV nonoccupational postexposure prophylaxis (HIV nPEP) [see Chapter 23, "Human Immunodeficiency Virus (HIV)"]

- Can be offered up to 72 hours after sexual assault
- Consultation with a Pediatric Infectious Disease specialist is recommended
- See tables to assess risk for HIV acquisition as a result of abuse

Provide vaccination for Hepatitis B if the child is unimmunized or incomplete.

- If the assailant is known Hepatitis B surface antigen positive and the survivor has not been previously vaccinated, administer Hep B vaccine and HBIG.
- If the assailant is known Hepatitis B surface antigen positive and the survivor has been previously vaccinated, administer Hep B vaccine (booster dose).

Emergency Contraception (EC)

- Can be offered up to 120 hours after a sexual assault if the pregnancy test is negative (see Chapter 13, "Contraception").

Discharge Planning

- Ensure that all immediate medical and mental health needs are addressed and that the appropriate child protective services and law enforcement agencies have been informed of the situation.
- If there are identified concerns for self-harm or suicidal ideation, consult a psychiatrist.
- Assess that child or teen will be discharged to a safe environment (perpetrator is not in the home or possibly returning) and determine (by asking family) if there are any other children at the home at risk for abuse.
- Review what was done during the exam (exam findings, tests ordered, and what follow up care is needed) with the patient and caregiver.
- Validate the child's feelings by acknowledging that sexual abuse disclosures are difficult to make and take courage.
- Remind the child that they may need to share their story with individuals responsible for keeping them safe and need some form of medical follow up at a later date.
- Schedule follow up serologic testing for syphilis and HIV at 12 weeks post assault.
- Complete Hepatitis B immunization as indicated if the child is not previously immunized or serology indicates the need for a booster dose.
- Follow up pregnancy testing should be provided if the child misses a menstrual period.
- Follow up with infectious disease specialist if HIV nPEP is provided.
- Recommend HPV vaccination if the child is greater or equal to age 9 and has not yet received this vaccination.
- Follow up medical examination is recommended for all patients, **especially under the following circumstances**:
  - To obtain photodocumentation for an abnormal finding or injury (follow up ASAP, remember that injuries heal quickly)
  - To assess the healing of an injury
  - To better assess an unclear finding or have the finding assessed by a physician with expertise in child sexual abuse evaluations
  - If further testing for STIs is needed (especially if antibiotic prophylaxis was not given)
  - To ensure that kids who were provided medication in the ER completed the course prescribed
  - To ensure that mental health needs are being addressed

Tell the caretaker that investigators generally suggest a child who makes a disclosure of abuse not be asked questions about the abuse because they will likely be scheduled to speak with a trained child forensic interviewer at a Children's Advocacy Center.

- Speaking with a child forensic interviewer will provide the child the opportunity to tell what happened.
- The greatest way to be of support to a child during this process is to reassure the child that making a disclosure of abuse might be difficult but it is also courageous.

Children's Advocacy Centers, Rape Crisis Agencies, and hospital based pediatric child abuse pediatricians/child protection teams are resources that the healthcare provider can contact to help ensure that a child and family will receive services and counseling. These agencies can provide counseling for both children and caretakers, as well as offer guidance to families regarding the investigative response and legal processes that comprise a multidisciplinary approach to a child sexual abuse outcry.

SEX TRAFFICKING

Definition

Sex trafficking is defined by the *Trafficking Victims Protection Act of 2000* as "the recruitment, harboring, transportation, provision, obtaining, patronizing, or soliciting of a person for the purpose of a commercial sex act."

Sex trafficking involves the use of force, fraud, or coercion to make an adult engage in commercial sex acts.

- *Any commercial sexual activity with a minor, even without force, fraud, or coercion, is considered trafficking.*

Clinical Indicators

- Physical Signs and Symptoms
  - Sexually transmitted diseases, HIV/AIDS, pelvic pain, rectal trauma, and urinary difficulties
  - Pregnancy
  - Malnourishment: Child trafficking victims can suffer from retarded growth
  - Dental caries and rotted teeth
  - Infectious diseases like tuberculosis
  - Bruises, scars, and other signs of physical abuse and torture. Sex industry victims are often beaten in areas that won't damage their outward appearance, like their lower back
  - Tattoos
  - Appears to be deprived of food, water, and/or sleep
- Behavioral Signs and Symptoms
  - Fears making eye contact
  - Projects attitude of shame
  - Provides answers which may seem untrue/incorrect
  - Attempts to act older than appears
  - Provides False ID/Multiple IDs
  - Limits communication with health professionals
  - Presents for care with an overly controlling "boyfriend" or "family member"
  - Substance abuse problems or addictions either from being coerced into drug use by their traffickers or by turning to substance abuse to help cope with or mentally escape their desperate situations

- Psychological trauma from daily mental abuse and torture, including depression, stress-related disorders, disorientation, confusion, phobias, and panic attacks
- Feelings of helplessness, shame, humiliation, shock, denial, or disbelief

History

- In teens, screen for sex trafficking by asking
  - Have you ever been in a position where you've had to consider exchanging sex for something you wanted or needed (money, food, shelter, or other items)?
  - Has anyone ever asked you to have sex or perform sexual acts with another person in exchange for something you wanted or needed (money, food, shelter, or other items)?
  - Has anyone ever wanted to take sexual pictures or videos of you or post such pictures or videos on the internet in exchange for something you wanted or needed?
  - Tell me all the ways you get money.
- An affirmative answer to at least two of the following can significantly increase the odds of being the victim of sex trafficking (sensitivity of 92%/specificity of 73%)
  - History of broken bones, major cuts requiring stitches, or loss of consciousness
  - Running away from home
  - Drug and alcohol use within the past 12 months
  - Law Enforcement involvement
  - Multiple sexual partners (>5 partners)
  - History of STIs
- When obtaining a history, the limitations of confidentiality should be reviewed, including a discussion of the healthcare provider's role as a mandated reporter.

Assess the need to obtain forensic evidence based on time frame of events.

Physical Exam

Physical examination

- Assess for both acute and chronic medical conditions
- Assess dental health
- Assess for bruising, acute injury
- Assess for acute anogenital injury
- Assess for signs of STI

Laboratory testing

- Pregnancy, STIs, and HIV
- Urine and/or serum screening for alcohol and drug use, as clinically indicated

Management

Offer contraceptive options, with particular focus on long-acting reversible contraception
Offer prophylaxis for STIs and pregnancy.

Reporting

Physicians are mandated reporters of suspected child abuse and neglect. In states where sex trafficking is considered a form of abuse, a physician must make a formal report of suspected exploitation to law enforcement and to child protective services.

Healthcare providers should educate authorities that the child is a victim of exploitation, not an offender. If you think you have come in contact with a victim of human trafficking, call the Trafficking Information and Referral Hotline at 1.888.3737.888.

This hotline will help you determine if you have encountered victims of human trafficking, will identify local resources available in your community to help victims, and will help you coordinate with local social service organizations to help protect and serve victims so they can begin the process of restoring their lives.

For more information on human trafficking visit www.acf.hhs.gov/trafficking.

BIBLIOGRAPHY

Adams JA, Farst KJ, and Kellogg ND. Interpretation of medical findings in suspected child sexual abuse: an update for 2018. J Pediatr Adolesc Gynecol. 2018;31: 225–231

Adams JA, Harper K, Knudson S, Revilla J. Examination findings in legally confirmed child sexual abuse: it's normal to be normal. Pediatrics. 1994;94:310–317.

American Academy of Pediatrics. Red Book: 2021–2024 Report of the Committee on Infectious Diseases. 32nd ed. American Academy of Pediatrics; 2021.

CDC (2016). Updated guidelines for antiretroviral postexposure prophylaxis after sexual, injection-drug use or other nonoccupational exposure to HIV in the US: Recommendations from the US Department of Health and Human Services.

CDC 2021. https://www.cdc.gov/violenceprevention/sexualviolence/trafficking.html

Greenbaum, J, et al. "Child sex trafficking and commercial sexual exploitation: health care needs of victims." Pediatrics 2015; 135.3: 566–574.

Greenbaum VJ, Dodd M, McCracken C. A short screening tool to identify victims of child sex trafficking in the health care setting. Ped Emerg Care. 2018;34 (1):33–37.

Jenny C, Crawford-Jakubiak JE, & Committee on Child Abuse and Neglect. The evaluation of children in the primary care setting when sexual abuse is suspected. Pediatrics. 2013;132(2), e558–e567.

Jenny C, Pierce MC, (eds.). Child abuse and neglect: diagnosis, treatment, and evidence. St. Louis, MO: Elsevier Saunders, 2011.

Kellogg, N, Menard, S, Santos, A. (2004). Genital anatomy in pregnant adolescents: "normal" does not mean "nothing happened." Pediatrics. 113:e67–e69.

Kempe, C. Henry. Sexual abuse, another hidden pediatric problem: the 1977 C. Anderson Aldrich Lecture. Pediatrics. 1978;62:382–389.

McCann J, Miyamoto S, Boyle C, Rogers K. Healing of hymenal injuries in prepubertal and adolescent girls: a descriptive study. Pediatrics. 2007; 119:e1094–e1106.

McCann J, Miyamoto S, Boyle C, Rogers K. Healing of nonhymenal injuries in prepubertal and adolescent girls: a descriptive study. Pediatrics. 2007; 120:1000–1011.

National Sexual Violence Resource Center (NSVRC). Tools for Trauma-Informed Practices. https://www.nsvrc.org/projects/lifespan/tools-trauma-informed-practice.

Safeta.org. https://www.safeta.org/page/KIDSIntro

U.S. Department of Justice Office on Violence Against Women. A National Protocol for Sexual Assault Medical Forensic Examinations: Adults/Adolescents. www.ncjrs.gov/pdffiles1/ovw/241903.pdf

Workowski KA, Bachmann LH, Chan PA, et al. Sexually transmitted infections treatment guidelines, 2021. MMWR Recomm Rep. 2021;70(No. RR-4):1–187. DOI: http://dx.doi.org/10.15585/mmwr.rr7004a1

47

Sexual Activity

Y. Frances Fei and Melina L. Dendrinos

Background

- Sexual development begins at birth and is influenced by what the child or adolescent learns and observes from the environment
- Sexual activity is a common part of normal development in adolescents and young adults
  - 40% of adolescents aged 15–19 report a history of sexual intercourse, and 45% report a history of oral sex
- Teenage pregnancy rates have declined in the United States in recent years but remain higher than other industrialized countries
- Contraceptive and STI care are integral parts of sexual health care
- Important for health-care providers to talk to their patients about sexual health during routine visits
  - Especially for populations who are often overlooked, including patients with developmental delay, patients in same-sex relationships, and transgender or gender nonbinary patients

Key Points

- It is the role of the health-care provider to
  - Ensure that patients are provided with accurate information regarding sexual health and reproductive safety
  - Support parents and guardians in being involved in their child's sexuality education. Open communication starting from a young age can leave the door open for the future
  - Perform confidential interviews starting at ages 11–14
    - Establish rapport with a patient before asking private questions
    - Screen for inappropriate or risky behavior
    - Assess sexual history as part of the "HEADSS" questions: home, education/employment, activities, drugs/diet, sexuality, suicide, safety (see Chapter 20, "Gynecologic Exam")
- Sexual behaviors are very common in children and adolescents. In most cases, these are due to curiosity and not problematic
  - Concerning behaviors include
    - Actions associated with force or aggression
    - Actions occurring between children of widely different cognitive abilities
    - Actions that cause significant anxiety or discomfort in the child
- Providers should avoid judgment and heterosexual bias. Many adolescents explore their sexual and gender identities
  - Patients who identify as LGBTQ may be at higher risk for unsafe sexual practices

DOI: 10.1201/9781003039235-47

Sexual Development

Preadolescence

- Parents and health-care providers play important roles in educating children regarding what is and is not acceptable
- Children should learn about private parts and who is allowed to see or touch these private parts
  - Initially, encourage "No-Go-Tell": Say no, leave the person, and tell a trusted adult
  - As independence is gained, discuss stranger awareness and online safety
- Early interactions between parents and children regarding sexuality will determine the child's comfort in approaching parents with issues in future years
- Environment plays a key role in sexual education
  - Communication/displays of affection at home
  - Social media
  - Peers
- Infants and toddlers, aged 0–4
  - Children are curious about their own and other people's bodies
  - May start exploring private parts, showing private parts in public, desiring to be naked, and asking questions about bodies and bodily functions
- Preschool, aged 4–6
  - May start mimicking behavior they have seen on television or other adults, such as kissing and holding hands
  - May start talking about their private parts in public, purposefully touching private parts (i.e. masturbation), or exploring private parts with other children in their play group
- School-aged, aged 7–11
  - May become more modest and desire more privacy
  - May begin dressing in private, masturbating in private, and viewing sexual content in the media
  - May start having feelings of sexual attraction towards peers and become more curious about their own sexuality

Adolescence

- Peer relationships become more influential
- May start experimenting with sexual identity and sexual behaviors
- Comprehensive sexual education does not increase earlier sexual behavior and is effective in preventing pregnancy and STIs
- Counseling contraception, prevention of STIs, and safe relationships should be addressed by the provider at each office visit (see Chapter 12, "Contraception"; Chapter 48, "STI"; Chapter 21, "High-Risk Behaviors"; and Chapter 51, "Transgender and Gender Diverse Care")
- Patients may also want to discuss the sexual response and/or sexual dysfunction
- Early adolescence, aged 11–14
  - Begin to form "crushes" and early romantic relationships
  - Masturbation and sexual fantasies are common; sexual intercourse is still uncommon
  - Begin to draw away from parents, and parents may also pull back to allow their children to have more independence
  - Concern with pubertal changes, especially with physical appearance

- Start to consider sexual identity
- Mostly concrete in thinking, so providers should focus on current issues that are important to them (body image, weight, acne)
- Middle adolescence, aged 14–17
  - More concern with physical appearance
  - Start experimenting with relationships and sexual activity
  - Relationships with peers are very influential
  - Becoming more abstract thinkers and can imagine consequences of their behaviors, but often do not see themselves as susceptible
  - Providers should address self-esteem issues, harmful relationships, and risky behavior, focusing on healthy behavior and risk reduction, as well as discuss characteristics of a healthy relationship and ask teens to match features of their own relationship
- Late adolescence, aged 17–21
  - Begin to solidify sexual orientation and gender identity
  - Begin to think about the future and forming long-term relationships
  - Have more feelings of love, tenderness, and passion
  - Providers should discuss support systems, personal goals, and family expectations

Developmental Delay and Disability

- Patients with cognitive delay or physical disabilities are often thought of as asexual and not included in sexual education, but they have similar rates of sexual activity
  - Need to receive sexual education at an appropriate developmental level
  - Parents should discuss appropriate behavior and ways to protect from unwanted attention starting at a young age
  - Providers need to equip parents with resources
- Parents and/or patients may seek contraception due to suspected or known sexual activity
  - Reversible contraception should be used whenever possible
  - Involve patient in decision-making if possible
  - Many teens with medical disabilities are on teratogenic medications and need to be aware of the importance of avoiding pregnancy

Congenital Anomalies and Differences of Sex Development

- Diagnoses that may impact the appearance of the external genitalia and/or fertility potential and can be very overwhelming
  - Patients may be at very different stages of development when the diagnosis is made
  - A mental health professional can be very helpful in assessing needs and providing counseling
- Patients should be reassured that
  - Regardless of the presence of anomalies or chromosomal differences, they can choose gender identity
  - External and internal genitalia differ widely across the population
  - They can form relationships and participate in sexual education in the same manner as their peers

Resources for Parents and Adolescents

Books

- Harris R, Emberley M. (2008). *It's Not the Stork: A Book about Girls, Boys, Babies, Bodies, Families, and Friends.* Candlewick.
- Harris R, Emberley M. (2014). *It's So Amazing!: A Book about Eggs, Sperm, Birth, Babies, and Family.* Candlewick.
- Harris R. Emberly M. (2014). *It's Perfectly Normal: Changing Bodies, Growing Up, Sex Gender and Sexual Health.* Candlewick.

Websites

- Center for Young Women's Health: targeted information for adolescents regarding sexual health, also provides information on chronic diseases and congenital anomalies. www.young-womenshealth.org
- Go Ask Alice: Q&As regarding sexual behavior for young adults. www.goaskalice.columbia.edu
- Sex Positive Families: resources for sexual education for parents and caregivers, including age-appropriate reading list. http://sexpositivefamilies.com/
- Society for Adolescent Health and Medicine: additional resources including webpages, apps, and helplines. www.adolescenthealth.org/Resources/Clinical-Care-Resources/Sexual-Reproductive-Health/SRH-One-pager-for-Adolescents.aspx

BIBLIOGRAPHY

Guttmacher Institute. *Adolescent Sexual and Reproductive Health in the United States New York.* New York, NY: Guttmacher Institute; 2019 [Available from: https://www.guttmacher.org/fact-sheet/american-teens-sexual-and-reproductive-health.]

Marcell AV, Burstein GR, AAP Committee on Adolescence. Sexual and reproductive health care services in the pediatric setting. Pediatrics. 2017; 140(5);e20172858.

Monasterio E, Combs N, Warner L, et al. (2010). *Sexual Health: An Adolescent Provider Toolkit.* San Francisco, CA: Adolescent Health Working Group.

National Guidelines Task Force (2004). *Guidelines for Comprehensive Sexuality Education: Kindergarten-12th Grade* (3rd ed.). New York, NY: Sexuality Information and Education Council of the United States.

48

Sexually Transmitted Infections (STIs)

Olivia Winfrey and Wendy L. Jackson

Key Points

- Rates of many sexually transmitted infections (STIs) are highest in the adolescent population.
- Adolescents and young adults (15–24 years of age) make up one-fourth of the sexually active population; however, they account for half of the 20 million new STI cases every year.
- Factors influencing the increased risk of adolescents in acquiring STIs
  - Unprotected intercourse
  - Biologically susceptible to infection (cervical ectropion)
  - Multiple partners and/or limited duration of relationships
  - Barriers to utilization of health care
- In almost all states adolescents in the United States can consent for diagnosis and treatment of STIs without parental consent, although some states have age limitations (see the Guttmacher Institute for details).
- Providers MUST remember to obtain an age-appropriate confidential sexual history on all adolescents (see Chapter 20, "Gynecologic Examination," and Chapter 21, "High-Risk Behaviors").
- Expedited Partner Therapy (EPT) is a beneficial harm-reduction practice that allows for treatment of partners without patient visit; laws vary by state, so it is important to understand ability to prescribe locally.
- Detailed treatment guidelines for STIs can be obtained via CDC (cdc.gov).
- Detailed information for patients can be obtained via American Sexual Health Association. (ashasexualhealth.org)

Chlamydia trachomatis

- The most frequently reported bacterial infectious disease in the United States
- The highest rates for chlamydia are in adolescents and young adults ≤24 years of age
- Infected individuals are often asymptomatic and are only detected by screening
- Sexually active women should be screened at least annually or with each new sexual partner
- Sequelae of undiagnosed infection include pelvic inflammatory disease (PID), ectopic pregnancy, infertility, chronic pelvic pain
- If present in a pediatric patient, infection is secondary to sexual abuse, and the patient must be treated and referred for a sexual abuse evaluation (see Chapter 46, "Sexual Abuse")
- Possibly secondary to vertical transmission from mother to child/infant if diagnosed within first 3 years of life

Presentation

- Can be symptomatic or asymptomatic
- May have mucopurulent vaginal discharge, dysuria, urinary frequency, pelvic pain. Friable and edematous cervix may be seen on exam

DOI: 10.1201/9781003039235-48

Diagnosis

- NAAT (nucleic acid amplification testing) from vaginal, endocervical, or first-catch urine sample
  - Urine may detect up to 10% fewer infections. Specimen should not be a catheter sample
  - Vaginal swabs may be self-collected if the patient prefers. Sensitivity and specificity for diagnosis is the same compared to specimens collected by a clinician
  - Rectal and oropharyngeal infection in persons engaging in receptive anal or oral intercourse can be diagnosed by NAAT at the anatomic site of exposure
  - Those diagnosed with chlamydia should be tested for human immunodeficiency virus (HIV), gonorrhea, and syphilis

Management

- Children <45 kg
  - Erythromycin 50 mg/kg/day orally divided into four doses daily for 14 days
- Children >45 kg but are <8 years of age
  - Azithromycin 1 g orally in a single dose
- Children >8 years of age and adolescents
  - Doxycycline 100 mg orally BID for 7 days (preferred for the non-pregnant adolescent)
  - Azithromycin 1 g orally in a single dose
- Alternative regimen for adolescents only
  - Levofloxacin 500 mg orally daily for 7 days
- Abstain from sexual intercourse for 7 days after completed treatment AND until partner is treated
- If state law allows, should provide prescription or additional medication dose to the patient so that she may give to her partner (EPT)
- Most recent sexual partner should be referred for treatment as should any partner within prior 60 days
- Infected adolescents should be screened for reinfection 3 months after treatment
- Educate patient that short of abstinence, condom use for anal, vaginal, and oral sex is the most effective way to prevent infection

Hepatitis A (HAV)

- Incubation period on average is 28 days (15–50 days)
- Viral infection transmitted through the fecal-oral route
- Can be prevented with vaccination: Two doses (0, and 6–12 months)
- Vaccination candidates are as follows:
  - All children at 1 year of age and anyone seeking immunity
  - Those at risk for sexual transmission
  - Persons who use injection/non-injection illegal drugs
  - Individuals working in high-risk environments
  - Homeless population
  - Those with chronic liver disease, HIV, or clotting disorders
  - Individuals with direct contact to someone with HAV

Presentation

- Can be asymptomatic or symptomatic
  - Fever, malaise, anorexia, nausea, vomiting, abdominal pain, and diarrhea
  - May progress to dark urine and jaundice
- Symptoms more common in older children and adults
  - Often asymptomatic in children <6 years (only 30% have symptoms)
  - Symptoms usually resolve in 2–3 weeks
  - Older children may be symptomatic up to 6 months

Diagnosis

- Serologic testing: IgM antibody to HAV
  - Antibodies are present at the time of symptoms
  - Can be detected in serum for up to 6 months after infection

Management

- Supportive care
- No dietary/activity restrictions
- Hospitalization for dehydration associated with nausea/vomiting
- Use medications metabolized by the liver with caution
- Postexposure prophylaxis exists for those not previously vaccinated
  - Either administer single dose monovalent HAV vaccine or immunoglobulin (0.1 mL/kg) administer within 2 weeks of exposure
  - Immunoglobulin for
    – Children aged <6 months
    – Immunocompromised persons
    – Persons with chronic liver disease
    – Persons with contraindications to the vaccine

Hepatitis B (HBV)

- Incubation period is 6 weeks to 6 months
- Transmitted through the following
  - Percutaneous (needle sticks, blood products, tattooing, etc.)
  - Mucosal (sexual intercourse, infected mother to infant)
- The younger HBV is acquired, the higher the risk for chronic infection (90% of infected infants and 30% of infected children <5 years of age will develop chronic HBV)
- 15–25% of those with chronic infection progress to death related to cirrhosis or hepatocellular carcinoma
- Can be prevented with vaccination: Three doses (birth, 1–2 months, and 6–18 months)
- Vaccination candidates are as follows
  - All unvaccinated children and adolescents
  - When sexual abuse is identified, initiate vaccination in previously unvaccinated children

- Those at increased risk of infection (e.g. those attending STI clinics)
- Persons with a history of an STI
- Persons with multiple sexual partners
- Persons having sex with an injection-drug user
- Persons engaging in illegal drug use
- Household members, sex partners, drug-sharing partners of a person with chronic HBV
- Persons on hemodialysis, receiving blood clotting factor concentrates, or occupational exposure to blood
- Persons in drug treatment/long-term correctional facilities

Presentation

- Can by asymptomatic or symptomatic
- Flu-like symptoms including anorexia, malaise, nausea, vomiting, abdominal pain, joint aches, fever, fatigue, and sometimes rash

Diagnosis

- Diagnosis is made with serology (see Table 48.1)
- For acute hepatitis: HbsAg and IgM anti-HBc establish the diagnosis

TABLE 48.1

Interpretation of Serologic Test Results[a] for HBV Infection

	Serologic Marker			
HBsAg	Total Anti-HBc	IgM Anti-HBc	Anti-HBs	Interpretation
−	−	−	−	Never infected
+[b]	−	−	−	Early acute infection; transient (up to 18 days) after vaccination
+	+	+	−	Acute infection
−	+	+	−	Acute resolving infection
−	+	−	+	Recovered from past infection and immune
+	+	−	−	Chronic infection
−	+	−	−	False positive (i.e., susceptible); past infection; "low-level" chronic infection[c]; passive transfer to infant born to HBsAg-positive mother
−	−	−	+	Immune if concentration is >10 mIU/mL, passive transfer after HBIG administration

Abbreviations: Anti-HBc = antibody to hepatitis B core antigen; anti-HBs = antibody to hepatitis B surface antigen; HBsAg = hepatitis B surface antigen; IgM = immunoglobulin M; mIU/mL = Milli-international units per milliliter.

Source: From https://www.cdc.gov/vaccines/vpd/hepb/index.html.

a Symbol for a negative test result, "−"; symbol for a positive test result, "+."

b To ensure that an HBsAg-positive test result is not false-positive, samples with repeatedly reactive HBsAg results should be tested with an FDA-cleared neutralizing confirmatory test.

c Persons positive for only anti-HBc are unlikely to be infectious except under unusual circumstances involving direct percutaneous exposure to large quantities of blood (e.g., blood transfusion and organ transplantation).

Management

- Acute infection
  - Supportive therapy
- Chronic infection
  - Antiviral agents and immune modulators
- Postexposure prophylaxis (PEP)
- ***Candidates for PEP-Postexposure Prophylaxis** (see* Table 48.2*)*
  - Vaccinated and HBsAg positive source: No treatment required
  - Vaccinated individuals with no documentation of vaccine response and HBsAg positive source: Single dose of Hepatitis B vaccine
  - Currently receiving Hepatitis B vaccine series and HBsAg positive source: Hepatitis B immune globulin (HBIG) and complete vaccine series
  - Unvaccinated and HBsAg positive source: Hepatitis B immune globulin (HBIG) and initiation of Hepatitis B vaccine within 24 hours. Recommended administration within 7 days if percutaneous exposure and 14 days if sexual exposure
  - Inadequate response after the previous vaccine and HBsAg positive source: Hepatitis B vaccine booster. If unavailable, vaccinate as soon as possible and administer HBIG within 14 days of sexual contact (7 days if percutaneous exposure)

TABLE 48.2

Guidelines for Postexposure Prophylaxis[*] of Persons with Nonoccupational Exposure[†] to Blood or Body Fluids That Contain Blood, by Exposure Type and Hepatitis B Vaccination Status

Source of Exposure	Unvaccinated Person[§]	Previously Vaccinated Person[¶]
HBsAg-Positive Source Percutaneous (e.g., bite or needlestick) or mucosal exposure to HBsAg-positive blood or body fluids *or* Sex or needle-sharing contact with an HBsAg-positive person *or* Victim of sexual assault or abuse by an assailant who is HBsAg positive	Administer hepatitis B vaccine series and HBIG	Complete hepatitis B vaccine series and HBIG, if vaccine series not completed *or* Administer hepatitis B vaccine booster dose, if previous vaccination without testing[**]
Source with Unknown HBsAg Status Percutaneous (e.g., bite or needlestick) or mucosal exposure to potentially infectious blood or body fluids from a source with unknown HBsAg status *or* Sex or needle-sharing contact with person with unknown HBsAg status *or* Victim of sexual assault or abuse by a perpetrator with unknown HBsAg status	Administer hepatitis B vaccine series	Complete hepatitis B vaccine series

Sources: CDC. CDC guidance for evaluating health-care personnel for hepatitis B virus protection and for administering postexposure management. MMWR Recomm Rep 2013;62(No. RR-10); CDC. Postexposure prophylaxis to prevent hepatitis B virus infection. MMWR Recomm Rep 2006;55(No. RR-16).

Abbreviations: HBIG = hepatitis B immune globulin; HBsAg = hepatitis B surface antigen.

[*] When indicated, immunoprophylaxis should be initiated as soon as possible, preferably within 24 hours. Studies are limited regarding the maximum interval after exposure during which postexposure prophylaxis is effective, but the interval is unlikely to exceed 7 days for percutaneous exposures or 14 days for sexual exposures. The hepatitis B vaccine series should be completed. These guidelines apply to nonoccupational exposures.

[†] These guidelines apply to nonoccupational exposures.

[§] A person who is in the process of being vaccinated but who has not completed the vaccine series should complete the series and receive treatment for hepatitis B as indicated.

[¶] A person who has written documentation of a complete hepatitis B vaccine series and who did not receive postvaccination testing.

[**] No booster dose is needed for persons who have written documentation of hepatitis B vaccine series with serologic response.

- Vaccinated and unknown HBsAg source: No further treatment
- Currently receiving Hepatitis B vaccine series and unknown HBsAg source: Complete vaccine series
- Unvaccinated and unknown HBsAg source: Initiate Hepatitis B vaccine immediately within 24 hours. Recommended administration within 7 days if percutaneous exposure and 14 days if sexual exposure

Hepatitis C (HCV)

- Incubation period from 2 to 26 weeks (average 2–12 weeks)
- Transmitted through the following
    - Direct percutaneous exposure to infected blood (injection drug use, needlesticks, birth to infected mothers, and prior to 1992-from donated organs and transfusion of blood products)
    - Rarely associated with medical procedures, contaminated personal hygiene items, tattooing, or sexual intercourse
- No available vaccine
- Screening
    - Universal screening for everyone 18 years old and older, as well as pregnant patients unless <0.1% prevalence of the condition
    - Illegal drug use, either current or remote history
    - Transfused blood from an individual with HCV
    - HIV positive patients
    - Maternal HCV at time of birth
    - Persistently elevated liver enzymes (specifically ALT)
    - Long-term hemodialysis
    - Needlestick resulting in exposure to HCV positive blood
- Chronic infection develops in 75–85% after acute infection
- Patients are not clinically ill, thus are unaware of illness and may transmit to others

Presentation

- Can be asymptomatic or symptomatic
- Symptoms may include decreased appetite, fever, fatigue, abdominal pain, clay-colored stools, nausea, vomiting, dark urine, joint pain, and jaundice

Diagnosis

- Serologic testing: Anti-HCV (if anti-HCV positive, confirm with HCV RNA)

Management

- CDC recommends people with hepatitis C have the following
    - Medical evaluation by primary care clinician or specialist (e.g. in hepatology, gastroenterology, or infectious disease) for chronic liver disease including treatment and monitoring
    - Treatment with direct acting antivirals (DAA), ribavirin, interferon, and peginterferon
    - Hepatitis A and B vaccination
    - Screening and brief intervention for alcohol consumption

Herpes Simplex Virus (HSV)

- Genital herpes is a recurrent, lifelong viral infection
- There are two types: Herpes simplex virus (HSV)-1 and HSV-2, both can infect the genital tract
- Most HSV infections are transmitted asymptomatically by persons unaware of their infection
- Asymptomatic viral shedding and recurrences are more likely in HSV-2

Presentation

- Primary HSV
  - Painful grouped vesicles, may last up to one week
  - Symptoms of local pain, itching, dysuria, constitutional symptoms (fever, myalgia, malaise, headache)
- Non-primary first episode
  - Fewer symptoms and lesions
- Recurrent HSV
  - Vesicles or ulcers without constitutional symptoms
- Appearance is typical (vesicle/ulceration on erythematous base)

Diagnosis

- HSV NAAT assays of a sample taken from the unroofed base of ulcer are most sensitive
- Viral culture (diagnostic standard) or PCR (higher sensitivity especially CNS infection, a blood test should not be performed for mucosal ulcer diagnosis) to confirm the diagnosis
- Serology is available but not recommended; only type-specific IgG-based assays should be requested

Management

Pediatric/Non-Sexually Active Adolescent Patients

- Sexual abuse must be considered as etiology
- If the history of oral cold sores and has Type 1 HSV, less likely to be secondary to sexual abuse; despite this, some type of investigation needs to be conducted by the health-care provider or referral to appropriate child advocacy center to evaluate for and ensure there has been no inappropriate sexual contact (see Chapter 46, "Sexual Abuse")

Sexually Active Patients

- Screen for syphilis, gonorrhea, chlamydia, bacterial vaginosis, and trichomonas
  - May be too uncomfortable at initial presentation to complete
  - Consider interval testing at follow-up visit after resolution of acute herpetic lesions

Pediatric Treatment (<12 Years)

- First Episode (mild to moderate)
  - Acyclovir oral: 40–80 mg/kg/day divided in 3–4 doses/day, maximum dose: 1,200 mg/day; for 7–10 days

OR
- Famciclovir oral (children weighing ≥45 kg): 250 mg TID for 7–10 days
  OR
- Valacyclovir oral: 20 mg/kg/dose BID, maximum dose: 1,000 mg/dose; for 7–10 days
- Recurrent episodes
  - Acyclovir oral: 20 mg/kg/dose TID; maximum dose: 400 mg; for 5 days
    OR
  - Valacyclovir: Treatment must be started with prodromal symptoms or manifestation of lesion
    - Patient weight <50 kg: Oral: 20 mg/kg/dose BID; maximum dose: 1,000 mg; for 5 days
    - Patient weight ≥50 kg: Oral: 1,000 mg once daily for 5 days
- Suppressive therapy
  - Acyclovir oral: 20 mg/kg/dose BID; maximum dose: 400 mg/dose
    OR
  - Valacyclovir oral: 20 mg/kg/dose once daily; maximum dose: 1,000 mg

Treatment for Adolescents (>12 Years)

- First clinical episode (mild to moderate)
  - Acyclovir oral: 400 mg TID for 7–10 days; treatment can be extended
  - Acyclovir oral: 200 mg 5×/day is effective, however not recommended due to frequency of dosing
    OR
  - Famciclovir oral: 250 mg TID for 7–10 days; treatment can be extended
    OR
  - Valacyclovir oral: 20 mg/kg/dose BID, maximum dose: 1,000 mg; for 7–10 days
- First clinical episode (severe)
  - IV Acyclovir 5 mg/kg/dose every 8 hours for 5–7 days *OR* 5–10 mg/kg/dose every 8 hours for 2–7 days, followed with oral therapy to complete at least 10 days
- Recurrent episodes
  - Acyclovir oral: 800 mg BID for 5 days *OR* 800 mg TID for 2 days
  - Acyclovir oral: 200mg every 4 hours (while awake) for 5 doses/d or 400 mg TID for 5 days is effective, however not recommended due to frequency of dosing
    OR
  - Famciclovir: Treatment must be started within 1 day of prodromal symptoms or manifestation of lesion
    - One-day regimen: Oral: 1,000 mg BID
    - Two-day regimen: Oral: 500 mg once as a single dose, followed 12 hours later by 250 mg BID for a total of 2 days
    - Five-day regimen: Oral: 125 mg
      OR
  - Valacyclovir: Treatment must be started with prodromal symptoms or manifestation of lesion
    - Patient weight <50 kg: Oral: 20 mg/kg/dose BID; maximum dose: 1,000 mg; for 5 days
    - Patient weight ≥50 kg: Oral: 1,000 mg once daily for 5 days
- Suppressive therapy (≥6 recurrences/year)
  - Periodically (once/year) discontinue treatment and reassess need for continuation

- Acyclovir oral 400 mg BID
  OR
- Famciclovir oral 250 mg BID (duration not established)
  OR
- Valacyclovir oral 1 g/day (can consider 500 mg daily but likely less effective if ≥10 episodes/year)
- *NOTE*: Immunocompromised individuals need specific dosing (see CDC guidelines)

Local Care

- Sitz baths TID to QID to keep the area clean and enhance voiding
- Avoid soaps
- Increase fluids to keep the urine dilute and less irritating
- Use of topical 2% lidocaine gel to ulcerated areas may minimize burning with urination; discontinue if aggravates symptoms
- May need to place indwelling catheter if urinary retention occurs Narcotics may be required for pain management

Counseling

- Recurrences, asymptomatic shedding, and sexual transmission are likely
- Episodic therapy can shorten the duration of recurrent episodes
- Important to inform current/future partners before sexual relationship
- Daily Valacyclovir effective in reducing transmission of HSV-2
- Highest rate of transmission occurs with active lesions or during prodrome, but the virus can be transmitted in an asymptomatic state
- Seek treatment at the first sign of infection to decrease viral shedding
- Always use latex condoms due to subclinical infections
- Abstain from any sexual activity during outbreaks, either oral or genital

Herpetic and any ulcerative lesions may increase HIV transmission, offer HIV testing. HSV can be transmitted perinatally to the infant, risk is highest if acquired during later in pregnancy, outbreaks are treated during pregnancy; suppression starts at 36 weeks gestation; symptoms/signs or prodrome in labor necessitates Cesarean delivery.

HUMAN IMMUNODEFICIENCY VIRUS (HIV) (see Chapter 23, "HIV")

HUMAN PAPILLOMAVIRUS (see Chapter 11, "Condyloma Acuminatum")

Neisseria gonorrhoeae

- Among females, the highest rates are in adolescents and young adults ≤24 years of age
- Up to 80% of infections in females are asymptomatic
- If present in a pediatric patient, infection is secondary to sexual abuse, and patient must be treated and referred for a sexual abuse evaluation (see Chapter 46, "Sexual Abuse")
- Can be vertically transmitted during childbirth

Presentation

- Can be symptomatic or asymptomatic
- May have mucopurulent vaginal discharge, irregular vaginal bleeding, vaginal pruritus, pelvic pain
- Friable and edematous cervix may be seen on exam

Diagnosis

- NAAT (preferred) from vaginal, endocervical, or first catch urine sample
  - Vaginal swabs may be self-collected if the patient prefers. Sensitivity and specificity for diagnosis is the same compared to specimens collected by a clinician
  - Culture if NAAT unavailable
- May need to do a culture on rectal, oropharyngeal, or conjunctival samples as not all NAAT are FDA approved for those sites
- Must obtain culture if concerned for treatment failure to obtain antibiotic sensitivities

Management

- Children ≤45 kg
  - Ceftriaxone 25–50 mg/kg, not to exceed 250mg IM, IV, or IM
- Children >45 kg and >8 years of age can be treated as adults
  - Ceftriaxone 500 mg IM as a single dose if weight <150 kg
  - Ceftriaxone 1 g IM as a single dose if weight ≥150 kg
- If Cephalosporin allergy
  - Gentamicin 240 mg IM **AND** Azithromycin 2 mg orally in a single dose
- If unable to give Ceftriaxone
  - Cefixime 800 mg orally in a single dose
    NOTE: If chlamydia infection **has not been excluded**, should treat with Doxycycline 100 mg orally BID for 7 days. During pregnancy, Azithromycin 1 g, as single a dose is recommended
- Abstain from sexual intercourse for 7 days after treatment completed AND until partner is treated
- If state law allows, should provide prescription or additional medication dose to the patient so that she may give to her partner (EPT)
- Most recent sexual partner should be referred for treatment as should any partner within prior 60 days
- Infected adolescents should be screened for reinfection 3 months after treatment
- If gonorrhea is present, should test for HIV, chlamydia, and syphilis
- Educate patient that short of abstinence, condom use for anal, vaginal, and oral sex is the most effective way to prevent disease

Pelvic Inflammatory Disease (PID) (see Chapter 37, "PID")

Syphilis

- Syphilis facilitates transmission of HIV
- Many adolescents may have had undetected chancres and unaware of infectivity
- Screening is important in those with multiple partners, history of gonorrhea, chlamydia

Presentation

- Divided into three stages of active disease and two stages of latent disease
- Stage 1: Primary syphilis
  - Non-tender ulcer or chancre with a raised border at site of inoculation within 3 weeks of exposure
  - Often undetected as it is non-tender
  - Resolves spontaneously in 3–6 weeks
- Stage 2: Secondary syphilis
  - Occurs within weeks to months in 25% of untreated patients
  - Symptoms include malaise, fever, headache, adenopathy, and condyloma lata
  - Maculopapular rash involves palms/soles
    Latent syphilis: Positive serology but no clinical manifestations
  - *Early latent*: Infection acquired within the preceding year
    - Need evidence of one of the following within that time frame:
      - Sexual debut
      - Documented seroconversion or at least fourfold increase in titer
      - History of primary or secondary syphilis symptoms
      - History of the sexual partner with infection
  - *Late latent*: Infection acquired >1 year prior, or for an unknown duration
    - Patients with late latent syphilis cannot transmit infection
- Stage 3: Tertiary syphilis
  - Final stage that takes years to develop
  - Occurs in 25–40% if left untreated
  - Characterized by neurologic, cardiovascular, and skeletal abnormalities
  - Neurosyphilis can occur at any stage of infection. Symptoms may include cranial nerve dysfunction, meningitis, stroke, and hearing loss
  - Spirochetes can cross the placenta and cause congenital syphilis

Diagnosis

- Serologic tests – Need 1 nontreponemal and 1 treponemal
  - Can perform either test type first
  - If first test is positive, perform the second test to confirm the diagnosis
  - If first is negative, stop
  - May take 2–4 weeks for test to become positive
- Nontreponemal tests, reported as a titer of antibody
  - Venereal Disease Research Laboratory (VDRL)
  - Rapid plasma reagin (RPR)
- Treponemal tests, reported as reactive or nonreactive
  - Fluorescent treponemal antibody absorption (FTA-ABS)
  - *T. pallidum* particle agglutination assay (TPPA)
  - *T. pallidum* enzyme immunoassay (TP-EIA)
- Need CSF studies to diagnose neurosyphilis

Management

- Penicillin G is preferred treatment. Dosage and length of treatment depends on stage and clinical signs
- Late latent and tertiary stages require a longer duration

- Infants and young children diagnosed with syphilis need evaluation to determine if it is acquired or congenital. For complete evaluation and treatment guidelines consult with CDC

Primary and secondary syphilis
- Children and Adolescents
  - Benzathine penicillin G 50,000 units/kg IM in a single dose, up to the adult dose of 2.4 million units

If penicillin allergy
- Doxycycline 100 mg orally BID for 14 days
  OR
- Tetracycline 500 mg orally QID for 14 days

Latent syphilis
- Early latent
- Same treatment as for primary and secondary syphilis, as above
- Late latent
- Children and Adolescents
  - Benzathine penicillin G 50,000 units/kg IM, up to the adult dose of 2.4 million units, administered weekly for 3 weeks.
- For penicillin allergy, use the same dosing as for primary and secondary syphilis, but a total treatment course of 28 days

Tertiary syphilis (no CNS involvement)
- Benzathine penicillin 2.4 million units IM administered weekly for 3 weeks.

Follow-Up

Primary and secondary syphilis
- Re-examine clinically and with serology at 6 and 12 months post treatment
- Compare titers. A fourfold decrease in titer (change in 2 dilutions) is required to demonstrate an acceptable response to therapy
- Persistent symptoms and at least fourfold increase in nontreponemal titer persisting >2 weeks is failed treatment or reinfection
  - If need to retreat – Benzathine penicillin G 2.4 million units IM once weekly × 3 doses
- Test for HIV
- If titers do not decrease fourfold, may be treatment failure, though this is unclear
  - Need additional clinical and serologic follow-up
  - If additional follow-up is not possible, should retreat – Benzathine penicillin G 2.4 million units IM once weekly × 3 doses
  - Evaluate CSF
  - Check HIV status

Latent syphilis
- Repeat nontreponemal test at 6, 12, and 24 months
- Need CSF exam to evaluate for neurosyphilis if one of the following is present
  - Sustained at least fourfold increase in titer
  - Initial high titer (≥1:32) does not decline at least fourfold after 12–24 months of therapy
  - Signs or symptoms of syphilis develop
- If CSF exam is negative, should retreat

Management of sexual contacts

- Primary, secondary, early latent
  - Treat those exposed within 90 days presumptively
  - For those exposed >90 days prior, treat on serology or presumptively if follow-up is uncertain
- Late latent
  - Evaluate partners clinically/serologically
- All patients with syphilis should be tested for HIV, gonorrhea, chlamydia, trichomonas

Trichomonas (see Chapter 60, "Vulvovaginitis")

Tubo-Ovarian Abscess (see Chapter 52, "Tubal Mass," and Chapter 37, "Pelvic Inflammatory Disease)

For a summary of treatment recommendations, see Table 48.3.

TABLE 48.3

Common Infections and First-Line Treatments

Infection	Treatment
Chlamydia	Children ≤45 kg: Erythromycin 50 mg/kg/day (max 2 g/day) PO divided into 4 doses for 14 days
	NOTE: Data are limited on the effectiveness and optimal dose of azithromycin for the treatment of children <45 kg)
	Children >45 kg and <8 years of age Azithromycin 1 g PO in a single dose
	Children >45 kg and >8 yo and adolescents: Doxycycline 100 mg PO BID for 7 days is the first choice; alternative Azithromycin 1 g orally in a single dose
Gonorrhea (uncomplicated vulvovaginitis, urethritis, pharyngitis, proctitis)	Children ≤45 kg: Ceftriaxone 25–50 mg IM/IV in single dose, not to exceed 250 mg IM
	Children >45kg and >8 years of age can be treated as adults:
	<150 kg: Ceftriaxone 500 mg IM in single dose
	≥150 kg: Ceftriaxone 1 g IM in single dose
	NOTE: If chlamydia infection has not been excluded, treat with Doxycycline 100 mg PO BID ×7 days
Herpes (first clinical episode)	<12 years: Oral Acyclovir 40–80 mg/kg/day divided TID or QID for 7–10 days; maximum daily dose: 1,200 mg
	≥12 years: Oral: Acyclovir 400 mg TID for 7–10 days; treatment can be extended beyond 10 days if healing is not complete
	NOTE: Other medications available, see text
Herpes (recurrent)	<12 years: Oral Acyclovir 20 mg/kg/dose TID for 5 days; maximum dose: 400 mg
	≥12 years: Oral Acyclovir : 800 mg BID for 5 days *or* 800 mg TID for 2 days
	Other medications available, see text
Herpes (suppressive)	<12 years: Oral Acyclovir 20 mg/kg/dose BID; maximum dose: 400 mg
	≥12 years: Oral Acyclovir 400 mg PO BID
	Other medications available, see text
Trichomoniasis	<45 kg: Metronidazole 45 mg/kg/day PO TID for 7 days; maximum dose: 2000 mg
	≥45 kg: Metronidazole 500 mg PO BID for 7 days
Syphilis (primary, secondary)	Children: Benzathine penicillin G 50,000 units/kg IM in a single dose, up to an adult dose of 2.4 million units
	Adolescents: Benzathine penicillin G 2.4 million units IM in a single dose

BIBLIOGRAPHY

American Sexual Health Association. https://www.ashasexualhealth.org/

Centers for Disease Control and Prevention. Sexually transmitted infections treatment guidelines, 2021. MMWR. July 23, 2021; 70(4) and https://www.cdc.gov/std/treatment-guidelines/STI-Guidelines-2021.pdf

Guttmacher Institute. https://www.guttmacher.org/state-policy/explore/overview-minors-consent-law#

Heston S, et al. Syphilis in children. Infect Dis Clin N Am. 2018; 32: 129–144.

Killebrew M, Garofalo R. Talking to teens about sex, sexuality, and sexually transmitted infections. Pediatr Ann. 2002; 31:566–572.

Lexicomp: Acyclovir (systemic): Drug information. UpToDate. Retrieved December 5, 2021, Available from https://www.uptodate.com/contents/acyclovir-systemic-drug-information

Lexicomp: Famciclovir: Drug information. UpToDate. Retrieved December 5, 2021, Available from https://www.uptodate.com/contents/famciclovir-drug-information

Lexicomp: Penicillin G benthazine (long-acting intramuscular): Drug information. UpToDate. Retrieved December 5, 2021, Available from https://www.uptodate.com/contents/penicillin-g-benzathine-long-acting-intramuscular-drug-information

Lexicomp: Valacyclovir: Drug information. UpToDate. Retrieved December 5, 2021, Available from https://www.uptodate.com/contents/valacyclovir-drug-information

49

Substance Abuse

Christine Osborne and Sarah K. McQuillan

Key Points

- Substance use by adolescents has an enormous impact on their health and well-being
- Impairs healthy growth and development, is associated with risky behaviors such as unprotected sex and dangerous driving, and contributes to the development of many other health problems
- Alcohol, marijuana, and tobacco are still the most widely used substances by children and adolescents before grade 12
  - 68% have tried alcohol, with more than half being drunk at least once, and 90% reporting binge-drinking behavior
  - 45% have reported using marijuana
  - 41% have tried cigarettes
- Daily use of marijuana has been steadily increasing among adolescents and since 2015 has even surpassed daily cigarette use in this population
- There has also been a recent dramatic increase in vaping by adolescents
- Opioids have now become the most used illicit drug after marijuana
- The earlier teens start using substances, the greater their chances of continuing to use substances and developing substance use problems later in life

Risk Factors

Family Factors

- Family history of substance use, dependence, or both
- Dysfunctional parenting style
- Extreme permissiveness or authoritarianism
- Conflicted families

Problem Behaviors

- Antisocial behavior
- Negative affect, low adaptability, and impulsivity
- Aggressiveness
- Early sexual experience
- Attention deficit disorder (ADD)

DOI: 10.1201/9781003039235-49

School Factors

- Early school failure
- Incomplete homework and truancy
- Lack of commitment to education
- Association with substance using peers
- Early onset of substance use
- History of sexual abuse

Community Factors

- Ready availability of alcohol and other drugs
- Tolerance for the use of alcohol or illegal drugs
- Overpopulated, disorganized, and deteriorating neighborhoods

Protective Factors

Parental Support

- Close communication with parents
- Positive parental support
- Lack of substances in the household

High Self-Esteem

- Assertiveness, social competence, school success, regular church attendance, and a strong sense of right and wrong

Interventions

Pediatric care providers tend to underestimate the prevalence of adolescent substance use. Discussing substance use should be done, preferably with a validated tool, with all patients to ensure that no one falls through the cracks. In the advent of COVID and reduction in in-person visits, the ability to determine confidentiality can be more challenging in a virtual appointment. Ensuring confidentiality before embarking on motivational interviews is paramount.

Motivational Interviewing

- Open-ended questions
  - "How does drinking on the weekends affect getting your homework done?"
- Reflective listening
  - "It sounds like you are very upset about the recent break-up with your girlfriend. I wonder whether you are more likely to drink when you are upset?"
- Affirmations
  - "Deciding not to go that party sounds like a good choice. It may have been difficult to avoid drinking if you went."
- Summary statements
  - "It is important to be able to hang out with your friends. Are there other activities you do with that group?"

- Eliciting change talk
    - "What are some of the things you would like to change?"

SBIRT

Recommended by the American Federal Substance Abuse and Mental Health Services Administration (SAMHSA) as part of all routine health care.

- S: Screening (using a validated tool, see below)
- BI: Brief intervention
    - For adolescents who do not use substances
        - Support and reinforce this decision and other related healthy behaviors
    - For adolescents who report infrequent use
        - Focus on encouraging them to change their behavior to support their health
        - Clear advice to stop using
        - Brief information on the negative effects of using
        - Discussion of a plan to stop using
        - Recognition and encouragement of other strengths and positive behaviors
- RT: Referral to Treatment
    - For adolescents who report frequent, or high-risk use
        - Multidisciplinary treatment group
        - Range from motivational interviewing, individual, group, or family counseling to intensive outpatient, hospital, or residential treatment
        - Adolescent medicine and/or psychiatry should be involved

Screening Tests

CRAFFT test

- Screening test for alcohol and other drug abuse with questions developmentally appropriate for teenagers
- A score of ≥2 indicates risk. A score of ≥4 should raise suspicion of substance dependence
    - C: Have you ever found yourself in a CAR driven by someone (including yourself) who was "high" or had been using alcohol or drugs?
    - R: Do you ever use alcohol or drugs to RELAX, feel better about yourself, fit in?
    - A: Do you ever use alcohol or drugs while you are by yourself, ALONE?
    - F: Do you ever FORGET things you did while using alcohol or drugs?
    - F: Do your FAMILY or FRIENDS ever tell you that you should cut down on your drinking or drug use?
    - T: Have you ever gotten into TROUBLE while you were using alcohol or drugs?

Marijuana screening

- The American Academy of Pediatrics endorses asking each patient at each health maintenance, specialty, and urgent care visit
    - "In the past year, how many times did you use marijuana" and providing structured response categories (never, once or twice, monthly, weekly or more)
- Can obtain a reliable indicator of the level of risk for a mild, moderate, or severe marijuana use disorder

SUBSTANCES

Alcohol

- Alcohol is the substance most commonly used by teens.
- Adolescent drinking patterns tend to be episodic and heavy.
  - More than 90% of alcohol consumed by teens is in the context of a binge drinking – Having five or more drinks in a row on one or more occasions in the prior 2 weeks
  - It is important that teens know what quantifies as binge drinking, consider signage in offices
- Alcoholism should be suspected in young people who
  - Are often intoxicated or experience withdrawal symptoms from chronic or recurrent alcohol use
  - Tolerate large quantities of alcohol
  - Attempt unsuccessfully to cut down or stop alcohol use
  - Experience blackouts attributable to drinking; or those who continue drinking despite adverse social, educational, occupational, physical, or psychological consequences or alcohol-related injuries
- Programs using a harm reduction philosophy have successfully lowered risky alcohol use.

Health Consequences

- Early and heavy alcohol use in adolescence impairs memory function by damaging the developing hippocampus
- Adolescents who drink heavily are more likely to have
  - Poorer school performance
  - Be involved in motor vehicle accidents, fights, and unintentional injuries than their peers
  - Risky sexual behaviors that could result in early pregnancies, STIs, etc.
- Alcohol use in pregnancy can result in fetal alcohol syndrome and other behavior effects
  - There is no safe level of alcohol use during pregnancy

Tobacco

- Cigarette smoking is the leading cause of preventable disease and mortality in the United States.
- Smoking is usually initiated in adolescence.
  - The age of smoking debut for 90% of people is between the ages of 11–16
  - Initiation associated with: Low socioeconomic status, low level of parent education
- Those who smoke ten or more cigarettes a day may benefit from nicotine replacement therapy and/or bupropion hydrochloride in conjunction with behavioral techniques, but data is limited in adolescents.

Health Consequences

- Nicotine produces structural and chemical changes in the brain that increase the risk of future alcohol and other drug addiction, panic attacks, and depression
- Thromboembolic events with estrogen-containing contraceptives
- Pregnancy-associated risks, i.e. ectopic pregnancy, low birth weight infants
- Future risk of lung diseases and cancers

Vaping

- While rates of tobacco use have fallen dramatically since the 1990s, electronic cigarettes have become increasingly popular among adolescents
- Vape devices (electronic cigarettes/e-cigs) are handheld devices designed to deliver liquefied nicotine (and sometimes marijuana) as well as flavoring chemicals via vapor instead of smoke
- Reasons for increase uptake include
  - Small sleek shape and
  - Ability to use the device surreptitiously (some look like a USB flash drive)
  - Flavors such as cotton candy and bubble gum

Health Consequences

- Adolescents associate little risk of harm with vaping.
- Because e-cigarettes have only been marketed for ~10 years and because the products are rapidly changing, scientific data are limited and will continue to emerge.
- Toxicants and carcinogens have been found in e-cigarette solutions and emissions.
- Both fine and ultrafine particulate matter can be inhaled into the lungs and enter the systemic circulation.
  - Can cause vaping-associated lung injury, which includes "abnormalities on chest imaging"
  - Other specific lung diseases associated include
    - Acute eosinophilic pneumonia
    - Diffuse alveolar damage
    - Organizing pneumonia
    - Lipoid pneumonia
- Studies support that nicotine dependence affects the areas of the brain that control executive function, memory, and mood.
- The lithium batteries used in many e-cigarette devices can explode, and the explosions have resulted in severe burns and fires.

Marijuana

- Tetrahydrocannabinol (THC) and cannabidiol (CBD) are the two most common cannabinoids.
  - THC has psychoactive properties and can induce a sensation of euphoria and significantly alter perception, alertness, coordination, mood, and energy.
  - CBD is devoid of psychoactive properties.
- An increasing group of people using this drug daily is adolescent girls.

Health Consequences

- Cannabis use during adolescence is associated with a permanent reduction in intellectual capacities, motivation, and lifetime achievement.
- Associated with a 2–5× increase in odds of developing chronic mental health disorders such as depression, anxiety, and schizophrenia later in life.
  - This may be due to the disruption in endogenous dopamine secretion and changes in gray matter, triggering lack of motivation and mental health symptoms.

- Although marijuana is considered less addictive than other psychoactive substances such as nicotine, cocaine, or heroin, it remains highly addictive.
  - Users often develop symptoms of withdrawal, which include
    - Irritability
    - Sleep difficulties
    - Loss of appetite
    - Nausea
    - Abdominal pain
    - Usually starting within 1 or 2 days after last use and can extend to 4–8 weeks

Marijuana use and Gynecological Conditions

Pain Conditions

- Some studies have suggested that cannabinoids could be a promising treatment for pelvic pain associated with endometriosis, and dysmenorrhea.
  - Interactions of the endocannabinoid system, which may decrease inflammation, neuropathic, and nociceptive pain.
  - Evidence remains insufficient to support the effectiveness of the use of cannabinoids for pain conditions in children and adolescents.

Menstrual Management

- Regular use of marijuana can disrupt the hypothalamic release of gonadotropin-releasing hormone, leading to a reduced production of estrogen and progesterone and a subsequent increase in the frequency of anovulatory cycles.
- Cannabinoids and oral contraceptives are both metabolized in the liver by cytochrome p450 (CYP) enzymes.
  - No evidence for decreased effectiveness of the oral contraceptive pill with concurrent marijuana use.
  - Can impact other medications such as certain anti-inflammatory agents, such as Naprosyn, as well as several antidepressant and antipsychotic medications.

STIs, Pregnancy

- Marijuana use during adolescence has been shown to be an independent risk factor for sexually transmitted infections.
- There are increased rates of unplanned pregnancies in young women who use marijuana.
- The use of marijuana during pregnancy and lactation is not recommended.
  - Can lead to low birth weight, hypertensive disorders of pregnancy, spontaneous preterm birth, and offspring cognitive and behavioral problems.

Opioids

The nonmedical use of prescription (Rx) opioids by adolescents now surpasses the use of all other illicit substances except marijuana; more than 10% of high school seniors reported the use of Rx opioids for nonmedical purposes.

Health Consequences

- Adolescents who develop opioid addiction are at high risk of associated complications including transition to injection drug use and fatal overdose.

- Compared with their non-using counterparts, these adolescents are almost 4× as likely to report sexual intercourse in the past 3 months.

Management

- Treatment of substance abuse should only be undertaken by a provider experienced in the nuances of mental health diseases and with special licensing.
- It is not recommended to attempt treatment with methadone or buprenorphine in the general PAG clinic.
- If you are suspicious of opioid abuse, also consider referral for naloxone.

A brief list of other substances increasing in abuse by adolescents

- Ecstasy (MDMA, Molly)
- Gamma-hydroxybutyrate (GHB, liquid X, g-juice)
- Rohypnol (roofies, forget pill)
- Ketamine (Special K, Vitamin K, Kit Kat)
  - Can lead to hallucinations, permanent memory loss, thought difficulty, and mood changes
- Inhalants (volatile hydrocarbons like toluene, gasoline, solvents, glue, spray paint)
  - Cause seizures, hypoxemia, and arrhythmias
- Heroin
- LSD, PCP
  - Can lead to violence, injuries
- Methamphetamine (crystal meth, ice, or crank)
  - Causes violence, hallucinations, and memory loss

RESOURCES

The best local resources are parents. Encourage parents to be role models for kids.

- https://www.cdc.gov/ncbddd/fasd/features/teen-substance-use.html#first-ref
- https://pcssnow.org/

BIBLIOGRAPHY

Center for Disease Control and Prevention. Substance use screening and implementation guide: no amount of substance use is safe for adolescents. *Subst Abuse.* 2020. https://www.aap.org/en-us/Documents/substance_use_screening_implementation.pdf. Substance Use Screening and Implementation Guide.

Chadi N, Levy S. What every pediatric gynecologist should know about marijuana use in adolescents. *J Pediatr Adolesc Gynecol.* 2019; 32(4):349–353.

Kelpin SS, Rusteikas SG, Karjane NW, Svikis DS. Screening for at-risk alcohol and drug use in the antenatal period: how do young women compare with older adult women? *J Pediatr Adolesc Gynecol.* 2019; 32(3):325–329.

Levy SJL, Williams JF. Substance use screening, brief intervention, and referral to treatment. *Pediatrics.* 2016; 138: el–el5.

SAMHSA-HRSA Center for Integrated Health Solutions. SBIRT: *Screening, Brief Intervention, and Referral to Treatment Opportunities for Implementation and Points for Consideration.* SAMHSA-HRSA Center for Integrated Health Solutions 2021.

50

Toxic Shock Syndrome (TSS)

Patricia Amorado and Kathryn Stambough

Definition

An illness characterized by high fever, sunburn-like rash, desquamation, hypotension, and abnormalities in multiple organ systems typically from a Gram-positive infection.

Key Points

- Classically associated with tampon use due to vaginal colonization with *Staphylococcus aureus* and production of toxic shock syndrome (TSS) toxin-1
- Sources of non-menstrual TSS include surgical wound colonization, burns, nasal packing, post-influenza pneumonia, postpartum infections, insulin pump infusion sites, or an unidentifiable source. Other gynecologic sources include diaphragm and contraceptive sponge use
- Most common bacteria is *Staph aureus*, which can be associated with *Streptococcus pyogenes*
- MRSA has been frequently reported
- Menstrual-associated TSS has decreased since FDA issued standardized absorbency labeling of tampons and encouraged users to employ the lowest absorbency tampon compatible for their flow

Presentation/Diagnosis (CDC Criteria)

- Fever: Temperature greater than or equal to 102°F (38.9°C)
- Rash: Diffuse macular erythroderma (typically spreads from trunk to extremities)
- Desquamation: 1–2 Weeks after rash onset
- Hypotension: Systolic blood pressure less than or equal to 90 mmHg in adults or less than 5%ile by age for children less than 16 years
- Multisystem involvement (must involve three or more organ systems)
  - Gastrointestinal: Vomiting or diarrhea at onset of illness
  - Muscular: Severe myalgia or elevation of creatine phosphokinase (CPK) at least 2× the upper limit of normal
  - Renal: Blood urea nitrogen (BUN) or creatinine elevation at least 2× the upper limit of normal with pyuria in the absence of urinary tract infection
  - Hepatic: Total bilirubin, ALT, or AST elevation at least 2× the upper limit of normal
  - Hematologic: Platelets less than 100,000/mm^3
  - CNS: Disorientation or alterations in consciousness without focal neurologic signs when fever and hypotension are absent

Laboratory Criteria for Diagnosis

TSS by S. pyogenes has positive blood cultures in up to 90% of cases and is identified more in immuno-compromised patients.

- Negative results on the following tests, if obtained
  - Cerebrospinal fluid cultures
  - Serologies for Rocky Mountain spotted fever, leptospirosis, or measles

Probable Diagnosis

- Meets the laboratory criteria and in which four of the five clinical criteria described above are present

Confirmed Diagnosis

- Meets the laboratory criteria and in which all five of the clinical criteria described above are present, including desquamation, unless the patient dies before desquamation occurs

Management

The seven R's of management

1. Recognition
2. Resuscitation
3. Removal of the source of infection
4. Rational choice of antibiotics
5. Role of adjunctive treatment
6. Review progress
7. Reduce the risk of secondary cases in close contacts and reinfection of patient

It is imperative to recognize the most common signs of TSS early, especially if there are known sources of infection, and begin treatment immediately.

- Hospitalize patient and immediately perform basic resuscitation efforts including IV fluid resuscitation and hemodynamic support
- Remove the source of infection (tampon, wound debridement, etc.) as soon as possible as the disease spreads quickly
- Order appropriate laboratory tests: Complete blood count, complete metabolic panel, coagulation tests, CPK level, blood cultures, cultures from any suspected source of infection (blood, rectum, vagina, oropharynx, nares, urine)
- Send Gram stain of vaginal swab
- Send vaginal swab for PCR TSST-1 testing
- Order serology for Rocky Mountain spotted fever, leptospirosis, measles (must return negative for TSS diagnosis)
- Begin rational choice of empiric antibiotic therapy that includes antistaphylococcal antibiotics
  - Oxacillin and third-generation cephalosporin
  - If suspecting MRSA, need vancomycin

- Consider the role of adjuvant therapy
  - Clindamycin, but must be used with other antibiotics
  - Although some studies utilize intravenous immunoglobulin (IVIG), benefits remain controversial
- Review progress including the need to tailor therapy to culture results. Intravenous antibiotics should be continued until clinical improvement and usually for at least 7 days before transitioning to oral antibiotics
- Reduce the risk of recurrence
  - Recurrence rate as high as 30%
  - Consider prophylaxis for close contacts with risk factors (e.g. mother-baby where one has known disease) which can include penicillin V, rifampicin, OR cephalexin
  - Avoidance of superabsorbent tampons
    - Tampon absorbency should match the volume of the current menstrual flow
    - Tampons should be changed every 4–6 hours and not be used overnight
    - In individuals with a history of TSS, tampon use should be avoided for at least 6 months
    - The presence of TSST-1 antibodies may be protective

BIBLIOGRAPHY

Burnham JP, Kollef MH. Understanding toxic shock syndrome. Intensive Care Med. 2015; 41:1701–1710.

CDC guidelines, https://wwwn.cdc.gov/nndss/conditions/toxic-shock-syndrome-other-than-streptococcal/case-definition/2011/

Curtis N. Toxic shock syndrome; under-recognised and undertreatment? Arch Dis Child. 2014; 99(12):1062–1064.

Patel BN, Hoefgen HR, Nour N, Merritt DF (2020). Chapter 16: Genital Trauma. In Emans SJ, Laufer MR, DiVasta AD, eds., *Pediatric & Adolescent Gynecology* (7th ed.). Wolters Kluwer.

Wilkins AL, Steer AC, Smeesters PR, Curtis N. Toxic shock syndrome—the seven Rs of management and treatment. J Infect. 2017; 74(S1):S147–S152.

51

Transgender and Gender Diverse Care

Frances Grimstad

Definitions

- The term "transgender" indicates a person who holds a gender identity that does not match that which they were assigned at birth, which is typically designated by secondary sex characteristics.
- By contrast, a "cisgender" person's identity and expression align with that which was assigned to them at birth.
- *Gender incongruence* is persistent incongruence between gender identity and anatomic sex characteristics from birth, with the absence of a confounding mental health condition.
- *Gender dysphoria* is discomfort that may arise in some individuals from the incongruence between their gender identity and anatomic sex characteristics from birth.

Key Points

- Approximately 0.6% of the US population identifies as transgender or gender diverse (TGD).
- TGD communities also encompass those who do not identify as a binary gender (e.g. male or female) but rather use terms like "nonbinary" and "genderqueer" to describe an experience of gender that transcends traditional normative gender experiences.
- Due to the stigma and trauma imposed upon them by the medical community, most TGD people are not "out" to their providers, which ultimately impairs the quality of care that they receive.
- It is important to offer medical care in a gender- and sexuality-neutral way, so that patients feel safe to disclose sensitive information and have their comprehensive medical needs met.
- A significant component of gender-affirming medical care is using the correct terminology and knowing how to apply it appropriately.
- In TGD youth, affirming identities improves mental health outcomes and quality of life.

Evaluation

Create a welcoming clinical setting

- Intake paperwork should capture a patient's chosen name, appropriate pronouns, and sexual orientation
- Electronic medical records should also reflect the above so that all staff will use the correct name and pronouns for each patient
- Patients should be surveyed repeatedly over time, as these indicators can change. For example, "I am Dr. X and I use she/her pronouns. How do you like to be addressed?"
  - Doing this for every patient at every visit normalizes the process and avoids singling out TGD patients

DOI: 10.1201/9781003039235-51

History

Past Medical History

- Social gender affirmation: How the patient chooses to present themselves in terms of dress, mannerisms, and social interactions to relay gender identity and for how long
- History of puberty-blocking therapies
- Use of gender-affirming hormones therapies (GAT) such as exogenous estradiol, testosterone, or antiandrogens
- History of hirsutism, virilization, or other intersex traits

Surgical History

- Especially of any gender-affirming surgeries such as hysterectomy, top surgery, or bottom surgery

Reproductive History

- For those who have uterus/ovaries
  - Age at menarche; menstrual pattern prior to puberty blockers, gender-affirming hormone therapy
  - Any bleeding while on blockers or gender-affirming hormone therapy
- For those who have penis/testes
  - Age at pubarche
- Desire for future fertility or family building or desire to undergo fertility preservation

Sexual History

- Sexual preferences
- Sexual activity
  - Use anatomy-driven, open-ended questions to elicit the most comprehensive information
    - "What body parts do you come in contact with during sex?"
    - "What body parts do you touch when you are intimate with someone?"

Physical Examination

- Check height, weight, blood pressure
- Utilize terms that patients use for their anatomy throughout the exam
- Genital exam is not required
  - For those with pelvic complaints, ensure exam is offered in a safe gender-affirming fashion. Offer noninvasive techniques (external exam only, self-swabs, abdominopelvic ultrasound) first and allow the patient to participate in the exam.

Management

- Counsel every patient on risks, benefits, and expected outcomes, including timing, prior to treatment
- If you do not provide puberty-blocking or gender-affirming hormone therapy, make the appropriate referral to a pediatric specialist with expertise in this area

Puberty Blocking Therapy

Criteria for initiation (as per the World Professional Association for Transgender Health Standards of Care Version 7)

- A qualified mental health provider (MHP) has confirmed that adolescent has long lasting and intense gender nonconformity or dysphoria that worsened with the onset of puberty without any coexisting psychological/medical/social problems that could interfere with treatment; and that the adolescent has the capacity to give informed consent to treatment.
- The adolescent has been informed of the effects and side effects of treatment and has given informed consent/parent or guardian has consented and supporting.
- The medical provider agrees with an indication for treatment, has confirmed that puberty has started (Tanner stage 2), and has confirmed there are no medical contraindications to treatment.

Typical therapy

- Leuprolide: 3.75 mg IM monthly or 11.25 mg IM every 3 months
- Histrelin implant: 50 mg subcutaneous implant every 15–18 months
    - Superior suppression of endogenous testosterone
- Progestins have also been used in high doses in those assigned male at birth

If a patient is not able to use puberty blockers, may offer menstrual suppression agents for those assigned female at birth

- Transmasculine patients typically will prefer non-estradiol methods
- Counsel that no method is perfect, but some are better than others at menstrual suppression
- Consider need for pregnancy prevention when choosing a method

Follow-up

- Every 3 months: Height, weight, Tanner stage, blood pressure
- Every 6–12 months: LH, FSH, estradiol, testosterone, vitamin D
- Every 1–2 years: CMP, lipids, glucose, Hgb A1C, DEXA, bone age as indicated per baseline health of youth

Gender-Affirming Hormone Therapies (GAT)

Offered to patients only by medical professionals who have expertise in the medical treatment of TGD youth.
   Criteria for initiation (as per the Endocrine Society and WPATH Standards of Care Version 7)

- Qualified MHP has confirmed the persistence of gender dysphoria without coexisting psychological, medical, or social problems that could interfere with treatment, and the adolescent has sufficient mental capacity to estimate consequences and weigh benefits/risks of planned treatment and give consent.
- The adolescent has been informed of the effects and side effects of treatment and has given informed consent/parent or guardian has given informed consent.
- The medical provider agrees with an indication for treatment and has confirmed no medical contraindications.
- Typically initiated at age 16 (with parental consent in countries where 18 is the age of majority).
    - Can be considered in younger patients on a case-by-case basis, never prior to the onset of natural puberty
    - Little evidence to support use in those younger than 13.5

Testosterone Pubertal Induction

- For induction in those on concomitant/following puberty-blocking therapy
  - Testosterone esters 25 mg/m^2 IM/SQ every 2 weeks (half if weekly, double if every 4 weeks)
  - Escalate dose every 6 months
  - Target dose for adult 100–200 mg every 2 weeks
- For postpubertal youth, doses can be increased more rapidly
  - 75 mg IM/SQ every 2 weeks for 6 months
  - Then 125 mg every 2 weeks
  - See Table 51.1 for additional treatment regiments
- Follow-up
  - Every 3 months: Height, weight, Tanner stage, BP
  - Every 6–12 months: LH, FSH, testosterone, CBC, lipids, vitamin D
  - Every 1–2 years: DEXA, bone age (until age 25–30 or peak bone mass achieved)
- Risks associated with treatment
  - Very high risk of erythrocytosis (hematocrit >50%)
  - Moderate risk of severe liver dysfunction, coronary artery disease, cerebrovascular disease, hypertension, breast, or uterine cancer
- Masculinizing effects
  - Skin oiliness/acne, fat redistribution, cessation of menses, clitoral enlargement, and vaginal atrophy within first 1–6 months
  - Facial/body hair growth, scalp hair loss, increased muscle mass and strength, and deepening of voice in 6–12 months
  - Max effects reached in 4–5 years

TABLE 51.1

Testosterone Dosing for Those >16 Years Old and Have Already Undergone Endogenous Puberty

Medication	Low Dose Start	Standard Start	Mid	Max
IM/SQ testosterone cypionate/ethanate	20 mg q week[a]	50 mg q week	75 mg q week	100 mg q week
Testosterone patch	1–2 mg q PM	4 mg/patch q PM	6 mg/patch q PM	8 mg/patch q PM
Testosterone 1% gel	12.5–25 mg q AM[b]	50 mg q AM	75 mg qAM	100 mg q day
Testosterone 5% cream	10 mg	50 mg	75 mg	100 mg
Testosterone pellets[c]	X	X	10 (75 mg each) pellets	

Adjust dose every 2–3 months to achieve desired changes and/or bring midrange testosterone to 400–700 ng/dl.

[a] Can do q2 week dosing.

[b] To minimize contact transfer, it should be placed and left to dry for a minimum of 2 hours and washed at a later time if there is a plan for close skin-skin contact.

[c] Newer formulation, dosing recommendations may evolve. Usually only started once someone is stable on testosterone (range of pellets used 6–12).

Estrogen Pubertal Induction

- After puberty-blocking treatment
  - Oral 17 β-estradiol 5 μg/kg/day and increasing the dose every 6 months
    - Can consider 10/15/20 μg/kg/day
    - Adult dose 2–6 mg/day
  - Transdermal 17 β-estradiol 6.25–12.5 μg/day
    - Can consider 25/37.5 μg/day
    - Adult dose 50–200 μg/day

- For postpubertal youth, the dose can be increased more rapidly
  - Oral 17 β-estradiol 1–2 mg/day and increased every 6 months
  - See Table 51.2 for additional treatment regiments
- Follow-up
  - Every 3 months: Height, weight, Tanner stage, BP
  - Every 6–12 months: LH, FSH, estradiol, total testosterone, vitamin D
  - Every 1–2 years: DEXA, bone age (until age 25–30 or peak bone mass achieved); prolactin, A1C, lipids as needed
- Risks associated with treatment
  - Very high risk of thromboembolic disease
  - Moderate risk of macroprolactinoma, breast cancer, coronary artery disease, cerebrovascular disease, cholelithiasis, hypertriglyceridemia
- Feminizing effects
  - Decreased sexual desire/spontaneous erections in the first month
  - Redistribution of body fat, decrease in muscle mass and strength, softening of the skin, breast growth, and decreased testicular volume in next 3–6 months
  - Decreased sperm production and sexual dysfunction are variable
  - No voice changes
  - Max effects in 2–3 years

TABLE 51.2

Estrogen/Antiandrogen/Progesterone Dosing for Those >16 Years Old and Have Already Undergone Endogenous Puberty

Type	Medication	Low Dose Start	Standard Start	Mid	Max
Estrogen	17-beta Estradiol oral/ sublingual	1 mg/day	2 mg/day	4 mg/day*	8 mg/day
	Estradiol patch	50 μg	100 μg	200 μg	400 μg
	Estradiol valarate intramuscular**	5 mg IM every week	10 mg IM every week	15 mg IM every week	20 mg IM every week
	Estradiol cypionate**	0.5 mg IM every week	1 mg IM every week	1.5–2 mg IM every week	2.5 mg IM every week
Antiandrogens	Spironolactone	X	50 mg/day	100 mg/day	200 mg/day
	Finasteride	X	5 mg/day	X	X
	Dutasteride	X	0.5 mg/day	X	X
	GnRH analogs	See Puberty Blocker section for dosing			
Progesterone	Provera	X	2.5 mg/day	5 mg/day	10 mg/day
	Micronized progesterone	X	100 mg/qHS	150 mg/qHS	200 mg/qHS

Adjust dose every 2–3 months to achieve desired changes and/or bring testosterone to <55 ng/dl.

* When dosing >2 mg recommend to split dosing twice a day.

** Can be combined and dosed every 2 weeks.

Gender-Affirming Surgeries

- Should be offered by qualified surgeons who are specifically trained to perform these procedures
- Criteria for inclusion for sterilizing procedures (genital affirmation surgeries)
- Persistent, well-documented gender dysphoria
- Legal age of majority
- Typically recommend continuous GAT for >12 months (however this may depend on the surgeon, the patient, and the surgery)

- Has successfully and continuously lived in new gender full time >12 months
- Any significant medical or mental health concerns are well controlled
- Has demonstrated knowledge of all practical aspects of surgery
- Has demonstrated competence and knowledge of the permanent nature of the procedure and has already pursued fertility preservation if desired

Transmasculine procedures include

- Hysterectomy (ovary sparing preferable if patient consents)
- Metoidioplasty or phalloplasty ("bottom surgery")

Transfeminine procedures include

- Vaginoplasty ("bottom surgery")

Criteria for inclusion for all other surgeries

- Persistent, well-documented gender dysphoria
- Typically done after the legal age of majority but may be done earlier with parental consent. Chest surgeries have been shown to have an improvement in well being in adolescents.
- Typically recommend continuous GAT for >12 months (however this may depend on the surgeon, the patient, and the surgery)
- Has successfully and continuously lived in new gender full time >12 months (however this may depend on the surgeon, the patient, and the surgery)
- Any significant medical or mental health concerns are well controlled
- Has demonstrated knowledge of all practical aspects of surgery

Transmasculine procedures include

- Mastectomy ("Top surgery")

Transfeminine procedures include

- Breast augmentation ("top surgery")
- Facial feminization surgery
- Thyroid chondroplasty

Reproductive Health Concerns

Fertility

- Should be discussed prior to initiation of gender-affirming hormones or surgeries
- All standard of care options for fertility preservation should be discussed and offered
  - Sperm banking, oocyte or embryo cryopreservation
  - Ovarian and testicular tissue cryopreservation
    - Under research protocols at this time
    - Only option for those planning puberty blockers followed by GAT
- If GAT has been initiated
  - Most data shows ovarian function is preserved on testosterone
    - Testosterone is discontinued prior to attempted oocyte retrieval
    - Persons can discontinue testosterone and carry a pregnancy

- Data shows estrogen can decrease fertility even after discontinuance. However, persons have successfully discontinued estrogen and produced sperm
  - As such cryopreservation before hormones is recommended

Breakthrough Bleeding on Testosterone

- Can be due to standard causes of abnormal uterine bleeding (See Chapter 1, "Abnormal Uterine Bleeding").
- Also can be due to breakthrough bleeding as seen on other menstrual suppression hormones.
- Ensure testosterone dose is within the cisgender male range
  - Consider increasing dose for menstrual suppression if determined safe
  - Verify no skipped/missed doses
- All forms of progestins, estrogens, and estrogen/progestin combinations that are used for menstrual suppression can be used to induce menstrual suppression in persons on testosterone.
  - GnRHa and danazol can also be used concomitantly with testosterone.

Contraception

- Testosterone is not an FDA-approved form of contraception for those with uterus/ovaries
  - All forms of contraception can be offered to persons on testosterone (see Chapter 12, "Contraception")
  - Clinicians should strongly consider LARC methods, including intrauterine devices, for all patients who need highly effective contraception
- Estrogen is not an FDA-approved form of contraception for those with testes

Post Vaginoplasty Care

- Patients who have undergone penile inversion vaginoplasty require ongoing vaginoplasty dilation. Similar complications to other vaginoplasties can arise including nonhealing granulation tissue, webbing, strictures, and fistulas
- The neovagina has no endogenous hormonally responsive cleansing
  - Discharge less likely to be infectious more likely to be retained sebum, lubrication, desquamating cells
  - Regular douching is may be helpful

BIBLIOGRAPHY

Grimstad F, Boskey ER, Taghinia A, Ganor O. Gender-affirming surgeries in transgender and gender diverse adolescent and young adults: a pediatric and adolescent gynecology primer. J Pediatr Adolesc Gynecol. 2021; 34(4):442–448. https://pubmed.ncbi.nlm.nih.gov/33852937/

Guidelines for the primary and gender-affirming care of transgender and gender nonbinary people. UCSF Transgender Care Program. 2016. https://transcare.ucsf.edu/guidelines

Hembree WC, Cohen-Kettenis PT, Gooren L, et al. Endocrine treatment of gender-dysphoric/gender-incongruent persons: an endocrine society clinic practice guideline. J Clin Endocrinol Metab. 2017;102(11):3869–3903.

52

Tubal Mass

Swetha Naroji

Key Points

- Tubal masses in premenarchal patients are most likely torsion
- Paratubal cysts are hormonally sensitive, strongly associated with PCOS
- IV antibiotics are an effective first-line treatment for tubo-ovarian abscesses (TOA)
- Consider medical management for ectopic pregnancy if not contraindicated

Types

Premenarchal tubal masses: Rare

- If simple: Cyst likely
- If complex: Likely torsion (see Chapter 36, "Ovarian/Adnexal Torsion")

Postmenarchal tubal masses

- Simple: Paratubal cyst (correlates with puberty)
- Complex: Torsion (see Chapter 36, "Ovarian/Adnexal Torsion"), Hydrosalpinx, Tubo-ovarian Abscess (TOA), Ectopic pregnancy

Diagnosis

History

- Reproductive-puberty onset, menarcheal status, sexual activity, menstrual irregularities
- History of hirsutism/acne
- Symptoms of pain, onset, and duration
- Prior history of masses noted on imaging

Physical Exam

- Height, weight
- Skin – Hirsutism
- Abdomen – Pain, masses

Imaging/Labs

- Premenarchal
  - Abdominal pelvic ultrasound

DOI: 10.1201/9781003039235-52

- Postmenarchal
  - Abdominal pelvic sonogram (transvaginal if sexually active – not necessary)
  - If sexually active → pregnancy test, sexually transmitted infection testing, pelvic exam
  - If positive pregnancy test → presumes ectopic pregnancy

Management

Simple cysts

- Serial ultrasound if asymptomatic until size >5 cm
- Laparoscopic cystectomy for large >5 cm or persistent cysts
- Rule out/treat PCOS

Tubal torsion (see Chapter 36, "Ovarian/Adnexal Torsion")

- Laparoscopic approach with conservation of tube preferred
- Perform cystectomy at diagnosis if indicated

Hydrosalpinx

- May be associated with torsion or pelvic inflammatory disease (PID)
- Does not require drainage or other treatment unless found as part of an infertility workup
  - Refer to Reproductive Endocrinology/Infertility, consider salpingectomy to improve assisted reproductive treatment (ART) outcomes

TOA

- Recommend inpatient management for at least 24–72 hours
- STI testing
  - Often associated with preceding PID (gonorrhea and chlamydia rarely isolated from abscess fluid)
  - May be spontaneous resulting from infection with upper genital tract organisms
- IV antibiotics as for pelvic inflammatory disease (see Chapter 37, "Pelvic Inflammatory Disease")
- If the patient does not clinically improve with IV antibiotics, or the mass is >7 cm, consider surgical drainage via laparoscopy
  - If available locally, interventional radiology may be able to drain, alleviating symptoms and identifying pathogens to inform medical management
- If still poorly responding despite adequate surgical and medical management, consult Infectious Disease for further recommendations

Ectopic pregnancy

- Should be highly suspected in any sexually active adolescent with a positive pregnancy test
- Diagnosis
  - Visualization of complex mass in adnexa with gestational sac or embryo with heartbeat
  - Serum hCG rising abnormally on serial evaluations q48 hours without evidence of intrauterine pregnancy
- Management
  - Surgical
    - Emergent surgical treatment in the hemodynamically unstable patient
    - Laparoscopic salpingectomy is preferred to salpingostomy if severe tubal damage

TABLE 52.1

Contraindications to Medical Management of Tubal Ectopic Pregnancies

Absolute Contraindications	Relative Contraindications
Intrauterine pregnancy or breastfeeding	Cardiac activity detected in ectopic pregnancy
Moderate-severe anemia, leukopenia, thrombocytopenia	High initial quantitative β HCG (>5000 mIU/mL)
Active pulmonary or peptic ulcer disease	>4 cm in size
Hepatic or renal dysfunction	Refusal to accept blood transfusion
Ruptured ectopic pregnancy	
Hemodynamically unstable	
Cannot follow up with providers	

- Medical (methotrexate)
  - If hemodynamically stable, unruptured, and without contraindications (see Table 52.1)
  - Patient must consent to immediate management and close outpatient follow-up
  - Additional lab tests prior to treatment: CBC, blood type, Rh status, AST/ALT, creatinine, quantitative β hCG
  - Rho (D) immune globulin (RhoGAM) is given if Rh negative (300 g IM)
  - Single-dose, two-dose, and fixed multiple-dose regimens available with close follow-up (see Table 52.2)
  - **If a patient presents with pelvic/abdominal pain during the course of treatment, assess clinically and check by ultrasound and CBC. If concern for rupture, surgical therapy**

TABLE 52.2

Methotrexate Regimens for Tubal Ectopic Pregnancies (Height and Weight in cm and kg then calculate Body Surface Area as m^2)

Single-dose:

1. Give one dose MTX (50 mg/m^2) IM on day 1
2. Measure β HCG on days 4 and 7
   a. Decrease >15%, β HCG weekly until nonpregnant level
   b. Decrease <15%, second MTX dose (50 mg/m^2) IM and start from step 1.
   c. If <15% after two doses, β HCG level increases or plateaus, consider surgery

Two doses:

1. Give first-dose MTX (50 mg/m^2) IM on day 1
2. Give second-dose MTX (50 mg/m^2) IM on day 4
3. Measure β HCG on days 4 and 7
   a. Decrease >15% → β HCG weekly until nonpregnant level
   b. Decrease <15% → third MTX dose (50 mg/m^2) IM on day 7, check β HCG on day 11
      i. Decrease >15% → β HCG weekly until nonpregnant level
      ii. Decrease <15% → fourth MTX dose (50 mg/m^2) IM on day 11, check β HCG on day 14
         A. Decrease >15% → β HCG weekly until nonpregnant level
         B. Decrease <15% → fourth MTX dose (50 mg/m^2) IM on day 11, check β HCG on day 14
4. If <15% after four doses, β HCG level increases or plateaus, consider surgery

Fixed multiple-dose:

1. Give MTX (1 mg/kg) IM on days 1, 3, 5, 7, give folinic acid (0.1 mg/kg) IM on days 2, 4, 6, 8
2. Measure β HCG on MTX days
   a. If decrease >15% → stop MTX and folinic acid, β HCG weekly until nonpregnant level
   b. If decrease <15% → continue regimen
3. If <15% after four doses, β HCG level increases or plateaus, consider surgery

BIBLIOGRAPHY

Rossi BV, Ference EH, Zurakowski D, Scholz S, Feins NR, Chow JS, Laufer MR. The clinical presentation and surgical management of adnexal torsion in the pediatric and adolescent population. J Pediatr Adolesc Gynecol. 2012 Apr;25(2):109–113. Doi: 10.1016/j.jpag.2011.10.006. Epub 2011 Dec 28. PMID: 22206683.

Tubal ectopic pregnancy: correction. ACOG Practice Bulletin No. 193. American College of Obstetricians and Gynecologists. Obstet Gynecol. 2019;133(5):1059. Erratum for: Obstet Gynecol. 2018;131(3):e91–e103.

53

Turner Syndrome (TS)

Ashli Lawson and Julie Strickland

Definition

A syndrome characterized by physical findings (such as short stature, signs of gonadal dysgenesis, cardiac defects, and psychosocial impairment) and complete or partial monosomy X with or without mosaicism.

Key Points

- Most common cause of primary amenorrhea in the United States
- Consider in any female with short stature and primary amenorrhea/delayed puberty
- Often accompanied by numerous comorbidities, such as cardiac defects, hearing loss, renal anomalies, and mental health disease along with gonadal failure, so a multidisciplinary approach is recommended
- Pregnancy contraindicated in patients with aortic root dilation >40–45 mm
- In patients with the presence of Y chromosome, gonadectomy is indicated due to risk of progression to gonadoblastoma and dysgerminoma

Diagnosis

Strong suspicion in

- Any female patient with
  - Unexplained growth failure or short stature
  - Pubertal delay
- Newborns with
  - Lymphedema of hands/feet
  - Thickened nuchal fold
  - Cardiac anomalies: Coarctation of the aorta, left-sided defects, hypoplastic left heart
  - Brachycephaly
  - Low hairline
  - Low-set ears
  - Micrognathia
  - Renal anomalies
- Children with
  - Short stature with declining growth velocity (<10 percentile for age)
  - Elevated follicle stimulating-hormone (FSH) level

DOI: 10.1201/9781003039235-53

- Any of the following physical characteristics
  - Any stigmata mentioned above in the newborn
  - Cubitus valgus
  - Nail hypoplasia
  - Hyperconvex uplifted nails
  - Multiple pigmented nevi
  - Characteristic facies
  - Short 4th metacarpal
  - High-arched palate
- Adolescents with
  - Absence of breast development by age 13
  - Pubertal arrest
  - Primary or secondary amenorrhea with elevated FSH
  - Unexplained short stature

Evaluation

Physical Exam

- Height, weight, blood pressure
- Head and Neck: general appearance of ears, eye lids, neck, and hearing
- Breast: Tanner stage, shield chest, wide-spaced nipples
- Cardiac: Evaluate for arrhythmia or murmurs
- GU: Tanner stage, presence/absence of the vagina

Laboratory Evaluation

- Workup for primary amenorrhea (see Chapter 4, "Amenorrhea")

Peripheral blood karyotype

- If peripheral karyotype normal and still suspect TS, assess karyotype of the additional tissue site (e.g. skin)
- If karyotype results in TS + Y component, gonadectomy is recommended due to increased risk of gonadoblastoma and dysgerminoma

Management

Multidisciplinary approach to treatment includes

- Cardiac
  - Congenital heart defect in 30% (most commonly bicuspid aortic valve and coarctation of the aorta)
  - Hypertension is also common even in absence of cardiac anomaly
    - Physical exam with yearly blood pressure checks
    - Echocardiogram (even if normal antenatal echocardiogram)
      - If malformation present, needs cardiology referral
      - If no malformation, repeat evaluation at age 12–15 years to evaluate the aortic root

- Renal
  - Congenital renal malformation present in 30% (most commonly rotational and duplicated collecting system)
    - Renal ultrasound needed
- ENT
  - Auditory: Congenital outer ear malformation in 30–50% (low set); 50–90% will develop sensorineural hearing loss
    - Hearing assessment every 10 years if no sensorineural deficit or every 3–5 years if present)
  - Speech: Often have speech and language difficulties
    - Consult speech therapist
  - Vision: Strabismus, amblyopia, and ptosis are common
    - Ophthalmology exam recommended
  - Dental: Retrognathic mandible
    - Orthodontic exam by age 8–10 years due to consequences of the retrognathic mandible
- Endocrine
  - Thyroid dysfunction: 10–30% develop primary hypothyroidism
    - TSH/Free T4 should be checked at diagnosis and every 1–2 years
  - Short stature: Consultation with endocrinology
    - Measure height and weight and use TS-specific growth curves
    - Growth hormone may be prescribed by an endocrinologist until the acceptable height is achieved or bone age is about 14
  - Metabolism: Predisposed to obesity
    - Counsel on healthy lifestyle habits
    - Glucose intolerance: Increased risk of diabetes over a lifetime, but rare in childhood
      - No need for childhood screening
- Gynecology
  - Puberty
    - 90% will have a primary ovarian insufficiency
    - 30% will undergo spontaneous pubertal development
    - 2–5% will have spontaneous menses (with pregnancy potential)
      - Individualize estrogen use depending on presentation, growth, and goal
      - Transdermal estrogen should be started at the latest by age 15
        - Initiate at 1/6th of the adult dose (0.0125 mg, cut patch in half)
        - Increase every 3–6 months depending on breast and height growth
      - Add progestin around 12–24 months or with the first bleed
        - Cyclic medroxyprogesterone acetate 10 mg daily for 10 days or micronized progesterone 100 mg daily; can consider progestin IUD (see Chapter 40, "POI")
      - Combined oral contraceptive pills are neither used for pubertal induction nor as to the standard for hormone replacement
        - 35 mcg or more of estradiol pills in individual circumstances have been used for hormone replacement
      - If the patient does not have a gonadal failure, continue the annual assessment
  - Reproduction
    - STI prevention counseling on all patients

- – If menstruating and no signs of gonadal failure
  - – Discuss contraception as well as desires for fertility preservation and pregnancy planning
- – If with gonadal insufficiency and desiring pregnancy
  - – Discuss in conjunction with REI, MFM, and other specialists the risks and benefits of IVF or cryopreserved ovarian tissue (experimental, see Chapter 18, "Fertility Preservation") and oocytes
  - – Pregnancy is contraindicated in patients with aortic root dilation >40–45 mm due to the risk of aortic dissection and death
- – In patients who have XY mosaicism
  - – Gonadectomy is required due to the risk of progression to gonadoblastoma and dysgerminoma
  - – Timing should be individualized
- • Psychosocial
  - • Social, behavioral, and educational deficits have been noted
    - – Higher levels of anxiety, adjustment problems related to immaturity, poor social cognition, and visual-spatial deficits
    - – NO increase in mental retardation
    - – Estrogen therapy may mitigate deficiencies, but studies are inconclusive

BIBLIOGRAPHY

Dabrowski, E, et al. Turner syndrome with Y chromosome: spontaneous thelarche, menarche, and risk of malignancy. J Pediatr Adolesc Gynecol. 2020; 33(1):10–14.

Klein, KO, Phillips SA. Review of hormone replacement therapy in girls and adolescents with hypogonadism. J Pediatr Adolesc Gynecol. 2019; 32(5):460–468.

Saenger, P. Recommendations for the diagnosis and management of Turner syndrome. J Clin Endocrinol Metab. 2001; 86(7):3061–3069.

54

Urinary Tract Infection (UTI)

Shashwati Pradhan

Definition

- Infection of any part of the urinary system including urethra, bladder, ureters, and kidneys with infections involving the lower urinary tract (bladder and urethra) being the most common

Key Points

- Common occurrence in young children with 8% of girls having at least one urinary tract infection (UTI) by 7 years of age
- *E. coli* is the most common bacterial pathogen, accounting for 85–90% of all cases
- Consider UTI as a source of infection in any infant or child between ages 2 months and 2 years presenting with fever and no other identifiable source
- Both positive urinalysis and significant bacteriuria are necessary to diagnose a UTI

Diagnosis

- History
  - *Signs and symptoms*: Dysuria, hematuria, frequency/urgency, enuresis, fever, abdominal pain nausea/vomiting
    - *Internal dysuria/abdominal pain*: More likely to be UTI
    - *External dysuria/splash dysuria*: Consider genital exam as the vulvar cause may be more likely
  - *Previous UTI history*: Culture proven or empirically treated
  - History of constipation or bowel dysfunction, anatomic and functional urinary tract abnormalities, and spinal cord disorders
  - *Older patients consider sexual history*: STI testing and symptoms in partner
- Physical examination
  - *Vital signs*: Fever, tachycardia
  - *Abdomen*: Look for constipation, palpable bladder, costovertebral tenderness
  - *Back*: Stigmata of spina bifida, sacral dimpling, sacral agenesis
  - *Vulva*: Assess for
    - External lesions that could result in pain with urination (e.g. herpes, vulvitis)
    - Anatomic conditions that would cause urine trapping (e.g. Labial adhesions, cloacal malformations)

- Lab evaluation
  - Urinalysis/urine culture
    - While urine culture is the gold standard, it takes at least 18 hours to detect bacterial growth and 48–72 hours for antibiotic sensitivities – therefore, rely on clinical suspicion and result of urine dipstick
    - *Toilet-trained children*: Obtain a clean voided midstream urine sample
    - *Infants and small children*: Catheterized urine sample
      - Positive urinalysis
        - Nitrites are helpful only if positive (not good marker for UTI in children)
        - Leukocyte esterase (false positives common)
        - Positive for nitrite, leukocyte esterase, and microscopic examination for WBCs and bacteria
      - Positive culture:
        - *Clean catch*: >5 × 10⁵ CFU/mL
        - *Catheter sample*: >10⁴ CFU/mL
    - If sexually active, urine or endocervical testing for gonorrhea and chlamydia

Management

Treatment

- No difference in efficacy between parenteral and oral antibiotics
  - Parenteral management may be required for children too ill or unable to tolerate oral intake
  - Switch parenteral to an oral medication when clinical improvement is noted
- Antibiotics should be given with consideration for culture sensitivities, prior urine cultures, and local epidemiology
- For patients >2 months of age with uncomplicated UTI
  - First-generation cephalosporin (e.g. Cephalexin 50–100 mg/kg per day by mouth BID or trimethoprim-sulfamethoxazole 8–10 mg trimethoprim/kg in 2–4 equally divided doses)
  - provided local resistance to *E. coli* to this treatment is not >15%
- Duration of treatment
  - *Lower UTI*: 3–5 days in patients >age 3; 10 days in patients <age 3
  - *Upper UTI*: 7–14 days

Recurrence

- 80% of school-age girls have repeat UTI in 6 months

Instruct about improved voiding habits

- Place patient on voiding schedule, with voiding 3–5× per day
- Urinate with legs apart to prevent reflux of urine into vagina
- Avoid bubble baths or irritants to the perineum
- Wipe front to back after bowel movements
- If sexually active, instruct to void after intercourse

Special Considerations

- All children with a history of febrile UTI > 2 years of age should undergo renal and bladder ultrasound
  - It is a minimally invasive technique with easy identification of hydronephrosis, hydroureters, bladder wall abnormalities, and acute complications of UTI (renal or perirenal abscess)
- Inpatient with atypical or recurrent UTI or pyelonephritis a voiding cystourethrogram (VCUG) is recommended
  - VCUG is the gold standard for diagnosis and grading of vesicourethral reflux
  - *If VCUG positive*: Nuclear renal scanning with technetium-labeled dimercaptosuccinic acid (DMSA) scan is recommended 4–6 months after UTI

BIBLIOGRAPHY

American Academy of Pediatrics. (2018). Tables of Antibacterial Drug Dosages. In Kimberlin DW, Brady MT, Jackson MA, Long SS, eds., *Red Book; 2018 Report of the Committee of Infectious Diseases* (31st ed., p. 914). Itasca, IL: American Academy of Pediatrics.

Korbel L, Howell M, Spencer JD. The clinical diagnosis and management of urinary tract infections in children and adolescents. Paediatr Int Child Health. 2017; 37(4):273–279.

Okarska-Napierla, M, Wasilewska A, Kuchar E. Urinary tract infection in children: diagnosis, treatment, imaging – comparison of current guidelines. J Pediatr Urol. 2017; 13(6):567–573.

Pool NM, Kronman MP, Rutman L, et al. Improving antibiotic prescribing for children with urinary tract infection in emergency and urgent care settings. Ped Emer Care. 2010; 36(6):e332–e339.

55

Uterine Anomalies and Masses

Swetha Naroji

Key Points

- Common uterine pathology in adults (fibroids, adenomyosis, polyps, endometrial hyperplasia) is rare in adolescents
- Treatment aims at controlling symptoms until definitive surgery can be completed, if needed
- Pelvic US and MRI best imaging modalities; CT is not useful in most cases
- Consider Müllerian abnormalities when uterine tissue appears abnormal in adolescent

Normal Uterine Ultrasound Findings

Prepubertal

- Length 2–4.5 cm
- Minimal endometrium
- Fundus = Cervix size

Postpubertal

- Length 5–8 cm
- Prominent endometrium >4 mm
- Fundus > Cervix size

Evaluation

History

- Reproductive-menstrual status, cycle duration/frequency, cramping or pain in relation to cycle, flow intermenstrual bleeding
- Abdominal pain
- Signs or symptoms of hyperandrogenism
- Sexual activity

Physical Exam

- Abdominal examination
- Consider pelvic exam if sexually active
- Consider rectal exam in nonsexually active patients

DOI: 10.1201/9781003039235-55

Imaging

- Pelvic sonography (abdominal, consider transvaginal if sexually active)
- MRI if complex pelvic anatomy noted
- If Müllerian abnormality is noted, consider imaging for skeletal or renal abnormalities

Labs

- Pregnancy test

Management

Fibroids (leiomyomas)

- Rare in teenagers, generally asymptomatic, no treatment needed
- If symptomatic
    - May have pelvic pain/pressure, associated heavy periods
    - Medical/surgical guidelines for adolescents do not exist
        - Goal of management is the preservation of fertility/management of symptoms
        - Medical management
            - Combined hormonal therapy
            - Selective progesterone receptor modulators
            - Aromatase inhibitors
        - Surgical management
            - Myomectomy when symptoms are not controlled by other methods, or when causing cervical obstruction

Adenomyosis

- Rare in teenagers, definitive treatment is hysterectomy, so difficult to treat
- May present as heavy periods, severe dysmenorrhea, with a positive family history of adenomyosis/endometriosis
- Consider continuous oral contraceptives, hormonal IUD, or GnRH agonists followed by continuous OCPs if symptomatic
- Accessory cavitated uterine masses (ACUM) is more common than adenomyosis
    - It is a cystic form of adenomyosis
    - Presents with progressive dysmenorrhea unresponsive to medical management
    - Diagnose with MRI
        - Can be confused with noncommunicated uterine horn but appears more cystic
        - Cyst fluid high signal intensity on T1-weighted images
        - Cyst wall/uterine wall with low signal intensity on T2-weighted images

Polyps

- Rare in teenagers, presents with persistent bleeding
- May appear as thickened endometrium on the US
- If symptomatic, consider hysteroscopic polypectomy

Endometrial hyperplasia

- Rare in teenagers, associated with unopposed estrogenic state especially in patients with PCOS
- Presents with breakthrough bleeding despite hormonal management
- Requires endometrial biopsy or D&C for diagnosis
- Treatment involves progestins and continued monitoring until childbearing is completed
- Consider GYN oncology consultation

Müllerian papillomas

- Rare lesions that present as polypoid masses arising from the uterus/cervix on vaginoscopy for a workup of persistent bleeding
- Benign
- Definitive diagnosis based on biopsy
- Definitive management is with complete excision

Müllerian anomalies (See Pfeifer et al. 2021 for information on classification)

- Associated with other abnormalities – skeletal and renal – perform spine and renal imaging
- Bicornuate uterus
  - No complications in adolescence
  - Counsel may have increased risk of
    - miscarriage/spontaneous abortion
    - intrauterine growth restriction
    - preterm delivery
    - fetal malpresentation, i.e. breech
  - If have poor pregnancy outcomes, such as late trimester loss thought to be due to uterine anomaly, seek specialist care
  - Maternal Fetal Medicine
  - Relative contraindication for IUD
  - No treatment is needed
- Unicornuate uterus
  - Contraindication for IUD
  - May have increased dysmenorrhea, treat with other available options (see Chapter 14, "Dysmenorrhea")
  - Pregnancy counseling regarding increased miscarriage, preterm delivery, and fetal malposition
  - If associated rudimentary uterine horn, perform hemi-hysterectomy on the affected side only
    - Diagnose using MRI or hysteroscopy (only one tubal os noted)
- Uterine didelphys
  - Contraindication for IUD
  - Pregnancy counseling regarding potential of implantation in one or both horns, increased risk of miscarriage, preterm delivery, and fetal malposition
  - Generally associated with two cervices, will need Pap test from each cervix
  - Rule out other anomalies such as OHVIRA (obstructed hemivagina ipsilateral renal agenesis) that may need surgical correction
- Rudimentary uterine horn
  - If horn contains endometrium, can cause cyclical pain and retrograde menstruation
  - MRI is best imaging modality

- • Can attempt continuous hormonal suppression menstrual suppression until the patient is ready for definitive excision
- • Resection can be completed laparoscopically or via laparotomy
- • If associated with a non-rudimentary uterus that is not damaged during resection, the patient can attempt labor and a vaginal birth
- • If the horn is communicating, counsel regarding the potential for pregnancy in horn and risk of uterine rupture
- • Diethylstilbestrol (DES) abnormalities
  - • Secondary to in utero exposure (last known exposure in the United States in the early 1980s)
  - • T-shaped appearance of the endometrial cavity with constricting bands, hypoplasia, and synechiae
  - • Also can include cervical anomalies
    - – Fibrous ridges
    - – Hoods – Circular fold that partially covers the cervix
    - – Cock's comb – An irregular peak on the anterior border
    - – Hypoplasia
    - – Pseudopolyp
- • **Tumors**
  - • Tumors are incredibly rare in this population, and if present most likely malignant
    - – Adenosarcoma – Rare
      - – Large polypoid and can fill endometrial cavity/be intramural or both
      - – MRI imaging is helpful to plan management
      - – Surgical resection primary treatment total hysterectomy with bilateral salpingo-oophorectomy
  - • Embryonal rhabdomyosarcoma
    - – Atypical to be uterine primary, however on imaging may appear uterine
    - – May present as abnormal bleeding especially in prepubertal girls
    - – Associated with DICER 1 mutation
    - – Sensitive to chemotherapy, recommend organ sparing surgery when possible

BIBLIOGRAPHY

Breech LB, Laufer MR (2019). Chapter 35 Uterine and Cervical Masses. In Emans SJ, Laufer MR, DiVasta AD (eds), *Emans, Laufer, Goldstein's Pediatric and Adolescent Gynecology* (7th ed., pp 548–555). Philadelphia, PA: Wolters Kluwer.

Dietrich JE, Millar DM, Quint EH. Non-obstructive müllerian anomalies. J Pediatr Adolesc Gynecol. 2014 Dec;27(6):386–395. Doi: 10.1016/j.jpag.2014.07.001. Epub 2014 Jul 17. PMID: 25438707.

Itam SP 2nd, Ayensu-Coker L, Sanchez J, Zurawin RK, Dietrich JE. Adenomyosis in the adolescent population: a case report and review of the literature. J Pediatr Adolesc Gynecol. 2009 Oct;22(5):e146–e147. Doi: 10.1016/j.jpag.2009.01.067. Epub 2009 Jul 8. PMID: 19589704.

Pfeifer SM, Attaran M, Goldstein J, Lindheim SR, Petrozza JC, Rackow BW, Siegelman E, Troiano R, Winter T, Zuckerman A, Ramaiah SD. ASRM Mullerian anomalies classification 2021. Fertil Steril 2021 Nov;116 (5):1238–1251. https://doi.org/10/1016/j.fertnstert.2021.09.025

56

Uterovaginal/Müllerian Agenesis (Mayer-Rokitansky-Küster-Hauser Syndrome (MRKH))

Christine M. Pennesi, Yuan Yuan (Jackie) Gong, and Melina L. Dendrinos

Key Points

- Congenital absence or underdevelopment of uterus and upper vagina due to paramesonephric duct failure
- Uncommon condition (1 in 4,000–5,000 females)
- May be difficult to distinguish from imperforate hymen or transverse vaginal septum—be diligent to make the correct diagnosis (careful exam and imaging)
- Evaluate for associated anomalies
- Interdisciplinary support (involving psychology or social work/sexual health counselor) is important throughout the care

Differential Diagnosis

- Androgen insensitivity
- Low transverse vaginal septum
- Distal vaginal atresia
- Imperforate hymen

Presentation

- Primary amenorrhea (+/− cyclic abdominal pain), typically as a teenager
- Incidental finding on well-child examination or imaging

Diagnosis

History

- Typically present at age 15–18 years with primary amenorrhea
- Note timing of pubertal development
  - Age-appropriate onset of breast and pubic hair development
- History of other congenital anomalies (skeletal, renal, cardiac, auditory)
- Assess for symptoms of cyclic abdominal pain

DOI: 10.1201/9781003039235-56

Physical Examination

- Assess breast and pubic hair development (usually Tanner stages 4 and 5 at presentation)
- Visually inspect external genitalia (typical female external genitalia and presence of hymenal fringe with shallow vaginal indentation)
- Assess vaginal length with a lubricated cotton swab or single-digit exam
- Consider rectal exam if no prior pelvic imaging (palpable cervix/uterus excludes the diagnosis of MRKH)
- Avoid laparoscopy for purpose of diagnosis
- Evaluate for extragenital malformations (MURCS—**M**üllerian duct aplasia, **R**enal agenesis/ectopia, **C**ervicothoracic **S**omite dysplasia)

Labs

- FSH, testosterone (normal female)
- Karyotype (46, XX; no causative genetic mutations identified to date)

Imaging

- Pelvic ultrasound gold standard
- Consider pelvic MRI
  - If pelvic pain is present, to assess for the presence of Müllerian remnants with endometrium
  - When ultrasound equivocal and/or to assess spine and kidneys
- Renal ultrasound (if kidneys not yet assessed)
- Spine X-ray
- Consider echocardiography, audiometry, etc., based on history

---

Treatment

Creation of Neovagina

- For purpose of penetrative sex
- Timing of treatment is decided by the individual patient and should not be influenced by others, studies suggest after age 16 or in select younger patients
- Extensive counseling regarding advantages and disadvantages of each method is critical
- Options
  - Dilation
    - First line in all cases, most effective treatment of all options
    - Successful in more than 90% with the support of the team (gynecologist, sexual health counselor, pelvic floor physical therapist) in creating a functional vagina without post-procedure complications found with surgical neovagina creation
    - Thorough examination to evaluate for hymenal anomalies (i.e. septa) is important, as these can cause pain with dilation
    - Usually self-dilation, but a coital dilation is an option
    - Resulting vagina has normal sensation and lubrication for sexual function
    - Suggested dilation schedule
      - Initial appointment with a provider to teach on proper dilation technique (see Figure 56.1) using a mirror to show anatomic landmarks to the patient so she understands where her clitoris, urethra, vagina, and anus are located exactly

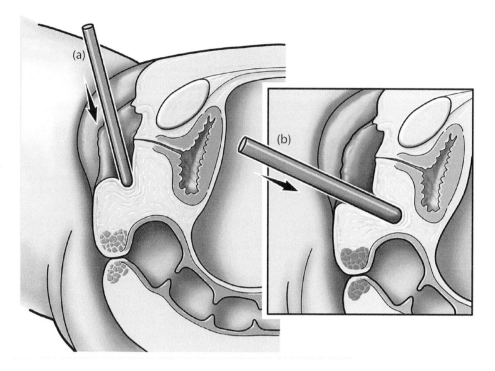

FIGURE 56.1   Vaginal dilation: (a) sagittal view of complete Müllerian agenesis, with vaginal dilator introduced into the vaginal dimple at a 45° angle. In this way, accidental dilation of the urethra can be avoided. (b) After initial insertion, the dilator is then dropped to a nearly horizontal angle, and gentle inward pressure is applied. (From Dwiggins M, Gomez-Lobo Congenital anomalies of the reproductive tract, in Sanfilippo JS, Lara-Torre E, Gomez-Lobo V, eds, Sanfilippo's Textbook of Pediatric and Adolescent Gynecology Second Edition. CRC Press, Boca Raton, 2020, with permission.)

- – Using dilators of the smallest size, place on the perineum and apply gentle pressure for 10–15 minutes 3× per day
- – Provide dilator instructions (https://www.seatllechildrens.org/pdf/pe1292.pdf or https://youngwomenshealth.org/2013/10/08/vaginal-dilator-instructions)
- – After 2 weeks, assess for progress and increase in dilator size
- – Continue for 8–12 weeks or until the vaginal length reaches 6 cm or is functional for satisfactory intercourse (may take up to 2 years)
- – Maintain with dilation or intercourse 3× per week to prevent stenosis
- • Surgery
  - – Requires dilation postoperatively for maintenance
  - – Various options
    - – McIndoe: Split-thickness skin graft
    - – Vecchietti: Laparoscopic traction dilation
    - – Davydov: Laparoscopic peritoneal lining pull through
    - – Williams vulvovaginoplasty: perineal vaginal "pouch"
    - – Bowel vaginoplasty: bowel graft
    - – Sheare: McIndoe without a skin graft
  - – Consultation with a surgeon with expertise in previous procedures recommended
  - – Complications are common (up to 15%) and include prolapse, dyspareunia, stenosis, increased discharge (bowel vagina)

Uterine Remnants

- Hysterectomy is recommended for patients with cervical agenesis and evidence of active endometrium
  - Risk of ascending infection from epithelialized endocervical tracts and high morbidity/mortality

Fertility and Family Building

- Ovarian function is normal and options include using oocytes with a gestational surrogate
- Uterine transplant experimental and only provided under a research protocol
- Adoption

Psychosocial

- Patients and their families cope with diagnosis in various ways, and feelings may change over time
- Patients should be offered interdisciplinary support throughout their care (including psychology, social work, sexual health counselor, connection with peer-support groups/mentors with MRKH diagnosis such as Beautiful You MRKH organization, www.beautifulyoumrkh.org)

BIBLIOGRAPHY

Choussein, S., Nasioudis, D., Schizas, D. et al. Müllerian dysgenesis: a critical review of the literature. Arch Gynecol Obstet. 2017;295:1369–1381.

Dwiggins, M., Gomez-Lobo, V. Congenital anomalies of the reproductive tract. In Sanfilippo, J.S., Lara-Torre, E., Gomez-Lobo, V., eds, *Sanfilippo's Textbook of Pediatric and Adolescent Gynecology* (2nd ed.). CRC Press/Taylor & Francis Group 2020, 48–69.

Müllerian agenesis: diagnosis, management, and treatment. ACOG Committee opinion no. 728. American College of Obstetricians and Gynecologists. Obstet Gynecol. 2018;131:e35–e42.

Oelschlager, Anne-Marie Amies, and Katherine Debiec. Vaginal dilator therapy: a guide for providers for assessing readiness and supporting patients through the process successfully. J Pediatr Adolesc Gynecol. 2019;32(4):354–358. Doi:10.1016/j.jpag.2019.05.002

57

Vaginal Bleeding in the Prepubertal Patient

Maggie L. Dwiggins

Key Points

- Differential diagnosis is broad; a targeted history and physical can often elicit etiology
- Must always rule out abuse as a cause
- Use of vaginoscopy is preferred, avoid in-office speculum examination due to discomfort and risk of injury to delicate unestrogenized tissue
- Most common causes in an emergency setting include foreign body and trauma; in an outpatient setting, the most common cause is nonspecific vulvovaginitis (75% of cases)

Differential Diagnosis

- Foreign body: Commonly toilet paper, can include small toys
- Trauma: Accidental (straddle injury), non-accidental (sexual abuse) (see Chapter 19, "Genital Trauma")
- Urethral prolapse: Donut-shaped or polypoid intralabial urethral mass, possibly more common with increased intra-abdominal or pelvic pressure (i.e. obesity, asthma, constipation)
- Vulvovaginal skin conditions: Atopic dermatitis, psoriasis, eczema, lichen sclerosus (see Chapter 59, "Vulvar Disorders"), nonspecific/pathogen-specific vulvovaginitis
- Endocrine dysfunction: Precocious puberty, isolated menarche (see Chapter 44, "Puberty"), hypothyroidism
- Neoplasms: Endodermal sinus tumor, granulosa cell tumor (see Chapter 35, "Ovarian Masses"), rhabdomyosarcoma, benign Müllerian papillomas, hemangiomas, lymphovascular malformations

Diagnosis

History

- Pubertal status: Thelarche/adrenarche
- Onset/duration of symptoms: Continuous, intermittent, once
- Heaviness of bleeding: Just wiping, spotting, passage of clots, pink vs bright red
- Recent or previous injury
- Recent viral illness: Especially of the upper respiratory tract
- Presence of skin findings: Vulvar and extragenital
- Hygiene practices: Independent toileting, bathing, use of lotions or perfumes
- Allergies

DOI: 10.1201/9781003039235-57

- Possibility of ingestion of exogenous hormones
- Family history of bleeding disorders

Physical Exam

- Height/weight
- Thyroid
- Breast: Tanner stage, axillary hair
- Skin: Presence of atopia, other skin conditions, café au lait spots, bruising, petechiae
- Abdomen: Enlargement
- Genital exam (see Chapter 20, "Gynecologic Examination"): Tanner stage, evaluate skin, evaluate for trauma, check for enlargement, palpable mass presence of bleeding/discharge/odor, presence of urethral prolapse
- Consider vaginal lavage: Visualization of bleeding or foreign body
- Rectal: Palpate foreign body or masses

Laboratory

- Tests are individualized based on physical exam findings and suspected diagnosis
  - Thyroid enlargement: Thyroid-stimulating hormone, prolactin
  - Easy bruising or petechia (family history of bleeding disorder): CBC, coagulation panel
  - Evidence of puberty: Hormonal evaluation (see Chapter 44, "Puberty")
  - Vaginal discharge/bleeding: Aerobic/anaerobic culture, testing for Shigella, sexually transmitted infections (STIs) testing as indicated

Imaging

- Tests are individualized based on the suspected diagnosis
  - Pelvic ultrasound with the transabdominal or transperineal approach
  - Pelvic X-ray for radiopaque foreign body
  - MRI and CT are rarely useful except in certain circumstances to evaluate suspected neoplasms

Management

- Foreign body
  - In-office vaginal lavage
    - Warm saline pushed through pediatric Foley catheter, IV tubing, or an other available tubing that has a blunt tip and can attach to a syringe
    - Careful to avoid touching the sensitive hymen
  - Vaginoscopy
    - When lavage is difficult or inconclusive, or if a heavy foreign body is suspected
    - Can be diagnostic and therapeutic
- Trauma (see Chapter 19, "Genital Trauma")
  - MUST rule out non-accidental abuse; history of injury does not match exam
  - *NOTE*: Straddle injuries typically involve the labia/vulva but are rarely penetrating to the vagina
- Urethral prolapse
  - Treat underlying cause if applicable (weight loss, manage cough/constipation)

- Topical estrogen cream 0.01% twice daily × 2–6 weeks
- Hygiene management with twice-daily sitz baths
- Vulvar skin disorders (see Chapter 59, "Vulvar Disorders," for other conditions and treatment)
  - Nonspecific vulvovaginitis
    - No pathogen, avoid treatment with antibiotics or antifungals
    - Counsel regarding hygiene: Wipe front to back, urinate with legs spread wide, daily plain water bath, avoid bubble baths or use of perfumed soaps/lotions
    - Use hypoallergenic emollients such as petroleum jelly, lanolin, or coconut oil to the vulva as needed
  - Specific vulvovaginitis
    - Most common pathogens are respiratory (group *A streptococcus, Streptococcus pyogenes, Haemophilus influenzae*) or enteric (*E. coli*, Prevotella, and Shigella) can be caused by MRSA (methicillin-resistant *Staphylcoccus aureus*) or STIs
    - Obtain cultures as warranted and treat with antibiotics based on results
    - Candida is very rarely isolated from the prepubertal vagina; so avoid treatment with nystatin, unless diaper rash is present
    - Hygiene recommendations same as earlier
- Endocrine
  - Primary hypothyroidism
    - Referral to endocrinology for hormone replacement
  - Precocious puberty/isolated premature menarche (see Chapter 44, "Puberty")
- Neoplasms
  - Benign
    - Müllerian papilloma: Excision and surveillance
  - Malignant
    - Ovarian carcinoma: Endodermal sinus, granulosa cell tumor (see Chapter 35, "Ovarian Masses")
    - Embryonal rhabdomyosarcoma: More common in the first two decades with bimodal distribution before age 2 years and after age 12 years
      - Upper vaginal tract and cervical more common in peripubertal ages
      - Exquisitely chemosensitive: Recommend primary organ sparing resection with neoadjuvant chemotherapy prior to the decision for removal of vital organs such as vagina, cervix, and uterus
      - Multidisciplinary approach recommended, including pediatric surgery, pediatric oncology, pediatric gynecology, and pediatric urology, as indicated
- Lymphovascular (see Chapter 59, "Vulvar Disorders": Hemangioma)

BIBLIOGRAPHY

Dwiggins M, Gomez-Lobo G. Current review of prepubertal vaginal bleeding. Curr Opin Obstet Gynecol. 2017;29(5):322–327.

Sugar N, Graham E. Common gynecologic problems in prepubertal girls. Pediatr Rev. 2006:27(6);213–23

58

Vaginal Tract Anomalies

Katherine Hayes

Key Points

- The genital exam is critical to identifying the type of anomaly and differentiating between patients with an imperforate hymen, labial adhesions/disorders, and those with vaginal tract anomalies.
- Pelvic ultrasound is the initial imaging method recommended for vaginal tract anomalies.
- It may be challenging to diagnose uterovaginal anomalies before puberty because of the small size of the prepubertal uterus, lack of endometrial stimulation, and the lack of distention of the vagina.

Evaluation

History

- Reproductive: pubertal status, presence/absence of menses, irregular periods or intermenstrual spotting, sexual activity, vaginal discharge
- Abdominal: pain, masses, tenderness
- GI: constipation, rectal pressure
- Family: genitourinary anomalies

Physical Exam

- Height, weight
- Presence of secondary sex characteristics
- Abdominal (masses, tenderness)
- Genital (identify the level of anomaly)
- Rectal (consider if young, palpate for vaginal masses/menstrual obstruction)

Imaging

Ultrasound gold standard first line

- Transabdominal to define hematocolpos/mucocolpos and identify structures
- Consider trans-perineal/trans-labial to help define the distance of collection to the perineum

Magnet resonance imaging (MRI) if difficulty visualizing the distance of the upper vagina to the perineum or if pelvic anatomy is confusing.

DOI: 10.1201/9781003039235-58

Management

- Imperative to accurately define the anatomy of the pelvic organs prior to any planned surgical correction (Figure 58.1).
- Simple incision and drainage of hematocolpos should not be performed as it is associated with a high rate of ascending infection/sepsis and scarring.
- Typically, obstructive vaginal anomalies are not surgical emergencies and the complexity of these conditions in combination with the risk of operative complications requires referral to a center with expertise in the management of these disorders.
- Allowing vaginal distention from the hematocolpos can increase the length of proximal vaginal tissue:
  - This can be mobilized to bridge the distance between the proximal and distal vaginal
  - Delaying surgery may thin the septum and decrease the risk of postoperative stenosis
- In cases where the surgical delay is needed and pain is an issue, menstrual suppression can be utilized (see Chapter 26, "Menstrual Suppression")
  - Combination oral contraceptive pills 30–25-mcg ethinyl estradiol/progestin pill continuously
  - Progestin-only pills (various combinations: 35-mcg norethindrone, 5–15-mg norethindrone acetate, 4-mg drospirenone)
  - Depot medroxyprogesterone acetate 150 mg intramuscularly every 12 weeks
  - GnRH agonist with add-back therapy 11.25 mg intramuscularly every 3 months or 3.75 mg every month with 5-mg norethindrone acetate daily

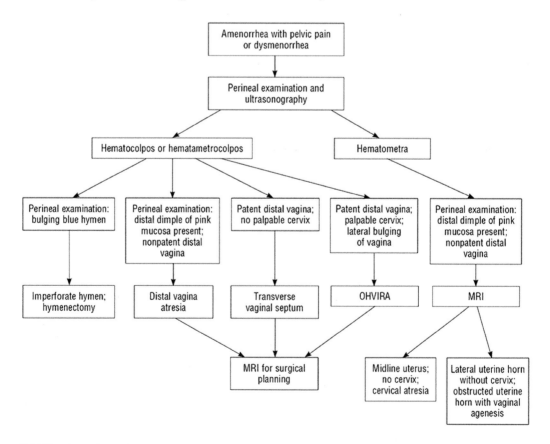

FIGURE 58.1 Diagnostic approach to a patient with an obstructed uterovaginal anomaly. (From Dietrich (2020), with permission.)

Indications for Expedited Surgery

- Urinary retention
- Severe uncontrolled pain
- Ascending infection in uterus and/or kidneys

Specific Anomalies

- Hymenal variants: imperforate, microperforate, cribriform, septate (see Chapter 24, "Hymenal Anatomy")
- Transverse vaginal septum
- Vaginal-cervical agenesis (see Chapter 56, "Uterovaginal Agenesis")
- Vaginal atresia
- Obstructed hemivagina and ipsilateral renal anomaly
- Longitudinal vaginal septum
- Urogenital sinus

Transverse Vaginal Septum

Embryology

- Disorder of vertical fusion: incomplete fusion between the Müllerian duct component of the vagina and the urogenital sinus
- Associated anomalies
  - Imperforate anus
  - Bicornuate uterus
  - Coarctation of the aorta
  - Atrial septal defect
  - Lumbar spine malformations

Clinical Presentation

- May present in neonatal, infant, or adolescent period
- Most frequently presents around menarche with a history of cyclic abdominal pain and primary amenorrhea
- Patients may present with urinary frequency, urinary retention, constipation or obstipation, or even rarely bowel obstruction
- Patients may complain of persistent spotting and/or vaginal discharge throughout the month if a microperforation is present or if spontaneous perforation of the septum occurs
  - Patients with a microperforation may not be diagnosed until late adolescence or even adulthood

Diagnosis

- Physical examination
  - Findings may vary depending on the location and the thickness of the septum
  - The septum may be
    - Low (incidence 14%): minimal to no lower vagina present, a bulge may be visualized if upper vagina is distended with blood or mucus and should be felt on rectal exam
    - Mid (incidence 40%): a portion of the lower vagina will be present, a bulge may be felt on rectal exam
    - High (incidence 46%): like mid-septums, a portion of the lower vagina will be present, a bulge may be difficult to feel on a rectal exam given the distance from the perineum

- In an adolescent or adult patient with menses, a speculum exam will reveal a blind-ending pouch without visualization of the cervix
- Imaging
  - Ultrasound, MRI
    - MRI can also help determine the thickness of the septum if unable to be measured on ultrasound and help identify the cervix and differentiate between the high septum and cervical atresia (see Chapter 56, "Uterovaginal/Müllerian Agenesis")

Management

- Risk of stenosis is high; therefore, surgical intervention is best performed when the patient will be committed to postoperative dilation
- Generally, a transverse incision is made through the septum to reach the upper vagina; the septum is then excised and the upper and lower vagina are anastomosed together with interrupted, dissolvable sutures (Figure 58.2)
  - A Z-plasty or Y-plasty technique should be utilized for septums greater than 1 cm in thickness to help decrease postoperative stricture formation
- The complexity of the surgery increases with the distance of the septum from the introitus as well as the thickness of the septum
- Allowing the upper vagina to distend with blood prior may help thin the septum
- Thick septums higher in the vagina may require extensive dissection and placement of an interposition graft with buccal mucosa or other materials (such as bowel)
- During the surgical correction, use of a catheter in the bladder and a double-gloved finger in the rectum can help identify the appropriate surgical plane
- Strong consideration should be given to the placement of a dilator postoperatively to help prevent stricture at the anastomosis site, especially with a thick septum that has more tension at the anastomosis

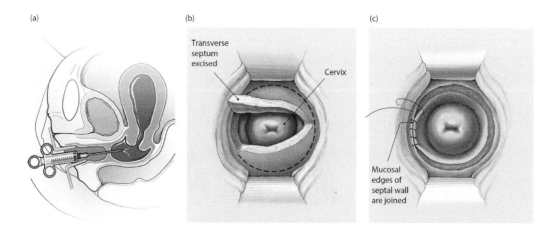

FIGURE 58.2 Transverse vaginal septum repair: (a) sagittal view of a transverse vaginal septum with accompanying hematocolpos, a spinal needle inserted into space with the aspiration of material to provide for clear evaluation of the anatomy. (b) A horizontal incision is made and carried down through the entire thickness of the septum, revealing the cervix and proximal vagina. The anterior and posterior leaflets are then cut circumferentially, flush with the vaginal wall. (c) The raw edges are then reapproximated with interrupted sutures. (From Dwiggins M, Gomez-Lobo V (2019). Congenital Anomalies of the Reproductive Tract. In Sanfilippo JS, Lara-Torre E, Gomez-Lobo V, eds., *Clinical Pediatric and Adolescent Gynecology* (2nd ed.). Boca Raton, FL: CRC Press, with permission.)

Distal Vaginal Atresia

Embryology

- Like a transverse septum, a disorder of vertical fusion: incomplete fusion of the Müllerian ducts and the urogenital sinus, leading to a fibrous band between the perineum and the normal upper vagina
- Distal vaginal atresia is associated with normal upper vagina, cervix, and uterus without the evidence of hymenal tissue at the introitus
- Infrequently associated with other anomalies but urinary tract anomalies, anorectal malformations, coarctation of the aorta, atrial septal defects, and lumbar spine malformations have been described

Clinical Presentation

- May present in neonatal, infant, or adolescent period
- Neonates or infants may present with urinary retention, constipation or obstipation, or persistent vomiting secondary to mucocolpos
- Most frequently presents around menarche with a history of cyclic abdominal pain and primary amenorrhea
- Adolescents may present with urinary frequency, urinary retention, constipation or obstipation, or even (rarely) bowel obstruction

Diagnosis

- Physical findings
  - Normal appearing external female genitalia
  - Vaginal dimple at introitus, occasionally a bulge may be visible with a very large hematocolpos
  - Rectal exam can reveal a palpable mass from the hematocolpos collected in the upper vagina
- Imaging: transabdominal/perineal ultrasound, MRI

Management

- Generally, a transverse incision is made through the atretic portion to reach the upper vagina, and the upper and lower vagina are anastomosed together with interrupted, dissolvable sutures often using a Z-plasty technique
- A catheter in the bladder and a double-gloved finger in the rectum can help identify the appropriate surgical plane between the urethra, bladder, and rectum to facilitate pull-through vaginoplasty
- The complexity of the surgery increases with the amount of the vagina that is atretic and may require an abdominal approach (open or laparoscopic) to mobilize the uterus and upper vagina
- If the upper vagina is more than 3 cm from the introitus, an interposition graft with buccal mucosa or other material (such as bowel) may be needed due to a high risk of postoperative stenosis
- Allowing the upper vagina to distend with blood and performing sequential dilations with a rigid dilator from below will thin the atretic portion and may prevent the need for an interposition graft
- A dilator should be used postoperatively to help prevent stricture at the anastomosis site if the obstruction is greater than 3 cm from the introitus

Obstructed Hemivagina and Ipsilateral Renal Anomaly (OHVIRA) (Figure 58.3)

Embryology

- Due to failure of lateral fusion of lower Müllerian ducts
- Associated with ipsilateral renal agenesis
- May have an ectopic ureter in the obstructed vagina

Clinical Presentation

- May present with dysmenorrhea if presents postpubertally, often worsening with each menses
  - May present with lateral bulging cystic mass at the introitus or an incidental hydrocolpos/hematocolpos posterior to the bladder
  - If an obstructed side has a spontaneous perforation, the patient may complain of persistent discharge throughout the month

Diagnosis

- Physical finding
  - Bulge on lateral sidewall due to hematocolpos
  - May have fistula draining obstructed menstrual blood
- Imaging: pelvic and renal ultrasound
  - When a solitary kidney is present, ectopic ureter should be ruled out, as it will be present in about 9% of cases and often drains into the obstructed hemivagina

Management

- Vaginoscopy can be utilized to visualize microperforation between vaginal canals
- Resect vaginal septum as much as possible (see transverse vaginal septum section)
- A spinal needle can be used to map the obstructed hemivagina and then a cut down can be performed on the needle to open the obstructed hemivagina and perform the unification of the two sides (see figure 58.3)

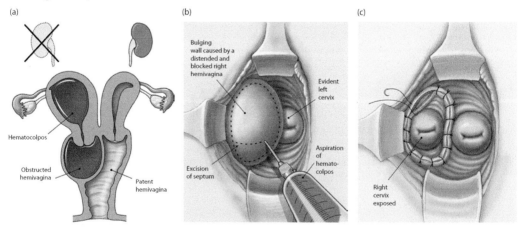

FIGURE 58.3   Obstructed hemivagina and ipsilateral renal anomaly: (a) vaginal view with distended right vaginal side-wall due to obstructed hemivagina, left cervix noted. Obstructed vagina can be drained with a spinal needle to allow for clear visualization of the anatomy. (b) A horizontal incision is then made along the obstructed vaginal sidewall, and septum excision is carried out circumferentially (dotted line). (c) After complete excision of the septum has been performed, the raw edges are then reapproximated using interrupted sutures. Two cervixes are clearly noted and the right hemivagina obstruction is completely resolved. (From Dwiggins M, Gomez-Lobo V (2019). Congenital Anomalies of the Reproductive Tract. In Sanfilippo JS, Lara-Torre E, Gomez-Lobo V, eds., *Clinical Pediatric and Adolescent Gynecology* (2nd ed.). Boca Raton, FL: CRC Press, with permission.)

Longitudinal Vaginal Septum

Embryology

- A failure of lateral fusion of the lower Müllerian ducts
- The upper Müllerian ducts may also fail to fuse
- Commonly associated with uterine didelphys, bicornuate uterus, or complete, septate uterus
- Associated renal anomalies are common

Clinical Presentation

- Patient may complain of continuous menstrual flow around tampon even on light bleeding days, difficulty using a tampon, or difficulty with intercourse
- If one side of the vagina is obstructed, the patient may present with cyclic pain (see OHVIRA section)

Diagnosis

- Physical findings
  - Septum can be missed with a speculum exam, as it will often just be pushed to one side
  - Careful exam will reveal two vaginal canals, one or two cervices may be present
- Imaging: Pelvic and renal ultrasound

Management

- If two patent vaginal canals are present, the septum does not need to be excised if the patient is not bothered
  - Patient must be educated about the possible traumatic tearing with coitus and/or delivery with childbearing
- If the patient desires removal, the procedure is completed vaginally
- The septum is visualized and separated from the anterior and posterior vaginal walls
  - Numerous techniques have been described with the use of sutures, monopolar electrocautery, bipolar electrocautery, harmonic scalpel, etc. with no consensus on best practice
  - Care should be taken to not damage the cervix, a small amount of septum should be left at the apex to avoid compromising cervical integrity

Urogenital Sinus

Embryology

- Arrested migration of the Müllerian ducts from the tubercles to the vestibule
- Results in a common channel for the vagina and urethra

Diagnosis

- Physical findings
  - A single opening between the phallus and anus
  - Labial fusion and clitoromegaly may be present
  - Anus may be orthotopic (low confluence) or displaced anteriorly (high confluence)
- Imaging
  - Retrograde genitogram to determine the level of the confluence and length of the common channel (see Chapter 45, "Radiologic Imaging for Gynecologic Conditions")
  - Ultrasound of the spine and kidneys

- Magnetic resonance imaging to help further define anatomy
- Endoscopy, including cystoscopy and vaginoscopy, may also be used to better define the anomaly before definitive surgical correction is planned

Management

- Given the complex nature of the anomaly, surgical correction should be performed with a multidisciplinary team that may include pediatric urology, pediatric surgery, and pediatric gynecology
- The procedure depends on whether the common channel starts above or below the sphincter
- May be completed as a staged procedure
- If present, underlying endocrinopathy, such as congenital adrenal hyperplasia, should be treated

BIBLIOGRAPHY

Dietrich JE (2020). Surgical Management of Reproductive Tract Anomalies. In Handa VL, Van Le L, eds. *TeLinde's Operative Gynecology* (12th ed., pp. 714–731). Wolters Kluwer.

Oelschalger AMA, Berger-chen SW. Management of acute obstructive uterovaginal anomalies: ACOG committee opinion, number 779. Obstet Gynecol. 2019; 133(6):e363–e371.

59

Vulvar Disorders

Atopic Dermatitis, Burns, Crohn's Disease (Vulvar Manifestations), Hidradenitis Suppurativa, Lichen Sclerosus, Nevi of Vulva, Psoriasis, Stevens-Johnson Syndrome (SJS) and Toxic Epidermal Necrolysis (TEN), Ulcers of the Vulva, and Vascular Anomalies of the Vulva

Tina Ho, Kaiane Habeshian, Kelsey Flood, Sameen Nooruddin, Laura Hollenbach, Kathryn Stambough, and Kalyani Marathe

ATOPIC DERMATITIS

Key Points

- Atopic dermatitis is a chronic inflammatory skin disorder that affects 10–13% of US children. It is characterized by skin barrier dysfunction and immune dysregulation.
- Atopic dermatitis is frequently associated with asthma and allergic rhinitis.

Diagnosis

History

- Intensely pruritic
- Infants usually have involvement of their cheeks, forehead, scalp, trunk, and the extensor aspects of their extremities
- In older children and adolescents, the disease is usually worst on flexural surfaces (e.g. neck, antecubital fossae, wrists, popliteal fossae)
- Sleep disturbance is common due to pruritus and can severely impair quality of life

Exam

- Acute: Weepy, erythematous patches and plaques +/– vesicles or crusting
- Subacute: Ill-defined, erythematous scaly patches, and thin plaques
- Chronic: Thickened, lichenified patches, and plaques +/– hypopigmentation or hyperpigmentation
- May be superinfected
- Typically spares the anogenital skin of children who wear diapers – However, may develop irritant or allergic contact dermatitis of anogenital skin

DOI: 10.1201/9781003039235-59

Differential Diagnosis

- Seborrheic dermatitis: Erythematous, hypopigmented, or hyperpigmented plaques with fine, yellow, greasy scale
- Tinea cruris: Annular plaques with central clearing and scale at the leading edge
- Candidiasis: Sharply demarcated, beefy red plaques with satellite lesions

Management

Atopic dermatitis

- Conservative management
  - Maximize skin hydration with frequent application of a fragrance-free cream or ointment at least twice daily and immediately after bathing
  - Bathe in plain, lukewarm water for 5–10 minutes using a gentle, fragrance-free soap or non-soap cleanser
  - Minimize scratching by trimming nails, wearing cotton clothing that limits access to involved skin, habit reversal therapy
- Steroid
  - Low-potency topical corticosteroid such as hydrocortisone 2.5% ointment twice daily for 2 weeks for mild flares
  - Medium-potency topical steroid such as triamcinolone 0.1% ointment twice daily for 2 weeks for moderate to severe flares
  - Higher potency topical steroids typically reserved for thick or lichenified plaques on the scalp, trunk, and extremities of older children and adolescents, whereas shorter courses of lower potency topical steroids should be used on the face, axillae, and anogenital skin
  - *NOTE*: Extreme caution should be exercised when using topical steroids in infants, especially on anogenital skin where occlusion can lead to increased systemic adsorption, hypothalamic-pituitary-adrenal axis suppression, and even death
- Other treatments, recommend consultation with dermatology for management
  - Tacrolimus 0.03 or 0.1% ointment and pimecrolimus 1% cream are nonsteroidal medications that are useful for maintenance in patients who flare frequently, as well as for long-term use in sensitive areas such as the axillae, inframammary, and anogenital skin
  - Second-generation antihistamines (e.g. cetirizine) may be helpful in patients who also have allergic rhinitis. Sedating antihistamines (e.g. diphenhydramine or hydroxyzine) may help with sleep.
- Culture if secondary infection is suspected
- Consider referral to dermatology for patients who have extensive, severe, or refractory disease, recurrent skin infections, suspected immunodeficiency, or failure to thrive

BURNS

Key Points

- Traumatic injuries to the skin or other tissues caused primarily by heat, electrical discharge, friction, chemicals, and radiation
- If scald burns are present in children, need to rule out child abuse

- Burns are classified by the depth of tissue injury. Traditionally burns were labeled as first through fourth degree; however, this has been replaced by the following system
  - Superficial: Limited to epidermal involvement
  - Superficial partial-thickness: Involves epidermis and parts of the dermis
  - Deep partial-thickness: Extend into deep dermis to damage hair follicles and glands
  - Full-thickness: Destruction of all dermal layers with injury of the subcutaneous tissue

Presentation

Appearance of classification of wounds are the following

- Superficial (epidermal)
  - Dry, red; blanches with pressure
  - Painful
- Superficial partial-thickness
  - Moist, red, weeping; blisters; blanches with pressure
  - Painful to temperature, air, and touch
- Deep partial-thickness
  - Wet or waxy dry
  - Blisters, easily unroofed
  - Variable in color
  - Blanching with pressure is delayed
  - Decreased sensation, may only feel deep pressure
- Full-thickness
  - Waxy white to grey to charred and black
  - Dry and inelastic
  - No blanching with pressure
  - Decreased sensation, may only feel deep pressure

Management

- For minor burns (superficial, superficial partial-thickness), treatment includes
  - Cooling with cold tap water within 3 hours of injury
  - Simple cleaning with mild soap and water
  - Dressings are not recommended for superficial burns
- For deeper minor burns that require a dressing
  - First layer of nonadherent gauze
  - Second layer of fluffed dry gauze
  - Final layer of elastic gauze that wraps the area
  - No consensus exists regarding dressings for genital burns
  - Dressing changes can range from twice daily to weekly; however, the majority can be changed daily
- Consider the application of a combination of topical estrogen and silver sulfadiazine cream
- For deep burns in the genital area: Consult with pediatric surgery and burn team

In the non-genital area

- Early wound excision is necessary for deep wounds in order to eliminate necrotic tissue and tissue prone to infection
- At the time of excision, wound coverage should also be done. This can include direct wound closure, skin grafts, tissue expansion, or tissue flaps depending on the extent of the wound and excision

Pain management is critical, especially if the burn is located in a sensitive area, which includes the genitalia area.

Acetic acid is a common substance used during colposcopy, and acetic acid burns can occur based on concentration and duration of application. Some studies have shown topical estrogen can be used for treatment.

Healing time for burns are the following

- Superficial: 3–6 days
- Superficial partial-thickness: 7–21 days
- Deep partial-thickness: >21 days; usually requires surgical management
- Full-thickness: Requires surgical treatment

CROHN'S DISEASE (VULVAR MANIFESTATIONS)

Key Points

- Crohn's disease (CD) is a type of inflammatory bowel disease that can affect any part of the gastrointestinal (GI) tract; histologically it is characterized by noncaseating granulomatous lesions
- Vulvar CD is an extra-intestinal manifestation and includes labial edema or induration, but the presentation of vulvar CD is quite heterogeneous
- The most common site of involvement outside the GI tract is the skin
- Vulvar involvement may be the sole initial presentation, especially in children; however, all children with cutaneous CD are eventually diagnosed with GI CD and thus should be followed by gastroenterology
- Clinical course of cutaneous CD may be different than the course of GI disease

Differential Diagnosis

- Infections (i.e. cellulitis, mycobacterial infections, actinomycosis, fungal infections)
- Bartholin gland cyst
- Perineal endometriosis
- Inflammatory processes (lichenoid eruptions, Bechet's, hidradenitis suppurativa [HS], sarcoid)
- Sexually transmitted infections (syphilis, herpes simplex virus, lymphogranuloma venereum, granuloma inguinale)
- Sexual abuse
- Lymphatic obstruction or lymphedema (primary or secondary)
- Foreign body
- Non-sexually acquired genital ulceration

Diagnosis

History

- May be diagnosed prior to, concurrent with, or after GI CD
- Pain, swelling or fullness, abscesses, ulceration, pruritus, discharge, and erythema are common symptoms; dyspareunia may be reported in adolescents
- Screen for GI symptoms: Abdominal pain, diarrhea, unintended weight loss
- Screen for gynecologic symptoms: Vulvovaginal pain, vulvar infections, pelvic pain, menstrual irregularities

Physical Examination

- Cutaneous lesions may either occur as
  - Direct extension of the GI tract disease (contiguous CD)
  - Distinct lesions with no connection to the GI tract (metastatic CD)
- Vulvar edema (with or without erythema), knife-cut ulcerations or fissures, draining fistulae, nodules, erythematous to violaceous plaques, perianal skin tags are classic findings
- Firm skin tags, verrucous nodules, and lymphangiectasias may occur secondary to chronic vulvar edema
- In children: Labial edema or induration is the most common presentation
- A full gynecological examination and examination of the buttocks is indicated; CD may be associated w/rectovaginal or rectovestibular fistulas

Laboratory tests and another workup

- Fecal calprotectin or lactoferrin levels may be elevated and serve as a screening test for GI inflammation
- Biopsy will demonstrate noncaseating granulomatous inflammation
  - Consider special stains to rule out infectious processes and foreign bodies
  - Due to pathergy, skin biopsy sites may not heal so some advocate for the noninvasive techniques initially (fecal studies, imaging, colonoscopy)
- Other considerations
  - Exclude rectovaginal fistulae
  - Screen for sexually transmitted infections
  - Patients should be referred to gastroenterology to undergo a workup for CD
- Imaging, i.e., pelvic MRI or ultrasound, may be helpful to establish the diagnosis and exclude other processes

Management

- Management should involve a multidisciplinary team: Gastroenterology, gynecology, dermatology, surgery, primary care
- Early treatment should be pursued to avoid anatomical distortion; however, often recalcitrant to treatment
- Currently no formal treatment guidelines, individualized approach is key
- Treatment of underlying CD is critical, regardless of whether or not there is GI involvement

Topical agents

- Steroids
- Tacrolimus

Oral antibiotics

- Metronidazole
- Tetracyclines
- Ciprofloxacin

Anti-inflammatory medications

- Steroids
- Cyclosporine
- Azathioprine
- Sulfasalazine
- 5-aminosalicylates
- Methotrexate

Biologics

- Tumor necrosis factor (TNF)-inhibitors
- Integrin inhibitors

Surgery: Excision – Uncommonly used, most vulvar manifestations are best managed by biologics

Prognosis

- Complete resolution is uncommon
- Course of skin disease does not necessarily parallel the course of GI involvement; GI symptoms may improve while cutaneous involvement persists
- Heightened awareness of this unique presentation may lead to earlier diagnosis and prevent morbidity

HIDRADENITIS SUPPURATIVA (HS)

Key Points

- HS is a chronic, intermittent inflammatory disease characterized by painful, potentially scarring inflammatory nodules, abscesses, and fistulae classically in the intertriginous regions
- Potentially debilitating chronic disease punctuated by fluctuations in the disease course
- Patients may be reluctant to discuss their symptoms with providers given embarrassment and misconceptions regarding the disease; therefore, providers should initiate discussion if exam demonstrates findings suggestive of HS
- Assessment of comorbidities is paramount as HS has many implications for patients' overall health and psychosocial well-being

Differential Diagnosis

- Abscess
- Folliculitis
- Crohn's disease
- Other infection (granuloma inguinale, tuberculosis, mycetoma)

Diagnosis

History

- Onset is usually after puberty
- Waxing and waning course
- Family history of HS is present in some patients
- Patients are often treated for recurrent bacterial abscesses prior to diagnosis of HS, for which patients may frequently seek care for in the emergency department
- Cases in prepubertal females should prompt consideration of genetic predisposition and investigation for hormonal imbalances (i.e. precocious puberty), although this is debated
  - First perform thorough investigation for signs of precocious puberty
  - Often associated with obesity

Physical Examination

- Characteristic lesions include inflammatory and noninflammatory nodules, double comedones, draining sinus tracts or fistulae, abscesses, scarring; malodor, and serosanguinous drainage may be present
- Common locations are intertriginous areas (inframammary skin, axillae, inguinal folds, buttocks, perineum, and in other skin folds), mons pubis, and central chest although ectopic HS may occur
- Fistulae to the urethra, bladder, or rectum can occur
- Hurley staging (see Figure 59.1)
  - Stage I: Recurrent nodules and abscesses with minimal scar
  - Stage II: One or limited number of sinuses and/or scarring within a region
  - Stage III: Multiple or extensive sinuses and/or scarring
  - Useful to document the progression of the disease and to determine treatment

Laboratory Tests

- Consideration of baseline erythrocyte sedimentation rate and C-reactive protein to assess inflammatory markers; longitudinal assessment may be useful in monitoring response to treatment
- Complete blood count may be helpful in patients with severe disease who may have concomitant blood dyscrasias (leukocytosis, thrombocytosis, anemia)
- Consider endocrinology evaluation if there is a concern for hormonal imbalances and referral for metabolic syndrome labs
- Biopsy and wound culture have limited usefulness, typically findings are normal

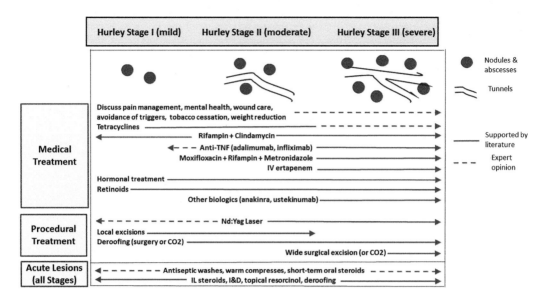

FIGURE 59.1 Overview of treatment strategies based on Hurley staging. I&D, Incision, and drainage; IL, intralesional; IV, intravenous; Nd:YAG, neodymium-doped yttrium-aluminum-garnet; TNF, tumor necrosis factor. (From Alikhan A, Sayed C, Alavi A, et al. North American clinical management guidelines for hidradenitis suppurativa: A publication from the United States and Canadian Hidradenitis Suppurativa Foundations: Part II: Topical, intralesional, and systemic medical management. J Am Acad Dermatol. 2019;81(1):91–101, with permission.)

Management

Patient education

- Patient support groups: HS Foundation
- Wound care
  - Avoid destruction of pustules as this may worsen disease
  - Keep clean to avoid secondary infection
- Counsel on weight loss, if applicable
- Counsel on smoking cessation, if applicable
- Consider referral for nutrition counseling
- Consider dairy avoidance, low glycemic index diet
- Consider supplementation for Hurley Stage I or II
  - Vitamin D if deficient, dosing based on need
  - Zinc gluconate 90 mg daily (can cause copper deficiency with long-term use)

Pain management

- Lidocaine, oral acetaminophen, oral NSAIDs preferred
- Use anticonvulsants such as pregabalin and gabapentin if pain not well controlled
- Use of narcotics is not recommended
- Referral to pain management

See Figure 59.1 for treatment management

Topicals

- Clindamycin 1% lotion
- Washes containing benzoyl peroxide, chlorhexidine, zinc pyrithione (dandruff shampoo)
- Dapsone

Antibiotics

- Typically have been used along with topical therapy
- Clindamycin and rifampin in combination 300 mg twice daily ×8–12 weeks
- Tetracyclines 500 mg twice daily
- Ertapenem as rescue therapy or surgical planning (given barriers to home infusions, antibiotic resistance, used only in extreme cases)

Hormonal

- Antiandrogen contraceptives (Yasmin, Yaz), spironolactone 100–150 mg daily have limited evidence
- Avoid progestin-only contraceptives that are thought to worsen HS
- Use of Metformin and Finasteride has been described

Biologics

- To be managed in severe cases by Dermatology
  - Includes Adalimumab, off-label use of Infliximab, and Etanercept

Systemic anti-inflammatory medications

- Systemic steroids (helpful for management of acute flares)
- Oral zinc gluconate 30 mg TID or 50 mg BID
- Data for other anti-inflammatory medications are not as robust and have been studied primarily in adults (i.e. methotrexate, apremilast)

Retinoids

- To be managed by Dermatology
  - Includes Acitretin, Isotretinoin, used with caution in reproductive aged females

Procedural interventions

- Intralesional steroid injection with Kenalog
- Laser hair removal/other laser interventions

Surgery

- Deroofing: Skin overlying sinus or abscess cavity is removed and base left untreated
- Wide local excision
  - Can result in a disease-free state
  - Caution if the large surface area is to be removed, especially in the anogenital region

- Incision and drainage should be undertaken with caution, as the scarred tract may create a nidus for further inflammation and recurrence rates approach 100%
  - May be useful to provide relief and allow for a smaller procedure to be performed

Comorbidities

- Acne
- Overweight and obesity
- Smoking (including second-hand smoke exposure)
- Hirsutism
- Pilonidal cysts
- Down syndrome
- Psoriasis
- Endocrine comorbidities (i.e. precocious puberty)
- Pain
- Psychosocial comorbidities (anxiety, depression)
- Inflammatory bowel disease

Prognosis

- Patients with early-onset HS may have more severe disease
- There is no cure to date; treatment should focus on controlling pain and preventing disease progression and scarring

LICHEN SCLEROSUS

Key Points

- Lichen sclerosus (LS) is a chronic multifactorial autoimmune scarring disorder that occurs in a bimodal distribution in childhood and in post-menopausal women.
- It most commonly affects the anogenital region.
- Contributing factors include irritants such as urine in the setting of hypo-estrogenated tissue.
- LS is often undiagnosed or misdiagnosed.
- Delayed or inadequate treatment can lead to permanent scarring, psychosocial complications, and a risk of vulvar squamous cell carcinoma (5% in adult women).
- Contrary to popular teaching, LS often does not resolve at puberty; although symptoms may improve, disease activity can persist.

Diagnosis

- The diagnosis is largely clinical. Skin biopsy is rarely required in children.

Symptoms

- Include pruritus, pain with urination and defecation, dyspareunia, blood in urine or stool, and constipation
- Vaginal discharge is not an expected feature of LS

Exam

- Symmetric ovoid white patches on the vulva
  - Classically involving the clitoral hood, extending across the labia majora and minora to the perineum and anus in a "figure of 8" distribution
  - Overlying "cigarette paper" wrinkling of the epidermis and a shiny appearance
  - Occasionally superficial ulceration will be noted
- Hyperkeratotic white papules, fissures, petechiae, and hematomas may be present
- Agglutination (resorption) of the labia minora, adhesions, burying of the clitoral hood, introital narrowing, and effacement of vulvar anatomy may be present in prolonged disease

Differential Diagnosis

Vitiligo

- Asymmetric white patches, classically *sparing* the clitoris

Vitiligoid LS

- Appears clinically like vitiligo but has symptoms of LS that improve with treatment and shows histologic features of LS on biopsy

Irritant contact dermatitis or atopic dermatitis

Nonspecific vulvovaginitis

Perianal itching associated with pinworm infestation

Management

- First-line treatment is with high-potency topical corticosteroids ointments (e.g. clobetasol ointment).
- The standard regiment includes steroid daily × 4–6 weeks, alternating days × 4–6 weeks, twice weekly × 1 month – exact regimen should be individualized.
  - Can consider de-escalation of the potency of steroids as opposed to taper
  - Follow-up every 4–6 weeks is recommended to monitor for improvement
  - Prolonged use of topical steroids can lead to persistent erythema, atrophy of skin with visible telangiectasias and small venules, and acne-like bumps in the surrounding skin
- Mid-to-low-potency topical corticosteroids and topical calcineurin inhibitors may be used for taper or maintenance.

Counsel on proper hygiene and toileting

- Avoid harsh substances including soap, wet wipes, bubble baths, and fragrances
- Sitz baths, dilute bleach baths, and Epson salt baths may help alleviate symptoms and flush out the skin
- Apply bland emollient or coconut oil to heal and protect the skin; the emollient barrier may help reduce dysuria.

Treat associated constipation with increased water and fiber intake and stool softeners

Relapses are common

LS can persist in adolescence and adulthood and long-term follow up is required

NEVI OF VULVA

Key Points

- Uncommon to find vulvar nevi in children; more likely in adolescents but the true prevalence is likely underestimated
- Most darkly pigmented vulvar lesions in this age group are lentigines (benign increase in melanin in the basal layer of the epithelium) or are benign nevi; vulvar melanoma in children is very rare
- Benign vulvar lentigines and nevi may appear atypical clinically, and nevi may exhibit atypia on histopathology, which can make them difficult to distinguish from melanoma
- Exhibit caution in deciding to biopsy due to the above factors

Types

Benign Nevi

Junctional nevi

- Small 2–10 mm diameter
- Flat with minimal elevation above the skin surface
- Involve only epidermal/dermal junction
- Uniform color from tan to black
- Well-demarcated, smooth contour
- Can be monitored every 6–12 months
- Consider biopsy for rapid and asymmetric changes in color, size, shape

Compound nevi: Arise from compound nevi or de novo

- May involve epidermis and dermis
- Size 4–10 mm diameter
- Uniform color/regular margins
- May become popular/polypoid/pedunculated
- Consider biopsy for rapid and asymmetric changes in color, size, shape

Melanoma

- Rare in children/teens especially on the vulva; most vulvar melanomas occur in the 7th decade
- One-fourth of vulvar melanomas may be amelanotic (nonpigmented); bleeding is a concerning sign
- Second-most common malignancy of the vulva in adults after squamous cell carcinoma

Risk Factors

Melanoma

- Congenital melanocytic nevi
- Dysplastic nevi

- Xeroderma pigmentosum
- Immunosuppression

Childhood genital lentigines

- Bannayan–Riley–Ruvalcaba syndrome (on the spectrum of PTEN hamartoma tumor syndrome; associated with lipomas, macrocephaly)
- Noonan syndrome with lentigines (formerly known as LEOPARD syndrome; associated with dark nevi all over the body, genital anomalies, short stature)

Diagnosis
History

- Duration of the lesion
- Change in lesion: Size, color, shape, borders
- Bleeding
- Family history of melanoma

Physical Examination

- Perform thorough skin examination including other nevi
- Identify lesion of concern

Management

- Nevi may gradually grow and evolve in children
- Rapid or sudden change, especially if asymmetric, or associated bleeding, is more concerning
- Exhibit caution when deciding to biopsy as results can lead to unnecessary interventions
  - Clinically monitoring with serial photographs is often a viable option
- Perform excisional biopsy for concerning lesions (rapidly growing/changing or bleeding)
- Shave biopsy amelanotic raised lesions
- When uncertain, refer to pediatric dermatology for opinion
- Follow up and manage based on microscopic dermatopathology results

Nevi arising with LS can mimic melanoma on histopathology. At the same time, melanoma may incite the development of LS in some patients. In these cases, a multidisciplinary approach to management is required, and the biopsy should be read by a pathologist who specializes in pigmented lesions.

PSORIASIS

Key Points

- Psoriasis is an immune-mediated, chronic inflammatory disease that classically presents with well-defined brightly erythematous, scaly plaques.
- 10% of patients with psoriasis will also have arthritis
- In patients with psoriasis involving visible areas of skin, 60% will also have anogenital involvement

Diagnosis

History

- Lesions that are rarely pruritic
- Can flare or be triggered by infection, especially group A *Streptococcus.*
- Koebner phenomenon: Skin lesions may be triggered cutaneous trauma (e.g. a scratch, irritants. and wiping in napkin psoriasis)
- Genital psoriasis may flare with intercourse and can cause dyspareunia.

Exam

- Sharply demarcated, round, erythematous plaques with overlying silvery-white scale frequently involving the scalp, elbows, knees, lumbosacral, and anogenital regions
- Inverse psoriasis predominantly affects intertriginous areas (e.g. axillae, inguinal folds, perineum, periumbilical, and inframammary skin)
- Very well-defined, shiny, brightly erythematous, fissured plaques with minimal to no scale (absent because of the increased humidity of this occluded area)

Differential Diagnosis

- Seborrheic dermatitis: Erythematous, hypopigmented or hyperpigmented plaques with fine, yellow, greasy scale
- Tinea cruris: Annular plaques with central clearing and scale at the leading edge
- Candidiasis: Sharply demarcated, beefy red plaques with satellite lesions

Management

- Mild-to-moderate cutaneous disease
  - Topical steroid such as hydrocortisone 2.5% ointment or triamcinolone 0.1% ointment can be used twice daily for 2–4 weeks
  - Disease severity, site of involvement, the thickness of the plaques, age of the child, and anticipated occlusion are all important considerations when selecting a topical steroid.
  - Calcipotriene 0.005% cream or ointment (vitamin D analogue) can be used simultaneously on anogenital skin to improve outcomes
- Severe or recalcitrant disease
  - Can add phototherapy, methotrexate, cyclosporine, systemic retinoids managed by Dermatology
- Referral to rheumatology if psoriatic arthritis is suspected
- Promote lifestyle modification in those with obesity or metabolic syndrome.
- Screen for depression and anxiety as moderate-to-severe psoriasis can result in poor physical, emotional, social, and school functioning

STEVENS-JOHNSON SYNDROME (SJS) AND TOXIC EPIDERMAL NECROLYSIS (TEN)

Key Points

- SJS and TEN are variants of a rare, acute, serious, and life-threatening skin reaction with mucosal involvement.
- Up to 70 % of patients with SJS or TEN develop genital lesions ranging from erosive ulcerative vaginitis, vulvar bullae, and vaginal synechia.

- Majority of cases are caused by a severe adverse reactions to medications
  - The highest risk medications include: allopurinol, trimethoprim-sulfamethoxazole (and other sulfa antibiotics), aminopenicillins, cephalosporins, quinolones, carbamazepine, phenytoin, phenobarbital, lamotrigine, and oxicam-type NSAIDs
- Infectious causes although rare, include mycoplasma pneumoniae (MIRM – mycoplasma pneumonia-induced rash and mucositis) and Herpes simplex infections.
- HLA-B gene variation is strongly associated with SJS/TEN.
- SJS has a mortality rate of 1–5%.
- TEN has a mortality rate of 30%.

Presentation

- Initially presents with fever and flu-like symptoms
- Skin involvement develops within few days after initial symptoms
- Early stage includes flat or slightly raised pink spots on the skin with dark-red centers that evolve into painful skin erosions that appear like a water burn
- Commonly a positive Nikolsky sign (sloughing of skin with mechanical force; however, this is not specifically diagnostic) is noted but is not specifically diagnostic
- Erosions typically start on the face and chest before spreading to other areas
- Skin erosions progress into large areas of epidermal detachment
- SJS is defined by <10% of total body surface area involvement
- TEN/SJS overlap involves 10–30% of total body surface involvement
- TEN involves >30% total body surface
- Involvement of oral and airway mucosal surfaces occurs in severe cases and can compromise respirations and swallowing
- Mucosal eye involvement can cause conjunctivitis and more severe ocular complications
- Severe skin and mucosal damage can lead to extreme body fluid loss and increase susceptibility to infections including pneumonia, sepsis, shock, and multisystem organ failure

Differential Diagnosis

- Autoimmune blistering diseases linear IgA (e.g. dermatosis and paraneoplastic pemphigus, pemphigus vulgaris, bullous pemphigoid)
- Acute generalized exanthematous pustulosis (AGEP)
- Disseminated fixed bullous drug eruption
- Staphylococcal scalded skin syndrome (SSSS)

Gyn Complications

- Erosions of genital mucosa
- Scarring
- Strictures/stenosis of urethra/vagnia
- Vaginal synechiae
- Urinary/Sexual dysfunction

Management

- In the acute stage, evaluation of disease extent/severity, removal of the offending drug, and initiation of supportive care especially with fluid and electrolyte resuscitation is imperative
- Specialized burn center treatment is essential to mitigate mortality in severe cases
- Patients need daily physical exams of genitalia, including periodic speculum exams, to monitor vaginal walls for stenosis

For vulvovaginal involvement therapies include

- Topical glucocorticoids applied to the external genitalia to prevent labial agglutination and/or intravaginal application to prevent vaginal stenosis
- Placement of vaginal molds to prevent adhesion formation in patients that are tampon users or sexually active
- Menstrual suppression to prevent the development of vaginal adenosis during the active phase of the disease
- Once disease process clears, consider continued speculum evaluation of vagina to assess for adenosis with biopsy of any lesion

Detailed drug history is crucial to help identify the etiology of SJS/TEN. Intradermal drug testing should not be performed due to the risk of recurrent SJS/TEN.

ULCERS OF THE VULVA

Key Points

- Although uncommon in the pediatric patient, always rule out sexual transmission as a cause of vulvar ulcers
- Typically exquisitely painful, supportive care necessary
- Culture for superinfection when clinically suspicious, use antibiotics only when indicated

Types

Infectious

- Coxsackievirus (hand, foot, mouth disease): Vesicles and erythematous, edematous papules on the buttocks, vaginal mucosa, oral mucosa, and palms/soles
- Varicella: Tender grouped vesicles or erosions on an erythematous base, usually in an immunocompromised patient

Sexually transmitted diseases

- Herpes simplex: See Chapter 48, "Sexually Transmitted Infections"
- Syphilis: See Chapter 48, "Sexually Transmitted Infections"
- Lymphogranuloma venereum: Painless vesicle or erosion on the vulva, vagina, or cervix (rarely observed) that precedes the development of tender inguinal, pararectal, and/or iliac lymphadenopathy that may ulcerate
- Chancroid: Papules and pustules on the vulva, cervix, or perianal skin that rupture to form painful, soft, ragged ulcers that bleed easily and may be associated with regional lymphadenopathy
- Granuloma inguinale (donovanosis): Painless, progressive, soft, friable beefy-red ulcers without regional lymphadenopathy

Systemic diseases

- Vulvar aphthae (non-sexually acquired genital ulceration or Lipschutz ulcer): Single or multiple, exquisitely painful well-demarcated deep ulcers with a fibrinous base and a surrounding erythematous halo on the labia minora, vestibule, and/or labia majora in a patient with a recent virus or viral symptoms
- Behcet's disease: Recurrent, sharply demarcated painful oral and genital ulcers in a patient with ocular disease and pathergy
- CD: See "Crohn's Disease (Vulvar Manifestations)" section

Autoimmune diseases

- Bullous pemphigoid: Tense subepidermal bullae that are pruritic and rupture to leave behind denuded areas of skin
- Linear IgA disease (chronic bullous disease of childhood): Pruritic vesicles and bullae in an annular arrangement on the lower trunk, buttocks, genitalia, and thighs
- Kawasaki disease: Perineal erythema or desquamation in a patient with prolonged, high spiking fevers
- Systemic lupus erythematosus: Erythematous plaques, erosions, or ulcers on the vulva, vestibule, or perianal skin

Cutaneous drug reactions

- Fixed drug eruption: Few cm round erosions on the vulva or perineum
- Erythema multiforme: Indurated plaques, target lesions, or painful erosions on the oral and anogenital mucosa, as well as the palms/soles and other parts of the body
- SJS/TEN (see section on painful full-thickness erosions in a patient with new medication exposure 7–21 days prior [see section regarding SJS/TEN for more information])

Diagnosis

- Thorough medical, surgical, family, social, and medication history
- Complete physical exam including external inspection of all mucous membranes (ocular, oral, vaginal, anal), hands and feet, and 100% of skin surface
- Appropriate testing for suspected bacterial and viral etiologies
- Consider complete blood count with differential, complete metabolic panel, erythrocyte sedimentation rate, C-reactive protein, serologies, fecal calprotectin, and/or antinuclear antibody
- If the disease is severe and diagnosis uncertain, a biopsy may be helpful
- If the patient has extragenital cutaneous manifestations, a skin biopsy may be performed under local anesthesia; however, most vulvar biopsies in children need to be done with general anesthesia

Management

Infectious

- Coxsackievirus (hand, foot, mouth disease)
    - Supportive care with topical emollients, ice, and sitz baths
    - Low-potency topical steroid and topical anesthetics may also be tried
    - Genital ulcers typically self-resolve in about 7 days

- Varicella
  - Start oral or intravenous acyclovir depending on the severity of infection
  - Avoid aspirin due to risk of developing Reye's syndrome

Sexually transmitted diseases

- Herpes simplex
  - See Chapter 48, "Sexually Transmitted Infections"
- Syphilis
  - See Chapter 48, "Sexually Transmitted Infections"
- Lymphogranuloma venereum
  - Treatment
    - Doxycycline 100 mg PO BID for 21 days *or*
    - Erythromycin base 500 mg PO QID for 21 days
  - Recent sexual partners should also be treated
  - Buboes may need to be aspirated to prevent rupture
- Chancroid
  - Treatment
    - Azithromycin 1 g PO in a single dose *or*
    - Ceftriaxone 250 mg IM in a single dose *or*
    - Ciprofloxacin 500 mg PO BID for 3 days *or*
    - Erythromycin base 500 mg PO QID for 7 days
  - Recent sexual partners should also be treated
  - Ulcers become less painful in 3 days and improve objectively within 7 days of treatment
- Granuloma inguinale (Donovanosis)
  - Treatment
    - Doxycycline 100 mg PO BID *or* trimethoprim-sulfamethoxazole 800–160 mg PO BID for 21 days or until ulcers have healed, whichever is longer
  - Ulcers should begin to improve within a few days of treatment

Systemic diseases

- Vulvar aphthae
  - Thorough review of systems to screen for Behcet's disease
  - Pain management with sitz baths, topical anesthetics, acetaminophen, ibuprofen, and opiates as needed
  - Super potent topical steroids or systemic steroids
  - Oral doxycycline, dapsone, colchicine, thalidomide, and TNF antagonists may be used in recurrent disease
- Behcet's disease
  - Refer to ophthalmology to evaluate for ocular involvement
  - Supportive care, including the use of sucralfate suspension
  - Ulcers usually heal spontaneously
  - Colchicine or dapsone may decrease frequency and severity of flares

Autoimmune diseases

- Bullous pemphigoid
  - Treatment with topical steroids, doxycycline and nicotinamide, dapsone, systemic steroids, azathioprine, and/or mycophenolate mofetil may be required depending on the severity of the disease

- Linear IgA disease
  - Treatment with topical steroids, sulfapyridine, dapsone, other antibiotics, systemic steroids, azathioprine, mycophenolate mofetil, and intravenous immunoglobulin may be used depending on the severity of disease
  - Usually remits prior to adolescence
- Kawasaki disease
  - Consult cardiology consult and echocardiogram
  - Has been associated with COVID-19 infections, consider consulting with infectious disease
  - Treatment with aspirin, intravenous immunoglobulin, possibly systemic steroids
- Systemic lupus erythematosus
  - Evaluate for the involvement of other organ systems
  - Treatment may include topical steroids and/or hydroxychloroquine

Cutaneous Drug Reactions

- Fixed drug eruption
  - Detailed medication history
  - Avoid causative agent
- Erythema multiforme
  - Supportive care
  - May consider long-term suppressive therapy with daily valacyclovir in patients with recurrent disease

VASCULAR ANOMALIES OF THE VULVA

Key Points

- These anomalies are rare, but proper diagnosis is important as involvement and treatment varies
- Can be broadly noted in two categories
  - Vascular tumors
    - Conditions of endothelial proliferation
    - More limited to the external genitalia
    - Include
      - Hemangiomas
      - Kaposiform hemangioendothelioma (KHE)
      - Kaposiform lymphangioendothelioma (KLE)
      - Tufted angioma
  - Vascular malformations
    - Congenital lesions of vascular dysmorphogenesis
    - Can involve internal genitalia including vagina and uterus
    - Complex combined vascular malformations may extend to include bladder, anorectum, buttocks, and lower extremity
    - Include
      - Capillary malformation (CM)
      - Lymphathic malformation (LM)
      - Venous malformation (VM)
      - Arteriovascular malformation (AVM)

- – Complex combined
    - – Capillary-lymphatic venous malformation (CLVM or Klippel Trenaunay syndrome)
    - – Complex lymphaticoarteriovascular malformation (CLAVM [Parkes Weber syndrome])

Characteristics

- Important to discern hemangiomas from vascular malformations:
- Vascular malformations comprise dysplastic vessels and fail to regress
- Hemangiomas
    - 1–2% of hemangiomas involve the genitalia
    - Infantile hemangiomas are not hereditary
    - More common in females, Caucasians, multiple births, and infants with low birth weight
    - If not present at birth, develop in the first month of life with rapid growth in the first six months
    - Are benign tumors of infancy and childhood and will rapidly grow during infancy and slowly involute by age 5
- When reticulated hemangioma noted on the lower extremity, buttock, or perineal area, consider whether or not this is a part of:
    - LUMBAR syndrome (**L**ower extremity hemangioma and other cutaneous defects, **U**rogenital anomalies, ulceration, **M**yelopathy, **B**ony deformities, **A**norectal malformations, **A**rterial anomalies, and **R**enal anomalies)
    - PELVIS syndrome (**P**erineal hemangioma, **E**xternal genital malformations, **L**ipomyelomeningocele, **V**esico renal anomalies, **I**mperforate anus, and **S**kin tag)
    - SACRAL syndrome (**S**pinal dysraphism, **A**nogenital anomalies, **C**utaneous anomalies, **R**enal and urologic anomalies associated with **A**ngioma of **L**umbosacral localization)
    - Evaluate with appropriate imaging

Diagnosis

Hemangiomas

- Presentation may range from a small almost negligible vascular papule to massive distorting tumors
- Radiologic evaluation and/or consultation with a pediatric surgeon which specializes in vascular malformations (dermatologic, vascular, or plastic surgeon) may aid in diagnosis
    - Ultrasound with color Doppler imaging is helpful
        - – Extremely operator dependent on the level of experience
        - – Can demonstrate a dense soft tissue mass with decreased arterial resistance and increased venous flow
    - MRI is very useful
        - – Often requires sedation
        - – Best utilized when the hemangioma involves multiple tissue layers
- Do not biopsy

Kaposiform Hemangioendotheliomas/Kaposiformendotheliomas

- Present as extensive ecchymotic cutaneous lesions
- Extremely aggressive
    - Can invade and cross multiple tissue planes

- Have characteristic clinical/radiographical patterns
- Can be associated with profound thrombocytopenia (Kasabach-Merritt phenomenon)

Vascular Malformations (VM)/Lymphatic Malformations (LM)

- Slow-flow lesions
- Growth may be exaggerated with puberty/pregnancy
- Can be associated with local soft tissue or skeletal overgrowth
- Appearance
  - VM may appear soft bluish compressible masses
  - LM the overlying skin may be normal with deep malformations, may be associated Lymphedema
- Can be associated with pain/bleeding, either spontaneous or due to trauma
- Diagnosis based on MRI with gadolinium contrast
  - LM are hyperintense on T2-weighted images from high water content (may have fluid-fluid levels)
  - VM are hyperintense of T2-weighted images with the enhancement of vascular channels on T1 images
  - Cross-sectional images may be helpful to obtain an accurate diagnosis
- CLVM (Klippel-Trenaunay syndrome)
  - A type of vascular malformation that most commonly involve the pelvis, trunk, and upper extremity
  - Associated with skeletal and soft tissue hypertrophy/anomalous venous drainage
  - Patients have bleeding, pain, infection, and often negative self-body image
  - May need aspirin therapy to decrease pain from associated phlebothrombosis
  - May need prophylactic antibiotic therapy for recurrent infections

---

Management

Hemangiomas

- Despite the size, the majority will regress with time
  - Typically completely regress or leave a small, predominantly fibrosed tumor, which may be removed at a later age if desired
  - Encourage expectant management rather than surgical intervention
    - May be difficult for the child and parents, who may need significant support and consultations during this process
    - Pictures are helpful to follow the progression of involution in the patient, as well as to show examples of similar hemangioma regression in other patients

Indications for treating hemangiomas during the growth phase

- Major expansion with disfigurement
- Functional compromise, necrosis, and ulceration

Treatment options during the growth phase

- Oral corticosteroids (Prednisone 2–3 mg/kg/day) with full dosages in the morning with food usually over a period of 6 weeks with slow tapering over two months
  - 70% of infants respond to prednisone

- Adverse effects: Cushingoid features, stunted linear growth, truncal obesity, hypertension, irritability, gastric ulcers
- Interferon alpha used after failure of corticosteroids (1–3 mU/m subcutaneous) given 3–7 times per week
  - Involution rate 75–80%
  - Adverse effects: Spastic diplegia can occur in 20% of patients, resolves with early drug discontinuation
- Propranolol (2–3 mg/kg/day divided in three doses)
  - Not FDA approved for the treatment of infantile hemangiomas
  - Improvement in hemangioma size within 24–48 hours of initial treatment and complete regression seen by 6 months of treatment
  - Wide variation in practices for initiation and monitoring of propranolol; consider baseline cardiology consultation and EKG prior to initiation
  - Adverse effects: Hypoglycemia, symptomatic hypotension
  - Consider giving doses with food to abate the hypoglycemic effect

Treatment options of ulcerated hemangiomas

- Topical antibiotics to prevent infection (metronidazole gel 7%, gentamycin cream, mupirocin)
- Topical lidocaine gel
- Pulsed dye laser to accelerate lightening and involution of superficial hemangiomas
- Surgical excision should be reserved for ulcerative and painful lesions refractory to medical management; often associated with residual scar
- Cryosurgery can be used to treat superficial hemangiomas

Kaposiform Hemangioendotheliomas/Kaposiformendotheliomas

- Antiangiogenic pharmacotherapy with systemic corticosteroid
- For initial treatment failure: Interferon or vincristine
- Surgical therapy not possible due to extensive anatomic involvement with most lesions

Vascular Malformations/Lymphatic Malformations

- Combination of sclerotherapy, and/or resection
  - Especially for recurrent infection, fluid leakage, swelling
  - Procedures should only be completed by skilled interventional radiologist or surgeon with experience treating vascular anomalies
- Recurrence is common, multiple treatments and/or surgeries are likely needed
- Complex lesions are best managed by a multidisciplinary team with significant experience in the treatment of vascular anomalies

BIBLIOGRAPHY

Alikhan A, Sayed C, Alavi A, et al. North American clinical management guidelines for hidradenitis suppurativa: a publication from the United States and Canadian Hidradenitis Suppurativa Foundations: Part I: Diagnosis, evaluation, and the use of complementary and procedural management. J Am Acad Dermatol. 2019; 81(1):76–90.

Alikhan A, Sayed C, Alavi A, et al. North American clinical management guidelines for hidradenitis suppurativa: a publication from the United States and Canadian Hidradenitis Suppurativa Foundations: Part II: Topical, intralesional, and systemic medical management. J Am Acad Dermatol. 2019; 81(1):91–101.

Barnhill RL, Albert LS, Shama SK, Goldenhersh MA, Rhodes AR, Sober AJ. Genital lentiginosis: a clinical and histopathologic study. J Am Acad Dermatol. 1990; 22(3):453–460.

Bohl TG. Vulvar ulcers and erosions: a clinical approach. Clin Obstet Gynecol. 2015;58:492–502.

Boxhoorn L, Stoof T., De Meij T., et al. Clinical experience and diagnostic algorithmic of vulvar Crohn's disease. Eur J Gastreoenterol Hepatol. 2017; 29:838–843.

Casey GA, Cooper SM, Powell JJ. Treatment of vulvar lichen sclerosus with topical corticosteroids in children: a study of 72 children. Clin Exp Dermatol. 2015; 40(3):289–292.

Egan CA, Bradley RR, Logsdon VK et al. Vulvar melanoma in childhood. Arch Dermatol. 1997; 133:345–348.

Fiorella L. Therapy of pediatric genital diseases. Dermatol Ther. 2004;17:117–128.

Granese R, Calagna G, Morabito G, et al. Vulvar involvement in pediatric Crohn's disease: a systematic review. Arch Gynecol Obstet. 2018;297(1):3–11.

Lee KC, Bercovitch L. Update on infantile hemangiomas. Semin Perinatol. 2013;37:49–58.

Lewis FM, Tatnall FM, Velangi SS, et al. British Association of Dermatologists guidelines for the management of lichen sclerosus, 2018. Br J Dermatol. 2018; 178(4):839–853.

Liy-Wong C, Pope E, Lara-Corrales I. Hidradenitis suppurativa in the pediatric population. J Am Acad Dermatol. 2015; 73(5 Suppl 1):S36–S41.

Mauskar MM, Marathe K, Venkatesan A, Schlosser BJ, Edwarfds L. Vulvar diseases: conditions in adults and children. J Am Acad Dermatol 2020;82:1287–1298.

Menter A, Cordoro KM, Davis DMR, Kroshinsky D, Paller AS, Armstrong AW et al. Joint American Academy of Dermatology-National Psoriasis Foundation guidelines of care for the management and treatment of psoriasis in pediatric patients. J Am Acad Dermatol. 2020;82:161–201.

Mikkelsen PR, Jemec GB. Hidradenitis suppurativa in children and adolescents: a review of treatment options. Paediatr Drugs. 2014;16(6):483–489.

Morris A, Rogers M, Fischer G, Williams K. Childhood psoriasis: a clinical review of 1262 cases. Pediatr Dermatol. 2001;18:188–198.

Murzaku EC, Penn LA, Hale CS, Pomeranz MK, Polsky D. Vulvar nevi, melanosis, and melanoma: an epidemiologic, clinical, and histopathologic review. J Am Acad Dermatol. 2014; 71(6):1241–1249.

Palamaras I., El-Jabbour J. Pietropaolo N., et al. Metastatic Crohn's disease: a review. JEADV. 22:1033–1043.

Paller A, Mancini AJ. *Hurwitz* Clinical Pediatric Dermatology. Elsevier; 2016.

Patel BN, Hoefgen HR, Nour N, Merritt DF (2020). Genital Trauma. In Emans SJ, Laufer M, DiVasta A, eds, *Pediatric & Adolescent Gynecology* (7th ed.). Wolters Kluwer.

Powell J, Wojnarowska F. Childhood vulvar lichen sclerosus. The course after puberty. J Reprod Med. 2002; 47(9):706–709.

Rock B, Hood AF, Rock JA. Prospective study of vulvar nevi. J Am Acad Dermatol. 1990;22:104–105.

Sand FL, Thomsen SF. Skin diseases of the vulva: infectious diseases. J Obstet Gynaecol. 2017;37:840–848.

Schroeder B. Vulvar disorders in adolescents. Obstet Gynecol Clin North Am. 2000; 27:35–48.

Vogel AM, Alesbury JA, Burrows PE, Fishman SJ. Vascular Anomalies of the female external genitalia. J Ped Surg. 2006;41:993–999.

Workowski KA, Bolan GA. Sexually transmitted diseases treatment guidelines, 2015. MMWR. 2015;64:1–137.

60

Vulvovaginitis

Judith Simms-Cendan

PEDIATRIC PATIENT

Key Points

- Typical complaint is discharge, dysuria, pruritis, or vulvar redness
- Most cases are 'nonspecific vulvovaginitis' without a specific infectious etiology
- Symptoms are frequently mistaken for yeast infection which is uncommon in a toilet-trained prepubertal girl
- Most nonspecific vulvovaginitis cases respond to hygienic and supportive measures
- In general, nonspecific cases have chronic history and bacterial/specific causes more acute presentations
- Bloody, malodorous discharge is most commonly due to vaginal foreign body

Definitions

- Vulvovaginitis: Symptoms that cause vulvar itching, irritation, burning in the setting of a vaginal discharge

Differential Diagnosis

- Nonspecific vulvovaginitis: Symptoms occur in the setting of normal flora
  - Normal flora
    - Aerobic: Staphylococcus epidermidis, enterococci, Escherichia coli, lactobacilli, Streptococcus viridans
    - Anaerobic bacteria: Peptococcus and bacteroides species
- Specific vulvovaginitis: Symptoms are caused by pathogens – most commonly respiratory/enteric
  - Respiratory: Group A β-hemolytic Streptococci (*Streptococcus pyogenes*), group B Streptococci β-hemolytic (*Streptococcus agalactiae*), *Neisseria meningitidis*, *Staphylococcus aureus*, *Haemophilus influenzae*, *Branhamella catarrhalis*, *Klebsiella pneumoniae*
  - Enteric: *E. coli*, Shigella, Yersinia
  - STIs
  - *Enterobiasis vermicularis* (pinworms)
- Yeast infections: Not common in prepubertal girls after toilet training, unless recent antibiotic use or poorly controlled diabetes or immunosuppression
- Lichen sclerosus (see Chapter 59, "Vulvar Disorders")

DOI: 10.1201/9781003039235-60

- Vaginal foreign bodies (toilet paper most common)
- Dermatosis (e.g. eczema, psoriasis, contact dermatitis, see Chapter 59, "Vulvar Disorders")

Risk Factors

- Anatomic and Physiologic Prepubertal Hypoestrogenic State
  - Thin, sensitive vulvar skin
  - Thin, atrophic vaginal epithelium more exposed due to lack of vulvar fat pads and pubic hair
  - Alkaline vaginal pH supports the growth of fecal and oropharyngeal bacteria
- Suboptimal Hygiene/Behavior
  - Poor hand washing
  - Inadequate cleansing of vulva after voiding or bowel movements
  - Exposure to vulvar irritants (e.g. dirt, sand, soaps, bubble baths)
  - Urine retained in the vagina when voiding with legs pressed together
  - Foreign body placement: Most commonly small bits of toilet paper
- Sexual Abuse (see Chapter 46, "Sexual Abuse, Sex Trafficking, and Rape")

Diagnosis

History

- Try to include direct questioning of child/patient
  - Perineal hygiene: Have patient demonstrate wiping after bowel movement: front-to-back or back-to-front
  - Ask about itching, scratching, pain (perianal itching – think pinworms)
- Ask about color, quantity, odor, and duration of discharge
  - Color of the discharge: White, yellow, green, purulent, or bloody
    - Bloody discharge: Think foreign body, Shigella, group A beta-hemolytic streptococci, trauma, vulvar scratching, condyloma, and rarely precocious puberty or tumor
    - Green discharge: Can be nonspecific but think of specific causes like Staphylococcus or Streptococcus, *H. influenzae*, gonorrhea, or foreign body
  - Does the discharge have any odor
    - Foul-smelling discharge: Associated with foreign body
- History of irritants
  - Bubble baths
  - Soaps and shampoos with strong odors (e.g. contact dermatitis)
  - Staying in damp clothing for long periods (pool/beach)
- History of atopic skin reactions/allergies
- History of recent upper respiratory/pharyngeal/skin infections in patient or family
- History of recent diarrheal illness
- Any clues/concerns about sexual abuse: Behavioral changes, nightmares

Physical Examination

- Skin
  - Look for psoriasis, eczema
  - Look for evidence bruising, trauma: Evidence of abuse

- Assess for secondary sexual characteristics: Breast budding/axillary hair (precocious puberty)
- Inspect external genitalia: Perineum, vulva, and vagina
  - Look for intense erythema, especially at vestibule (Strep and staph)
  - Look for discharge, depigmentation, excoriations, ulcers, condyloma, tumors
  - Use labial traction to allow better visualization of the vagina (see "Gynecologic Examination," Chapter 20)
  - Consider the use of knee-chest position to allow a complete assessment of vagina (see "Gynecologic Examination," Chapter 20)
  - May be able to visualize upper vagina and may be helpful to rule out the foreign body

Assessing Discharge

- Use small Dacron Calgiswab to obtain specimens (less irritating)
- Send for
  - Aerobic culture
  - PCR assay for gonorrhea, chlamydia, trichomonas if any concern of abuse
- Alternate technique: Use a small pediatric feeding tube attached to a syringe or catheter within a catheter technique (as described in "Gynecologic Examination," Chapter 20) to put one or two drops of fluid into the vagina and aspirate for specimens

Evaluating for Foreign Body

- Use a small pediatric feeding tube attached to a 20-ml syringe filled with warm water. Use labial traction to allow hymen to open and gently place a feeding tube through the vagina without touching hymen and try to flush out foreign body from vagina
- Consider the use of flexible office hysteroscope (e.g. Endosee, Cooper Surgical) if available

Management

Nonspecific Vulvovaginitis (75% of Cases)

- Educate caregiver and provide Patient Handout on Prepubertal Vulvovaginitis (North American Society for Pediatric and Adolescent Gynecology; www.naspag.org)
- Improved hygiene
  - Front-to-back wiping
  - Good hand washing
  - Urinate with legs apart to limit urine reflux into the vagina (consider sitting backwards on the toilet seat)
  - Avoid vulvar skin irritants (e.g. bubble baths)
  - Shampoo hair while washing in the shower to avoid sitting in dirty, soapy water
  - Avoid tight clothing; change out of wet bathing suits
- Sitz bath in warm tap water: 15 min 2–3 times daily
- Avoid soap to the vulva
- Pat vulva dry or dry with a blow dryer on a cool setting

- Apply protective barrier cream to the vulva, e.g., A&D ointment (Schering-Plough Healthcare Products, Inc, Memphis, TN, USA) or Aqua-phor® (Beiersdorf Inc, Hamburg, Germany)
- Consider low-potency topical steroids if significant irritation/redness

If No Response to Hygiene Management/Persistent Nonspecific Vaginitis

- Empiric treatment for enterobiasis (pinworms), mebendazole (100 mg), pyrantel pamoate (1 g, available without a prescription), or albendazole (400 mg). Repeat dose in 2 weeks
- Empiric treatment with amoxicillin, amoxicillin clavulanate or cephalosporin for 10 days
- Examination under anesthesia/vaginoscopy

Specific Vulvovaginitis

- See Table 60.1 for antibiotic dosing
- Consider topical emollient for skin irritation

ADOLESCENT PATIENT

Key Points

- Physiologic leukorrhea (normal estrogen-related desquamation of epithelial cells) is the most common discharge in pubescent girl
- The most common cause of vulvovaginitis in the adolescent is an infection, including yeast, bacterial vaginosis, or STI
- Vaginal discharge may be the presenting symptom for sexually transmitted diseases in the adolescent

TABLE 60.1

Specific Causes and Treatment of Vulvovaginitis

Pathogen	Bacteria	Antibiotic	Less than 20 kg	Greater than 20 kg
Skin/perineal flora	S. aureus, S. epidermidis, S. viridans, S. pyogenes	Ampicillin or Amoxicillin or Azithromycin *or Trimethoprim/** sulfamethoxazole	25 mg/kg q 6 h × 5–10 days 20 mg/kg q 12 h × 5–10 days *10 mg/kg × 1 day, 5 mg/kg × 4 days **5 mg/kg dose q 12 h × 5–10 days	500 mg q 6 h × 5–10 days 20 mg/kg q 12 h × 5–10 days 10 mg/kg × 1 day, 5 mg/kg × 4 days 5 mg/kg dose q 12 h × 5–10 days
Enteric	E. coli	Azithromycin	As above	As above
	Proteus vulgaris	Trimethoprim/ sulfamethoxazole	As above	As above
	Shigella	Amoxicillin	As above	As above
	Yersinia	Trimethoprim/ Sulfamethoxazole	As above	As above
	Enterococcus S. agalactiae	Ampicillin	As above	As above
Respiratory pathogens	Haemophilus influenzae S. pneumonia	Amoxicillin or Amoxicillin-clavulanate Cephalexin	As above 30 mg/kg/day Divided q 12 h for 7 days 25–50 mg/kg/day PO divided q 6–8 h for 10 days	30 mg/kg/day Divided q 12 h for 7 days 25–50 mg/kg/day PO divided q 6–8 h for 10 days

Pathogenesis and Risk Factors

Physiologic Changes

- Physiologic changes are not vulvovaginitis but cause patient/parent concern
  - Onset of puberty increases normal leukorrhea creating a physiologic discharge
    - Usually begins after the onset of breast development but prior to the onset of menstruation
  - Odor can be caused by increased sweat and normal bacteria in sweat glands

Noninfectious Vulvovaginitis

- Atopic reaction and folliculitis
  - Increased shaving, use of soaps and feminine hygiene products
- Increased sports, wearing of tight clothing causes irritation
- Friction injury due to insufficient lubrication during intercourse can cause irritation and discharge
- Retained tampons and condoms can cause malodorous vaginal discharge
- Partial obstruction of menstrual flow from a Müllerian anomaly can produce a bloody, foul-smelling discharge

Infectious Vulvovaginitis

- Vulvovaginal candidiasis
  - *Candida albicans*, *tropicalis*, and *glabrata* most common species
  - Colonization is normal, symptoms are from overgrowth
  - Uncommon unless history of antibiotic use, immunosuppression, diabetes, pregnancy
  - Poor hygiene can be a risk factor
- Bacterial vaginosis (BV)
  - Caused by *Gardnerella vaginalis*, Prevotella, Mycoplasma, Ureaplasma, Atopobium, Mobiluncus
  - Heavy menses, which alters vaginal pH, can trigger amine-producing bacterial overgrowth
  - Douching and sexual activity increase risk (but not considered an STI)
- Trichomonas (Trich)
  - Associated with an irritating vaginal discharge
  - Very common STI
  - Coinfection with BV is Common

Diagnosis

History

- Symptoms
  - Itching, burning, discharge, odor, duration
  - Intense pruritis and thick white discharge – Yeast
  - Malodorous fishy discharge – BV
  - Frothy, profuse, malodorous discharge – Trichomonas

- Menstrual history
  - Cycle length, duration, heaviness, the onset of discharge related to menses
  - BV symptoms can worsen after menses
- Hygiene history
  - Shaving, pads (deodorant), scented soaps/body wash, feminine hygiene washes
  - Frequency of pad/tampon changes during menses
- Sexual history (without parent or guardian!)
  - Coitarche, condom use
  - Number of partners/new partners
  - Pain with intercourse
  - History of childhood sexual abuse or sexual assault
    - Increases fear there is something wrong/dirty/infected
- Contraception use
  - Combined OCs can trigger vulvodynia in susceptible women (due to lowering of testosterone). Consider switching to levonorgestrel IUD
  - Depot medroxyprogesterone can cause atrophic vaginitis

Physical

- Examine external genitalia with a mirror so the patient can see, be engaged, and be less afraid
  - Note any inflammation, erythema, ulcers, lesions, signs of trauma
  - Look for signs of eczema, psoriasis, atopic reactions
  - Vulvar edema, excoriation erythema can be seen with yeast
- If the patient is never sexually active and/or cannot tolerate a small Pederson speculum
  - Consider a blind swab or patient performed swab for BV, yeast, STIs (if indicated)
  - Use saline-moistened cotton-tipped applicator or Dacron urethral swabs inserted just inside the hymenal ring to obtain specimens
- In addition to those who are sexually active, many adolescent patients who have not been sexually active, especially those who use tampons, can tolerate a speculum exam with a thin Pedersen speculum
  - Thick curd-like adherent clumpy discharge – Yeast
  - Thin white, frothy malodorous, fishy discharge – BV
  - Think trichomonas if
    - Frothy, yellow malodorous discharge with vulvovaginal irritation
    - Grossly visible punctate hemorrhages of the cervix (strawberry cervix)
- Commercially available swab molecular quantitative tests report candida species and test for bacteria causing BV in addition to STIs (trich, gonorrhea, chlamydia)
  - Particularly helpful if in doubt about the clinical diagnosis or if recurrent symptoms
  - Nucleic acid amplification testing is the gold standard for testing for *Neisseria gonorrhoeae, Chlamydia trachomatis, Trichomonas vaginalis*
  - Nucleic acid amplification testing for trichomonas is 3–5× more sensitive than wet mount. Vaginal swab and urine testing are both sensitive
- pH testing and wet mounts of vaginal discharge can give point-of-care information
  - pH > 4.5: Bacterial vaginosis or trichomoniasis
  - pH < 4.5: Physiologic leukorrhea or candida

- Wet mount
  - Saline prep
    - Clue cells (squamous cells with bacteria on borders): BV
    - Motile protozoa with flagella: Trichomonas
    - A lot of WBCs: Screen for STIs
  - KOH: Look for budding yeast or hyphae – Yeast

Management

Physiologic Discharge

- Education: Most teens are unaware of the cyclic nature and impact of hormonal changes on vaginal discharge; typically, self-limited condition
- Supportive: Encourage use of panty liners or shields
- Discourage use of douching attempts to clear normal process

Candidal Vulvovaginitis (CVV)

- Uncomplicated, initial treatments
  - Fluconazole 150 mg PO × 1. Can repeat in 3 days if severe infection (extensive vulvar erythema, edema, excoriation, fissure formation)
    - Often preferred by adolescents
  - Selected OTC treatments
    - Short course topical therapy preferred
      - Miconazole 4% vaginal cream, 5 g daily × 3 days
      - Miconazole 1200 mg suppository × 1 day
      - Clotrimazole 2% cream, 5 g daily × 3 days
  - Prescription intravaginal
    - Terconazole 80 mg supp × 3 days
    - Terconazole 0.8%, 1 full applicator (5 g) daily for 3 days
  - Consider a topical low-potency steroid if the patient has an erythematous, severely pruritic inflammatory response to the yeast
- Complicated, recurrent CVV
  - 100-mg, 150-mg, or 200-mg oral dose of fluconazole every third day for a total of 3 doses (day 1, 4, and 7)
  - Maintenance for recurrent CVV: Fluconazole 100 mg PO once/week for 6 months
  - Nonalbicans CVV
    - Terconazole 0.4% topically 7–14 days
    - Fluconazole does not work well for this
    - Boric acid capsules 600 mg per vagina once/day for 14 days
  - Consider screening for diabetes, HIV

Bacterial vaginosis

- First line
  - Metronidazole 500 mg twice a day for a 7 day
  - Metronidazole gel 0.75%, one applicatorful (5 g) intravaginally daily × 5 days
  - Clindamycin cream 2%, one applicatorful (5 g) intravaginally at bedtime for 7 days

- Second line
  - Clindamycin 300 mg twice a day for 7 days
  - Tinidazole 2 g orally for 2 days
  - Clindamycin ovules 100 mg vaginally at bedtime × 3 days
- Caution
  - Remind patients to avoid alcohol while taking nitroimidazoles: Up to 24 h after the last dose of metronidazole, and up to 72 h after the last dose of tinidazole
  - Metronidazole has a strong metallic aftertaste
  - Clindamycin cream and ovules contain oils that can break down latex condoms
  - Oral clindamycin can increase the risk of *Clostridioides difficile* colitis

Trichomonas vaginalis

- Metronidazole 500 mg 2 times a day for 7 days (see caution above) or Tinidazole 2 g orally in a single dose
- Repeat testing in 3 months
- Do STI testing and emphasize condom use. Trichomonas increases the risk of acquiring HIV
- Sexual partners must also be treated with the same medicine at the same time. Reinfection is common
- For resistant strains, consider ordering metronidazole susceptibility testing through the CDC

BIBLIOGRAPHY

Centers for Disease Control and Prevention. (2021). *Sexually Transmitted Diseases Treatment Guidelines*, July 22, 2021. https://www.cdc.gov/std/treatment-guidelines/default.htm

Loveless M, Myint O. Vulvovaginitis-presentation of more common problems in pediatric and adolescent gynecology. Best Pract Res Clin Obstetr Gynaecol. 2018; 48:14–27.

Zuckerman A, Romano M. NASPAG clinical recommendations: vulvovaginitis. JPAG. 2016; 29:673–679.

Index

Note: Page numbers in *italics* represent figures and **bold** indicate tables in the text.